Medicaid Reform and the American States

Medicaid Reform and the American States

CASE STUDIES ON THE POLITICS OF MANAGED CARE

EDITED BY

Mark R. Daniels

AUBURN HOUSE
Westport, Connecticut • London

Library of Congress Cataloging-in-Publication Data

Medicaid reform and the American States : case studies on the politics
  of managed care / edited by Mark R. Daniels.
     p. cm.
   Includes bibliographical references and index.
   ISBN 0–86569–263–7 (alk. paper)
   1. Medicaid. 2. Managed care plans (Medical care)—United States.
 I. Daniels, Mark Ross, 1952– .
 RA412.5.U6M427 1998
 368.4'2'00973—dc21   97–23657

British Library Cataloguing in Publication Data is available.

Library of Congress Catalog Card Number: 97–23657
ISBN: 0–86569–263–7

First published in 1998

Auburn House, 88 Post Road West, Westport, CT 06881
An imprint of Greenwood Publishing Group, Inc.

Printed in the United States of America

The paper used in this book complies with the
Permanent Paper Standard issued by the National
Information Standards Organization (Z39.48–1984).

10 9 8 7 6 5 4 3 2 1

To Nat and Noah True-Daniels

Contents

Figures and Tables

FIGURES

TABLES

Preface

After completing a manuscript on Tennessee's efforts to reform its Medicaid plan,[1] it occurred to me that Medicaid had slowly become one of my primary research interests. I had published previously a manuscript on Oklahoma's use (or misuse) of Medicaid funds for the institutionalization of emotionally troubled, dependent children.[2] What interested me most about the uses of Medicaid funds was the breadth and variety of Medicaid-funded programs and the abundance of organizational delivery systems. Comparing my knowledge of Oklahoma's and Tennessee's Medicaid programs, I concluded from this anecdotal data that a state's Medicaid program must be in large part a result of the state's unique political and economic resources.

For example, each state has considerable discretion concerning eligibility requirements, total enrollment, total cost (states add their own source revenue to the federal funds received according to a matching formula), types of services covered, and the level of payment for services received. In addition, each state has discretion concerning the type of health system used for the delivery of health services. States may also apply to the federal government for a waiver from Medicaid, substitute their own unique program, and continue to receive Medicaid funds for that program.

Starting under the administration of President Reagan, states have been increasingly given greater discretion in the administration of federally funded programs. In turn, each state's unique political and economic variables give rise to individually stylized approaches to the delivery of Medicaid services.

After serving as editor of the *SPAE Forum*, the newsletter of the American Society for Public Administration's Section on Public Administration Education, and also serving as editor for a symposium in the *International Journal of Public Administration*,[3] I finally felt enough self-confidence to begin an even more ambitious editorial project. I decided to edit a book containing examples of Medicaid reform from among the American state governments. After advertising the project in journals and newsletters, and sending invitations to public administration and health administration faculty across the country, I finally had sixteen chapter drafts and was fortunate to obtain a contract with a respected academic and commercial press, Greenwood Publishing Group, Inc.

I first wish to thank the authors of these cases who have worked with me on this project for almost three years. Thank you for your scholarship, and for your patience. I also wish to thank the editors of Greenwood Publishing Group for their editing and production assistance, and for their patience.

I must also point out my gratitude to Dr. Frank J. Thompson, Professor and Dean, School of Public Affairs, State University of New York–Albany, for encouraging and supporting my interest in health policy. Frank was my Ph.D. committee chairperson at the University of Georgia and has been a source of continued support throughout my career.

I also thank Dr. David Mason for his encouragement and support of this project, and for his generosity, humor, and friendship.

I have always remembered J. D. Salinger's character ''Franny''[4] and her observation that poets (and writers) are supposed to leave something beautiful after they get off the page. In this respect, I dedicate this book to my sons, Nat and Noah True-Daniels. They have helped me to discover the true meaning of life.

Of course, any errors occurring in this book are my responsibility.

NOTES

1. Mark R. Daniels, ''Implementing Policy Termination: Health Care Reform in Tennessee,'' *Policy Studies Review* 14, nos. 3/4 (1996): 353–374; Mark R. Daniels, ''Tennessee's TennCare Health Reform Program: Implications for Other State Governments,'' *New England Journal of Human Services* 13, no. 1 (1995): 12–19.

2. Mark R. Daniels, ''Organizational Termination and Policy Continuation: Closing the Oklahoma Public Training Schools,'' *Policy Sciences* 28 (1995): 301–316; Mark R. Daniels, ''The Politics and Economics of Dependent Children's Mental Health Care Financing: The Oklahoma Paradox,'' *Journal of Health and Human Services Administration* 16, no. 2 (1993): 171–196.

3. Mark R. Daniels, (ed.), ''Public Policy and Organization Termination,'' *International Journal of Public Administration* 20, no. 12 (December 1997). Contains five original refereed articles, including an ''Afterword'' by Peter deLeon, and an introduction, ''Theories for the Termination of Public Policies, Programs, and Organizations,'' by the author.

4. J. D. Salinger, *Franny and Zooey* (New York: Bantam Books, 1964).

1

Introduction: The Inconsistency and Paradox of American Health Care

MARK R. DANIELS

Medicaid is the primary means for providing medical care to the nation's indigent and disabled populations. Almost 13 percent of all Americans received some form of medical coverage, such as physician services or long-term nursing care, through Medicaid in 1992. The costs of Medicaid have risen dramatically: over $126 billion was spent in 1993 by both the federal and state governments on this program.

State governments have become alarmed by the growing share of their budgets consumed by Medicaid. For example, in Tennessee, over 1.4 million people are covered by TennCare, the state's Medicaid-financed health program, at an annual cost of $3.5 billion forecast for fiscal year (FY) 1997, of which $1.05 billion or 30% was derived from state operating revenue. Nationwide, over $100 billion is annually spent for Medicaid programs accounting for, on the average, 20% of a state's operating budget.

The growing emphasis on the uninsured, which includes the poor who do not qualify for Medicaid, has pressured state governments to find ways to increase Medicaid enrollments while simultaneously controlling the program's rapidly skyrocketing costs.

This book presents the efforts of sixteen states to reform their Medicaid programs through a system of "managed care": programs that seek to control or manage the use by patients of physicians and other health care services. Managed care is a type of prepaid health plan or insurance program in which those who are covered receive medical service in a coordinated fashion in order to eliminate unnecessary services. These sixteen cases are presented in the alphabetical order of each state.

Before turning to the experiences of these sixteen states, this chapter will first present an overview of the inconsistency and paradox of American health care.

Second, this chapter will review the development of Medicaid in order to provide a historical context for the presentation of the sixteen case experiences.
Third, a typology of managed care will be presented which will include an
orientation into the terminology of managed care. And, fourth, a summary assessment of the experiences of these sixteen states with managed care will be
made in order to prepare the reader for trends and patterns among the cases.

THE INCONSISTENCY AND PARADOX OF AMERICAN HEALTH CARE

Health care in the United States is characterized by inconsistency and paradox.[1] The United States commits greater financial resources to health care than
any other industrialized country, including Canada, Germany, the Netherlands,
Japan, and the United Kingdom.[2] Health care expenditures in the United States
broke the $2 billion-a-day level in 1991, and total expenditures in 1992 exceeded
$800 billion. But within this extraordinary spending lies inconsistency. An ex-
ample of this inconsistency is health insurance coverage. Of almost 219 million
Americans, 71.2% have private health insurance, 13% have publicly funded
health insurance, and 15.9% are uninsured.[3] U.S. health care for the most part
is a privately financed business transaction, with doctors, hospitals, and other
health care organizations selling products and services in the marketplace. About
58% of national health expenditures are paid for through private sector payments.[4] These payments are referred to as ''third-party'' payments, where, for
example, the physician is the first party, the patient the second party, and the
insurer-payer the third party. This third-party approach to paying for health care
affects the perception of consumers concerning who pays for health care: usually, someone other than the patient.

The 15.8% of Americans without health insurance number about 35 million.
Who are the uninsured? About three-fourths are employed, yet do not receive
or cannot afford health insurance through their employers. About 2 million are
uninsurable because of excluded or preexisting conditions. Thus, an inconsistency: the ability to pay for health care varies from patient to patient. Some
patients have adequate health insurance coverage, but 35 million have none
whatsoever.

The paradox of American health care is found within the concept of health
care efficiency. If efficiency is defined as the maximum utilization of resources,
then what kind of health care do Americans get from the highest priced health
care system in the world? Life expectancy in the United States ranks behind
that of Canada, Japan, and the United Kingdom, and more than a dozen countries
have lower infant mortality rates than the United States.[5] And, in a study of two
California public hospital emergency rooms, over half of all outpatient visits
were by uninsured patients who used the hospital as a family doctor because
physicians would not see them as patients.[6]

"Uniquely in the industrialized world," observes economist Uwe Reinhardt, "American health care exhibits opulent splendor and shocking deprivation side by side."[7] For example, new technology and surgical techniques enable medical centers to provide heart and lung transplants, and liver transplants are commonplace. At the same time, some individuals have no access to health care for routine services. For example, officials in the Tennessee Department of Health and Human Services recently investigated the death of a baby whose mother says she was denied health care by area hospitals.[8] It seems that because the mother's enrollment in an insurance plan could not be verified, she was denied service at several hospitals before she eventually received treatment. The mother claims that the delay in treatment contributed to her baby's death.

Publicly funded medical services are designed to lessen the inconsistency and paradox of American health care. The primary program for delivering health services to the indigent and disabled is Medicaid.

THE DEVELOPMENT OF MEDICAID

Of publicly funded health insurance, 84% is provided through the federally and state-funded Medicaid program. The program called Medicaid is actually a collection of programs that vary from state to state. Enacted into law in 1965, along with Medicare, Medicaid is funded with state and federal revenue and pays for acute care services and for long-term services for low-income households. However, the eligibility requirements and the range of available health services varies greatly among the 50 states.

Federal revenue for Medicaid is provided to states through matching grants for services and benefits that states have agreed to offer to specified populations. The federal government also matches additional payments that states decide to provide to cover a mix of services and benefits that vary from state to state. The federal match is from 50% to 70% of program costs. Some states pay for services on a fee-for-service payment system; however, the recent trend is for states to capitate costs or physician visits, or to have payments negotiated and monitored through a managed care payment system.

The ultimate cost of Medicaid-related services to a state depends upon six factors.[9] First, the range of available services (the more services offered, the higher the cost). Second, the type of reimbursement system used to pay providers (for example, fee-for-service versus managed care). Third, eligibility requirements which determine how many households will be enrolled in Medicaid. Fourth, the number of households below the poverty line in the state. Fifth, the rate of use and price of medical services in the state. And sixth, the number of elderly and disabled individuals enrolled in the program.

When Medicaid was implemented in 1966, the intent was to enable Medicaid patients to receive care and treatment identical with that received by patients covered by other third-party payers.[10] At that time, patients were accustomed to selecting their own physicians and having third-party payers pay on a fee-for-service basis. In other words, insurance companies would pay physicians on a treatment-by-treatment basis, with the patient paying a yearly deductible or co-payment. However, the Medicaid program required the physician to accept payment in full without holding the patient responsible for any part of the bill. This resulted in physicians having to accept less than full payment from Medicaid patients as opposed to full payment from patients with other third-party payers. Many physicians elected not to accept Medicaid patients. Physicians and other providers made a distinction between Medicaid patients and other insured patients.

This distinction resulted in two important outcomes: first, a restriction on freedom of choice of providers for Medicaid patients; and second, the development of packaged provider systems for Medicaid patients.[11] In the first outcome, the few physicians who would accept Medicaid's lower payments found that specializing in Medicaid patients could provide a volume adequate enough to assure profitability. These physicians soon earned the title "Medicaid docs," and their practices were surrounded with accusations of inefficiency and improper service usage and billing. In the second outcome, a system of coordinated service providers who would accept the lower Medicaid payments became in effect the first de facto Preferred Provider Organization (PPO), an outcome that predated current PPO systems.[12]

After a quarter century of experience with Medicaid, there are five significant problems and complaints:[13] (1) restricted access to mainstream providers of care; (2) excessive reliance on clinically and economically inappropriate sites of care; (3) lack of coordination in care delivery and lack of an identified regular source of primary care; (4) inappropriately high levels of certain types of care; and (5) indiscriminate and episodic seeking of care (i.e., "doctor shopping").

Altogether, these problems contribute to a subculture or syndrome of Medicaid: limited access resulting in episodic treatment patterns, in turn leading to a poor quality of care which is often inappropriate or inefficient. For example, most hospital emergency rooms would accept Medicaid patients; therefore, the most convenient and reliable source of treatment for Medicaid patients would be the emergency room. However, treatment there is much more expensive than in a doctor's office or clinic, and the treatment is emergency intervention instead of prevention or wellness examinations or checkups. The usage of emergency rooms by Medicaid patients for symptoms more appropriately treated in a physician's office or clinic also tended to drive up the cost of Medicaid.

The solution most often sought by state governments in response to the sky-rocketing cost of Medicaid is "managed care": a recent term used for programs that seek to control or "manage" the use by patients of physicians and other health care services. Much of the activity of managed care by state governments is a result of the Omnibus Budget Reconciliation Act of 1981 which, among many things, encouraged states to design alternative programs to Medicaid that would control costs and at the same time improve the access and quality of health care delivery systems. Subject to approval of the Health Care Financing Administration (HCFA), a state can apply for a waiver from the federally designed Medicaid program and substitute a program that the state has designed. Many of the states included in this book have successfully received such a waiver and have substituted their own Medicaid program, paid for with matching federal dollars.

A TYPOLOGY OF MANAGED CARE

Managed care is a type of prepaid health plan or insurance program in which the enrollees receive medical service in a coordinated manner to eliminate unnecessary services.[14] Usually, enrollees must have a primary care physician's or a utilization review person's approval before receiving care from a specialist and before being hospitalized on a nonemergency basis. There are a variety of managed care programs, ranging from Health Maintenance Organizations (HMOs) and PPOs to preadmission reviews required by some traditional health insurance companies. All have a common goal: to reduce health expenditures while maintaining the quality of care.

HMOs are organized systems that provide comprehensive health services to a voluntarily enrolled population for a fixed, prepaid, usually capitated fee, that is, a certain amount paid for each person enrolled, or a per capita (capitation) payment.[15] A set of health care benefits is provided, usually involving the services of physicians, other health care professionals, hospitals, and outpatient facilities all for a monthly payment, regardless of the number or the complexity of the services provided. The federal government thought that HMOs would control the costs of health care, and Congress passed the 1973 Health Maintenance Organization Act which provided financial incentives for the development of HMOs. The federal government favored HMOs for services paid through Medicaid (and Medicare). Businesses soon found them appealing for the same reason: HMOs seemed like a good way of putting a lid on rising costs.

HMOs use a number of utilization management practices to control unnecessary services and costs of health, including the following five features.[16] First, primary care physicians who act as "gatekeepers," who have the authority to approve a patient to see a specialist, but only after an initial examination. Second, concurrent utilization review of services that patients receive during treatment. Third, retrospective utilization reviews of services patients have received in order to audit treatment protocols and to establish baseline data for future reference. Fourth, prior authorization for patient care (for example, over the phone or computer approval before admission to a hospital). And, fifth, primary care physician profiles of the type of physician sorted for type of diagnosis and treatment plan (what kind of doctors do what for certain kinds of patients). Traditional insurance and PPOs also use the same kind of utilization management and physicians are now taught to expect utilization review for almost every patient they see.

PPOs are a coordinated system of health care provided to a defined group of people at a negotiated fee-for-service rate. As discussed above, Medicaid developed into a kind of PPO as a response to the discounted fee-for-service rate that the federal government was paying for services. PPOs have attracted much interest as a way to contain costs while retaining the patient's choice of physician and retaining the fee-for-service type of payment. The success of PPOs depends on the recruitment of cost-effective physicians and hospitals. This, in turn, assumes that in a geographical area of service there will be enough providers to create competition strong enough to negotiate discounted rates for services.

Even in rural parts of the nation, where competition among providers is minimal, the "gatekeeper" approach of primary care case management (PCCM) by a designated physician and third-party payer is usually in place. Even among profoundly rural areas where there are multiple counties without physicians (such as in parts of Texas and South Dakota), patients will still be given a designated primary care physician who will participate in PCCM with the third-party payer.

A typology of managed care programs used within the Medicaid context has been developed. The first (Type I) has a fee-for-service primary care gatekeeper; the second (Type II) has a risk-sharing primary care gatekeeper; and the third (Type III) has a HMO or Pre-Paid Health Plan (PHP).[17]

Under the Type I model, the fee-for-service (FFS) primary care gatekeeper, state agencies, or independent Health Insurance Organizations (HIOs) contract with Primary Care Physicians (PCPs) or with Primary Care Organizations (PCOs) to provide, broker or refer, and authorize all covered service to enrolled individuals. They are paid on a FFS basis, and usually also receive a nominal monthly case management payment per patient.

The Type II model, the risk-sharing primary care gatekeeper, is similar to Type I with the main difference being the method of gatekeeper payment. The main distinction between Type I and Type II is in the financial incentives—financial losses and gains—shared by the gatekeeper. These incentives may take the form of capitation payments which may result in a monthly cash loss if the costs of services provided exceeds the captitation income, or may result in a profit if the costs of services are brought in under the capitation income. Under Type II, Managed Care Organizations (MCOs) become the middle organization between the income source (state agency or HIO) and the PCP and referral providers. The way MCOs make money is by bringing the cost of services under the monthly capitated income.

Type III programs include those individuals enrolled in HMOs and other forms of PHPs that assume complete responsibility for all covered services. Enrolled individuals may have elected for coverage with the HMO or PHP or may have been required by state legislation to enroll. A state agency may negotiate a contract directly with the HMO or PHP or through an intermediary such as a HIO or MCO. The main distinction between Type III programs and

Type I and II is the total risk assumed by the HMO or PHP. Income is received by the HMO or PHP, and providers, payment rates, and ultimate financial risk are the exclusive responsibility of the HMO or PHP.

What are the effects of PCCM on the cost and uses of Medicaid dollars? Robert E. Hurley, Deborah A. Freund, and John E. Paul have studied 25 Medicaid PCCM programs enrolling approximately 1.25 million people.[18] Overall, these researchers find it hard to draw conclusions about the underlying changes in costs and uses of Medicaid under PCCM: are changes in cost and uses due to patient behavior, or to changes in the provider and the services available to the patient? For example, Hurley et al. found sharp reductions in emergency room usage for almost 80% of the programs studied. However, it could not be determined if this reduction is due to fewer beneficiaries needing emergency room services, or whether it is due to the restrictions or penalties involved in emergency room usage under PCCM. If PCCM results in beneficiaries first visiting their primary physician instead of seeking emergency room assistance, then PCCM is working as intended. However, if beneficiaries are being turned away from emergency rooms because nonemergency services are only delivered by the primary physician, and these beneficiaries subsequently do not receive any health services, then the PCCM is not working as intended. Costs may be decreasing from lower emergency room usage, but it is not clear from the data if beneficiaries are receiving appropriate care in the absence of emergency room visits.

Inpatient care also experienced a decline in the Hurley et al. study, and even small decreases in inpatient care can result in large savings, due to the high cost of inpatient services. At the time of the study, inpatient care was decreasing among all health programs due to increased utilization review and changes in medical procedures. Hurley et al. report mixed findings, and are cautious to attribute the decrease in inpatient services among beneficiaries to these Medicaid PCCM programs.

Similarly, the researchers were unable to draw conclusions about prescription and ancillary services use. While PCCM should result in higher physician visits and more prescriptions, the use and cost of prescription services did not increase. This could be due to the use of less costly generic drugs, or to a reduction in redundant or inappropriate prescriptions through PCCM.

Finally, Hurley et al. conclude that while there is no question about cost reductions in PCCM Medicaid programs, it is not certain to what these reductions are attributed. Are the savings a result of having beneficiaries treated with more medically appropriate services (seeing their primary physician for cold symptoms in place of an emergency room visit)? Or, are the savings a result of fewer services being rendered to beneficiaries (no emergency room visit, no service whatsoever)? Or, are the savings at the expense of providers who are delivering services at a lower, discounted rate and accepting lower (or in some cases, zero) profit margins? Managed care Medicaid programs cost less than their predecessors, but specific factors that lead to this decrease are less clear.

THE EXPERIENCES OF SIXTEEN STATES

It is within the above typology of managed care that the experiences of sixteen states will be presented in the chapters to follow. Some states use more than one of the managed care types, depending upon the availability of service providers across the state. Some states extend managed care to cover all health services, and other states cover only specialty health services. For example, Tennessee has slowly added mental health and retardation services to its TennCare program in order to extend managed care to all state-provided health services. South Dakota, however, has focused on managed care for prenatal and obstetric services due to the low birth weight and high morbidity and mortality rates of babies born within state-funded services.

Few states have allowed citizen participation in the design of the managed care health system. The one notable exception is Oregon, where ''town hall'' meetings were scheduled across the state to obtain feedback from consumers and health care providers about the design of the state program.

Table 1.1 summarizes and compares the important features of the managed care programs in these sixteen states. The first two columns indicate whether or not the state obtained a waiver from HCFA, and if so whether it is a statewide demonstration project or a local project. For example, Tennessee's waiver is for a statewide managed care program, while Alabama's is for a local HMO project in Mobile. Next, the type of PCCM is indicated. This is the primary type of PCCM selected by the state. Many of the Type II programs use MCOs for PCCM, and these MCOs may use independent physicians for PCCM; however, from the state's perspective the model selected is Type II. The sixth column indicates whether or not cost control has been achieved through the managed care system, and the seventh column indicates whether or not access to the state program was increased for uninsured individuals living in the state.

Of these sixteen states, just over half, or about 56%, have received waivers from HCFA for statewide managed care demonstration projects. Three states have waivers for more limited, local programs, like the HMO demonstration project in Mobile, Alabama. All together, about three-fourths of these states have some type of HCFA waiver. These waivers probably provide states with more discretion and control over their managed care programs than they could have through the federal Medicaid program.

Almost all the states select a Type II or Type III PCCM program. These programs allow the states to pay a capitated rate to a MCO or HMO and those organizations in turn administer the managed care program, not the states. The states provide the funding, but the MCOs and HMOs administer the programs and arrange for the delivery of services. Only the two most rural states (South Dakota and Texas) administer the programs and arrange for the delivery of services. Only in the two most rural states was Type I PCCM used. This is due to the low health provider-to-population ratio in rural areas, and the fact that

Table 1.1
Comparison of Medicaid Managed Care Programs of Sixteen States

	Waiver		PCCM			Cost	Increased
	State	Local	Type I	Type II	Type III	Control	Access
Alabama	no	yes			x	yes	no
Arizona	yes	no		x		no	yes
California	yes	no		x	x	yes	no
Delaware	yes	no		x	x	yes	yes
Florida	yes	no		x	x	yes	no
Kansas	no	no		x	x	yes	no
Maryland	yes	no		x	x	yes	no
Michigan	no	yes			x	yes	no
New York	yes	no		x		yes	no
Ohio	yes	no	x	x	x	yes	no
Oklahoma	yes			x	x	yes	no
Oregon	yes	no		x	x	yes	yes
S. Dakota	yes	no	x	x		yes	no
Tennessee	yes	no		x	x	yes	no
Texas	yes	no	x	x		yes	no
W. Virginia	no	yes		x	x	yes	yes

many counties in South Dakota and Texas have no doctors. In some cases, the designated Primary Care Physician might be 60 miles from the patient.

All states except Arizona report cost control results from managed care. Arizona is an unusual case because of its lack of experience with Medicaid prior to 1981. Arizona originally managed its demonstration program, AHCCCS, through a private sector MCO contract that turned out to be a disaster. Arizona's categorization as PCCM Type II in Table 1.1 refers to this early MCO arrangement; currently, the state administers the AHCCCS program. In addition, an unexpected high enrollment experienced by Arizona after the beginning of the 1981 demonstration project drastically increased costs. Without baseline data it is hard to assess the cost control features of the Arizona program.

One-fourth of all states obtained higher access levels of uninsured individuals as a result of their managed care programs. Reducing the number of uninsured individuals is one strategy of cost control for managed care programs. However,

Figure 1.1
Conclusions from Fifteen States with Medicaid Managed Care Systems

I. Medicaid programs using managed care systems are better able to control the costs of health care than the programs they have replaced, but it is hard to explain why.

II. The quality of care delivered through managed care is not adequately measured or monitored by the states; therefore, conclusions about the quality of health services are hard to make.

legislatures are suspicious of how more individuals can become eligible for health coverage and have this result in cost savings. For example, in Tennessee, the legislature did not believe that more people could be covered by a Medicaid-type program and have the managed care aspect of the program result in cost control. For this reason, the legislature demanded that the proposed enrollment cap be reduced as a requirement for funding. Subsequently, fewer people than intended are now covered by TennCare, allowing the percentage of individuals outside of managed care to be higher than planned.

Two major conclusions become apparent through the review of these sixteen cases (see Figure 1.1). First, Medicaid programs using managed care health systems control health care costs better than the systems they have replaced, but it is hard to explain why. Second, the quality of care delivered through managed care is not adequately measured or monitored by these states.

Conclusion I: Managed Care Programs and Cost Control

Although managed care began earlier in this century as a way of providing coordinated health services including prevention services to better guarantee the health of the insured, these fifteen states view managed care as a system of cost control. These states are interested in expanding health services to a larger population not so much to expand government services, but rather to extend control over health expenditures of residents who have no health insurance coverage. This focus on cost control slants the original intent of managed care, which was based on providing a population of enrollees with comprehensive and high-quality health services.

Most striking, however, is the lack of hard data or evidence that costs are being better controlled under managed care. Many of these states report that the growth of health expenditures has declined or has become stable as a result of the managed care programs. But despite the overriding goal of cost cutting and cost control, these states have not designed a system within which costs can be identified and monitored across time. For example, there are no patient tracking systems that identify diagnoses and treatment and costs. In Tennessee, skyrocketing costs have been trimmed, but whether this is due to managed care or just lower payments to providers is not clear. One way of cutting costs is, of course, to spend less. In Tennessee, less spending has meant lower reimbursements to physicians, hospitals, and other health care providers.

In the case of Arizona, costs dramatically increased at the beginning of AHCCCS. Arizona never participated in the Medicaid program, and the indigent could rely only upon county aid programs. When Arizona decided to apply to HCFA for a waiver and qualify for matching federal dollars, the indigent and working poor had access to a state health program for the first time. Whether Arizona's cost containment care program is controlling costs is difficult to assess, because there is little baseline data with which to compare current program costs.

Greater efforts need to be made in the accounting systems of these managed care programs in order to identify the main factors behind cost control. Data collection should be standardized in order to allow for comparison among the states. HCFA could require, through the waiver application process, a standardized accounting system that could be used for comparison data analysis.

Conclusion II: The Quality of Managed Care Is Not Adequately Measured

These fifteen states have difficulty demonstrating that their managed care programs have increased the quality of health services. While these programs have certainly increased the number of individuals covered, the overall quality of services has not been adequately measured. In the case of Tennessee, some former Medicaid patients felt they were better off under the old program than under the new managed care program. Because the quality of care delivered through managed care is not adequately measured or monitored by these states, conclusions about quality are hard to make. Anecdotal data from these cases suggests that quality of care has not increased through these managed care programs, and in many cases, seems to have declined.

SUMMARY

Has managed care accomplished its objectives of cost control and improved health care access and quality? The following cases present a mixed report, and reveal the difficulty with which health reform efforts can be evaluated. Greater monitoring and evaluation is needed, and state governments need to design better systems to assess the performance of their managed care health programs.

NOTES

1. Henry J. Aaron, *Serious and Unstable Condition: Financing America's Health Care* (Washington, D.C.: The Brookings Institution, 1991), 1.

2. Laurene A. Graig, *Health of Nations: An International Perspective on U.S. Health Care Reform*, 2nd ed. (Washington, D.C.: Congressional Quarterly Inc., 1993), 15–17.

3. Colin Winterbottom, David W. Liska and Karen M. Obermaier, *State-Level Databook on Health Care Access and Financing*, 2nd ed. (Washington, D.C.: The Urban Institute, 1995), 18.

4. Michael D. Reagan, *Curing the Crisis: Options for America's Health Care* (Boulder, Colo.: Westview Press, 1992), 13–14.

5. Ibid., 53.

6. Ibid., 40.

7. Ibid., 3.

8. Jon Coolidge, "Baby Death, TennCare Link Probed," *Commercial Appeal* (Memphis, Tenn.) (February 19, 1994).

9. Aaron, *Serious and Unstable Condition*, 65.

10. Robert E. Hurley, Deborah A. Freund, and John E. Paul, *Managed Care in Medicaid: Lessons for Policy and Program Design* (Ann Arbor, Mich.: Health Administration Press, 1993), 25.

11. Ibid., 26.

12. R. E. Hurley and D. Freund, "Determinants of Provider Selection or Assignment in a Mandatory Case Management Program and Their Implications for Utilization," *Inquiry* 25, no. 3 (1988): 402–410.

13. Deborah A. Freund, *Medicaid Reform: Four Studies of Case Management* (Washington, D.C.: American Enterprise Institute, 1984).

14. Marshall W. Raffel, and Norma K. Raffel, *The U.S. Health System: Origins and Functions*, 4th ed. (Albany, N.Y.: Delmar Publishers, 1994), 64 ff.

15. Ibid.

16. Ibid., 66.

17. Hurley, Freund, and Paul, *Managed Care in Medicaid*, 46–53.

18. Ibid., 98–104.

2

The Alabama Medicaid Reform Plan

RENE P. McELDOWNEY

INTRODUCTION

Our analysis of Alabama's Medicaid reform initiative focuses on the historical developments of federal and state events. The underlying framework of this investigation rests on the premise that state health care policy is influenced by three sets of factors: level of economic development, general political culture, and patterns of interest group activity.[1] The chapter will start by reviewing the 30-year evolution of the Alabama Medicaid Agency and the political influences which helped to shape its current programs and structure. The second half of this chapter will be devoted to the specifics of Alabama Medicaid Reform along with some of its outcomes and projected ramifications.

BACKGROUND

Historically, the Alabama Medicaid program has had a narrow base of political and constituency support. Despite being responsible for the overwhelming majority of in-state nursing home care, the agency still has a relatively poor public image of serving only minority and indigent clients. Prior to the implementation of the state Medicaid program, most of Alabama's eleemosynary health care was provided by an often inadequate and uncoordinated system of charitable activities and organizations. The resulting outcome was that many poor and disabled Alabamians often went without adequate health care and often died as the result of delayed or lack of treatment.

It was a full five years after the enactment of the 1965 federal Social Security Act before Alabama's Medicaid agency first "opened its doors." On June 30, 1967, the state's first female Governor, Lurleen B. Wallace, signed an Executive Order to institute the formation of Alabama's Medicaid program. The Order called for a divided system of operations. The Department of Pensions and

Security was to be responsible for determining Medicaid eligibility, while the Medical Services Administration (MSA) within the Department of Public Health would actually run the program. It is still somewhat unclear as to why this particular management structure was chosen. It appears to be more of a political consideration than an ardent belief that such structural arrangements are superior to the concise regulatory model. In any case, this division of essential operations eventually led to the first among many fiscal crises that was to haunt the agency throughout its 30-year history.

THE 1970s

Almost from its very inception, the Alabama Medicaid program has been plagued with a variety of difficulties. Upon opening its doors in January of 1970, the agency had 253,991 certified eligibles. By the same token, departmental documents show that later that same year the number of eligibles had risen to just over 313,000, an 18 percent increase. It is of little surprise, therefore, that by the start of its second year of operations, Alabama's Medicaid program was already experiencing its first among many financial emergencies. The rapid increase in the number of Medicaid recipients, coupled with the pent-up needs of a populace which has traditionally been without adequate health care, translated into an acute shortage of available funds. Reports indicate that an additional $6.5 million was needed to cover 1971 expenses, while more than a million dollars was still owed to hospitals and providers for 1970 services.[2]

The federal matching rate for Alabama's program in 1970 was approximately three to one; which means that the federal government supplies three dollars for every one dollar raised by the state. This rate remained relatively stable throughout the mid-1970s (see Table 2.1), as state appropriations steadily increased (see Table 2.2). The additional burden of a rapidly rising Medicaid population and the resulting unforeseen expenditures forced the state to find additional funds. Alabama's traditional anti-tax sentiment compelled lawmakers to raise additional funds through a variety of mechanisms. These included increases in state Medicaid appropriations, imprinter rental funds, insurance premium refunds, third-party collections, provider co-payment recoveries, and retroactive adjustments.[3]

Despite its continuing fiscal and organizational difficulties, the Alabama Medicaid Agency was not reorganized until the late 1970s. As a result of the shortcomings of the original organizational structure, the state's executive administration recommended that Medicaid operations be elevated to a cabinet post in 1977. This allowed the Medicaid Agency to be a completely separate entity which had direct access to the state's governor and budget operations. This new provision allowed the office to be headed by a single Commissioner who would have the responsibility for determining both Medicaid eligibility and overall operations.

Due to the ongoing financial difficulties, one of the first mandates of the new Commissioner was the implementation of a new cost containment program. To curtail rising Medicaid expenditures, agency officials outlined several new changes which included a retroactive claims process for the reimbursement of

Table 2.1
Medicaid Appropriations from the General Fund

Years	Millions
1978	57.062
1979	66
1980	93.9
1981	76
1982	90
1983	94.045
1983	95.819
1984	101.608
1985	103.696
1986	105.872
1987	101.692
1988	114.99
1989	122.014
1990	145.657
1991	129.465
1993	128.935
1994	139.511

pharmaceuticals, new limitations on the number of hospital days covered, and the formation of a new Medicaid fraud unit.[4]

The federal matching rate was also steadily decreasing during this same time period (Table 2.1). This forced state officials to take additional measures to make up for the funding shortfall. While the cost containment program was helping to control overall Medicaid spending, it was in no way able to compensate for the decreases in federal funding. The mechanism chosen by the state was a mass transfer of funds from various other governmental agencies, including the Department of Mental Health, the Department of Pensions and Security, and the Office of the Attorney General. These transfers marked the beginning of a dangerous pattern to cover state Medicaid funding shortages by raiding the budgets of other departments and government agencies. This practice became particularly acute during the late 1980s and 1990s when a series of funding difficulties began to jeopardize Medicaid operations.

Table 2.2
Medicaid Matching Funds, State/Federal (percent)

Years	State Funds	Federal Funds
1978	27.42%	72.58%
1979	27.42%	72.58%
1980	8.68%	71.32%
1981	28.67%	71.33%
1982	28.87%	71.13%
1983	28.87%	71.13%
1984	27.86%	72.14%
1985	27.86%	72.14%
1986	27.70%	72.30%
1987	27.59%	72.41%
1988	26.71%	73.29%
1989	26.90%	73.10%
1990	26.79%	73.21%
1991	27.27%	72.73%
1992	27.07%	72.93%
1993	28.55%	71.45%
1994	28.78%	71.22%
1995	29.55%	70.45%

THE 1980s

The 1980s were marked by rising health care costs and federally mandated expanded Medicaid services. But the real fiscal nemesis of this period was the cost of providing long-term care. Natural demographic changes coupled with advances in medical science were causing unprecedented increases in Medicaid nursing home expenditures. Long-term care began to account for more than 40% of benefit outlays, with projected costs due to increase throughout the foreseeable future.[5] Thus, new government policies were instituted to help curb this trend and ease the strain on other Medicaid services and programs. Among the policy changes were a moratorium on the number of new nursing home beds and more restrictive criteria for Medicaid nursing home assistance. These new policy actions had an almost immediate effect. The number of nursing home application denials increased from just 1% to nearly 15% in a year's time. The result was that the rise in Medicaid nursing home expenditures began to come into line as these new policies began to take hold.

The 1980s also marked the state's first quasi-experiment with managed care. In an effort to reduce costs and enhance rural health care, state Medicaid officials entered into a cooperative agreement to pilot-test a rural health maintenance program for Medicaid recipients.[6] The project was limited to Greene County, Alabama, which has historically had a disproportionate number of Medicaid beneficiaries and an acute lack of health care services. Unfortunately, the project was to be short-lived due to a variety of unspecified funding and logistical difficulties.

The crown jewel of the state's 1980s flirtation with managed care was the 1988 Maternity Waiver project. The overarching goal of this program was to combat Alabama's high infant mortality rate by developing a coordinated system of ongoing prenatal care. The mandate of the initiative was to ensure that "eligible pregnant women receive comprehensive, coordinated and case managed medical care appropriate to their risk status through a primary provider network."[7] In essence, the program operated by directing women to appropriate health care providers and then augmenting their care through a set of managed care case coordinators. These coordinators worked closely with the women to help ensure a healthy pregnancy. Their activities included a variety of measures including developing a plan of care, facilitating patient education classes, following up on missed appointments, and assisting with transportation needs. The Medicaid Waiver project was designed to eliminate the fragmented and insufficient care of the previous system while helping to ensure that recipients received a comprehensive set of medical and new-parent services. The care provided through this program was fashioned to be an interwoven network of services to help mothers and infants obtain a healthy start on life.

THE 1990s AND BEYOND

The success of the managed care maternity waiver was instrumental in advancing Alabama Medicaid managed care. Nationally, managed Medicaid programs were picking up political steam by demonstrating that states could provide high-quality health care at lower costs. Several states started to explore the concept as early as the late 1970s, but the bulk of Medicaid managed care programs did not appear on the horizon until overall expenditures began taking their toll on state budgets. As the previous section demonstrates, Alabama was no different in this regard. As its budget has become increasingly strapped by growing overall demands and reductions in federal spending, the Alabama state Medicaid agency has taken incremental steps toward establishing a statewide Medicaid managed plan.

During the early 1990s, Alabama's Medicaid agency pursued several different avenues toward establishing state Medicaid managed care. The majority of these efforts, however, were thwarted by more pressing political problems such as funding mechanism difficulties, provider opposition, and policy changes within the Health Care Financing Authority (HCFA). Due to increasing costs and limited resources, HCFA initiated new rules and regulations on how states could legally raise their portion of federally matched Medicaid funds. The overall objective of these new changes was to curtail federal government Medicaid spending and shift more of the responsibility back to the individual states. But to poor states like Alabama, these new rule changes marked a dramatic shift in the state's ability to fund its Medicaid program and sparked an intense search for ever more creative ways of raising funds that would be matched at the federal level.

THE DANCE FOR THE DOLLARS

One of the initial schemes Alabama used to increase its matching federal funds was through a type of voluntary hospital tax. Until 1992, all state-level Medicaid agencies were able to partially offset the direct costs of funding their Medicaid programs by collecting voluntary contributions from hospitals. Alabama benefited from this system because of its favorable federal matching rate. But, as federal budget officials began to see outlays for Medicaid matching funds rise to record-setting levels, HCFA officials were called into action to curtail rising costs. Agency analysts determined that the hospital contribution system was largely to blame for the increases and recommended that the program be cut in order to control costs. Thus, HCFA officials started to promulgate new rules and regulations designed to put a stop to voluntary hospital contributions, in order to stem the ever-increasing flood of federal Medicaid dollars to the states.

These policy changes were a major setback to the state of Alabama, which has a significant Medicaid population and a limited tax base. Efforts were made to partially make up for the hospital contribution shortfall through a federal compromise which allowed Alabama to secure additional funding through what was termed provider taxes. Specifically, the provision hammered out between state officials and the federal government allowed the state to increase its Medicaid matching contributions by requiring private hospitals to pay a case-adjusted $25 per patient day, and all nursing homes to pay $1,000 per bed.

As 1993 approached, state Medicaid officials experienced yet another emergency; a state budget shortfall of $20.6 million for 1993, and an anticipated $65 million shortage for fiscal 1994. As a result, the agency began to fall behind in its payments to providers and announced that it would be forced to cut payments by 15% across the board if a solution could not be found.[8] The Medicaid agency and Alabama hospitals were able to negotiate a legislative solution which effectively repealed the aforementioned provider tax and transfer program. Instead, the entire provider portion was to come from nonmandatory, intergovernmental transfers from the state's two leading teaching hospitals at the University of Alabama at Birmingham and the University of South Alabama in Mobile. The state also agreed to come up with an additional $10 million for 1994 but required that any remaining 1993 or 1994 expenditures were to come from reduced payments to hospitals and other providers.[9]

MEDICAID REFORM IN ALABAMA

The combined difficulties of federal Medicaid funding policy changes and severe state budget shortfalls prompted state officials to take another look at establishing a statewide Medicaid managed care program. After months of negotiations and meetings with various provider groups, Alabama state Medicaid officials decided that the wisest approach would be to start small, see what problems developed, and then proceed in establishing a larger statewide effort. The advantages of a smaller, well-defined initiative are considerable to a state which has a very low managed care market penetration (10%) and a high number of Medicaid recipients. There are many areas in Alabama which have a severe shortage of health care services and the logistical problems of trying to implement a statewide program of managed care delivery in regions which lack sufficient numbers of health care providers seemed inadvisable.

To overcome these difficulties, it was decided that the best approach for the state was to start with a five-year demonstration pilot project. By being able to select a specific site, agency officials maintained that they could better ensure adequate medical care delivery and avoid many of the pitfalls experienced by the other state Medicaid managed care programs. A smaller program would also facilitate direct comprehensive evaluation and provide greater opportunity to address problems at their beginning stages rather than at the crisis level. And finally, by going into an already established HMO market, the state felt that it could capitalize on the experience of an up and running health maintenance organization and avoid the numerous difficulties associated with trying to entice managed care companies to service areas with severe shortages of health care providers and economically poor population groups.

In general, the prospect of a setting up a Medicaid pilot project is seen by state officials as a giant step toward resolving the state's ongoing Medicaid funding difficulties. Rural states like Alabama, which have a significant number of poor and indigent, are at a distinct disadvantage when it comes to trying to establish statewide comprehensive Medicaid managed care. Experiences from early pioneering Medicaid managed care programs have documented how abuse and substandard care can run rampant without established networks of care and adequate government oversight.[10]

PROGRAM SPECIFICS

The State of Alabama has one of the most restrictive Medicaid programs in the nation in terms of eligibility, benefits to recipients, and payments to providers. For adults to qualify for coverage under Aid to Families with Dependent Children (AFDC), a family must have a child living in the home, one parent must be absent or incapacitated, and the family's annual income must be no more than 16% above the federal poverty level. AFDC eligibility levels for Alabama are currently at the federally mandated minimum.[11]

By introducing a Medicaid managed care pilot program, the Alabama Medicaid Agency believes that it has a unique opportunity to improve the above situation while helping to ensure the well-being of the state's poor and disabled. As stated in their Medicaid Waiver application, the broad goals of the program are: (1) To prove that, in certain communities, collaboration is more effective and cost-efficient than a competitive system; (2) To provide coordinated and accessible care to Medicaid recipients; (3) To expand education and outreach efforts, thereby improving Medicaid recipients' health and overall quality of life; (4) To provide service coordination for children with special needs and persons with disabilities; (5) To maintain quality of care under a formulary with the pharmacy program. In other words, the overall goal of the agency is to provide a more efficient and effective health care program at reduced costs.

The site chosen for the Medicaid pilot project is the city of Mobile and its surrounding county area. Located in the southern tip of the state, this county is very typical of urban areas within the deep south. Its current population base is about 400,000, with the more affluent populations living in the suburbs and outer areas. Most of the area's indigent are minority, female, and poorly educated. There are approximately 41,235 Medicaid recipients who are slated to be included in the Medicaid managed care pilot project. The projected demonstration project eligibles are as shown in Table 2.3.[12]

The types of problems facing managed care pilot project participants are, unfortunately, not unique. Like most states, Alabama's health-related problems relate to high rates of adolescent pregnancy, large numbers of low birth weight babies, high infant mortality rates, and low percentages of early childhood inoculations. Furthermore, over 50% of all Mobile County births are to Medicaid mothers, 18% of which are documented as having inadequate or no prenatal care. The prevalence and incidence of these problems is particularly high among teenage mothers.[13]

Table 2.3
Demonstration Project Eligibles

Category	no. Eligibles
AFDC	21,627
Low Income Children (SOBRA)	10,092
Low Income Pregnant Women (SOBRA)	1,799
Infants (0-1) of SSI Mothers	15
Aged	122
Blind	50
Disabled	7,494
Refugees	56
Total	41,235

As previously mentioned, Alabama's infant mortality rate is well above the national average. The state's 1993 infant mortality statistic was 10.3 deaths per 1,000 live births, which is nearly 3 percentage points above the national average of 8.6%. Racial disparities among infant deaths are even more striking. The infant mortality rate for African-American babies born in Alabama is nearly 17 deaths for every 1,000 live births. Nonwhite infants are also 2.1 times more likely to die before their first birthday than their Caucasian counterparts, and have a 26% chance of being born to a mother without a high school education.

State officials maintain that several factors need to be addressed in order to combat these abysmal statistics. Some of the more commonly cited factors include a fragmented health care delivery system, a shortage of primary care physicians willing to treat Medicaid patients, unreasonably restrictive eligibility requirements, and an overall lack of continuum of care. The managed care demonstration pilot project hopes to address this situation by establishing a coordinated network of care and preventive medicine. And because one of the primary expenses of the current fee-for-service Medicaid program is related to childbearing, one of the main objectives of the program will be to improve maternal and infant health.[14]

Mobile County has been part of Alabama's Maternity Waiver Program for a number of years. The existing waiver program is incorporated into the managed care pilot project. Project documents outline a continuous flow of care from the initial onset of pregnancy into early childhood. Once a positive pregnancy test has been documented, women who are potentially eligible for Medicaid are referred to an eligibility worker for application and enrollment. After enrollment has been accomplished, a case management worker then refers the women to an OB/GYN provider and continue to work closely with that provider to streamline the women's care throughout pregnancy and postpartum period (see Table 2.3). By targeting the Medicaid recipients during the early stages of their pregnancies, state officials predict that they can realize a significant decrease in overall costs while helping to improve the health and well-being of the state's maternal and infant population.

Another challenge before the state Medicaid agency was the selection and development of a provider network. Factors which influenced the process included: (1) location of the managed care facility; (2) adequate choice of health care providers; (3) number of non-Medicaid patients currently enrolled in the HMO; (4) profit/nonprofit status; (5) financial solvency; (6) regulation compliance history.

It was important to Medicaid officials that patients have ready access to health care services. Since reliable transportation is often a problem for the poor and disabled, the location of prospective HMOs was of primary consideration. Ideally, the facility should be easily accessible to public transportation, located in an area frequented by Medicaid recipients, have low- or no-cost parking, and provide a reasonably safe environment.

Federal Medicaid guidelines require that Medicaid patients have a choice of primary care physicians. The theory behind the traditional Medicaid fee-for-service system was that Medicaid patients would have access to any number of area physicians. In practice, however, patients often had a very difficult time in finding private physicians willing to take Medicaid recipients. This problem was particularly acute in obstetrics, where patients often made up to 20 telephone calls in order to secure an obstetrician. Thus, any HMO being considered for the project had to demonstrate that it had an adequate number of primary care physicians for the Medicaid populace to choose from, and the ability to provide obstetrical care.

One of the primary lessons learned from the states which originally implemented Medicaid managed care was that a managed care facility which treated a mix of Medicaid and non-Medicaid patients was preferable to an HMO which serviced only the Medicaid populace. Some of the reasons cited for this finding include the stigma associated with receiving treatment from a managed care program which is known to service only poorer population groups, the pressure that the middle class exerts in terms of maintaining certain levels of care and the improved attitudes of the health care staff. Many Medicaid officials indicate that by having a healthy mix of both Medicaid and commercial patients, overall quality and services are easier to maintain.[15] Commercial patients are more likely to have their complaints and dissatisfactions addressed and are less shy about voicing their objections to company officials and their employers.

The profit/nonprofit status of demonstration project HMOs was not of major importance in the selection process. However, for political reasons Medicaid officials agreed that all things being equal, a nonprofit HMO would be more preferable. Alabama is a provincial state in many ways, and there were fears that the idea of taxpayer money being used for stockholder gain might spur public opposition. In addition, because of the limited number of HMOs operating within the state, public attitudes toward the managed care industry are still somewhat suspect and agency officials believed that the overall success of their project would lie in part with their ability to avoid public opposition.[16]

A couple of Medicaid managed care states experienced several managed care organizations who were not financially solvent enough to adequately treat Medicaid patients, who have a history of using a disproportionate amount of health care services. The results were that inadequately funded managed care facilities often ended up closing their doors and leaving scores of Medicaid recipients without medical care and state Medicaid agencies scrambling to make up the losses. Alabama officials have sought to avoid such occurrences through protractive measures. They have chosen to adopt a three-tiered regulatory model which divides the responsibility of overseeing HMOs between existing state agencies. While the Alabama Medicaid Agency still has responsibility for the overall program, inspections and licensing functions are to be carried out by the state Department of Public Health while financial requirements are overseen by the state Department of Insurance.

The basic premise of a health maintenance organization is that it provides prepaid health care to a set of beneficiaries and thus incurs the financial risk for providing that care. Thus, most states have concluded that managed care is a type of insurance and thereby falls within the jurisdiction of state insurance department codes and regulations. Alabama falls in line with this philosophy and any managed care facility wishing to do business in the state of Alabama must meet state insurance department criteria and guidelines. In addition, the Alabama Medicaid Agency requires some additional safeguards for HMO pilot project participants. Managed care organizations wishing to take part in the demonstration project must post a performance bond with a corporate bonding company licensed by the Alabama Department of Insurance. The monetary amount of this bond must be equal to one and one-half months' capitation payment. The Trustee must also be a national bank or other independent trust entity approved by the Commissioner of the Alabama Medicaid Agency, and the funds are to be clearly earmarked as a specific security for the five-year duration of the demonstration project.[17]

The difficulties associated with implementing a Medicaid managed care program can be considerable. The Alabama Medicaid Agency ultimately has the responsibility for monitoring the provision of Medicaid services, and the implementation of the managed care demonstration project does not lessen this requirement. Legally, the agency has an obligation to monitor the delivery of Medicaid services and oversee quality improvement activities. The regulatory history of any pilot project HMO is therefore of primary consideration to the agency. Medicaid officials maintain that working with managed care organizations which have a good regulatory history lessens the burden of possible punitive regulatory actions and helps lend to the success of the overall program. As a rule, managed care organizations which are used to abiding by state and federal guidelines have good working relationships with regulatory officials, which is a distinct advantage in working out program details and problem solving.

THE PROVIDER NETWORK

After presenting program specifics and weeks of negotiations, state officials decided to contract with only one area managed care organization; what the federal government terms "a sole source provider." This decision was a rapid departure from how Medicaid managed care is usually delivered. Because patient provider choice is such a fundamental aspect of the federal Medicaid program, most states engage several managed care companies to treat their Medicaid recipients. However, given the unique characteristics of the Medicaid provider network in Mobile County, state Medicaid officials decided to enlist the services of only one HMO. It was reasoned that a collaborative, sole-source provider would be better able to provide services in a cost-effective and coordinated manner than a system of competing health maintenance organizations. In addition, the state Medicaid agency maintained that a single-source system would also reduce the costs associated with duplication of program administration, education, tracking systems, and the possibility that a Medicaid recipient might "fall through the cracks."

The managed care company chosen to participate in the Mobile pilot project consists of a closed panel network of providers which have historically provided health care services to the bulk of Mobile's Medicaid population. The University of South Alabama Hospital (USAMC) has been the dominant provider of hospital care for the Medicaid population for over a decade. It has also worked closely with Medicaid officials through the 1988 Maternity Waiver project and in trying to meet the health needs of Mobile and its surrounding county areas. USAMC also has had an exclusive managed care contract with a successful nonprofit HMO (PrimeHealth) for the past ten years.

In 1983, the University of South Alabama identified a critical need to develop a commercially insured payer base in order to support and maintain its College of Medicine, teaching mission, hospital (USAMC), and Health Services Foundation. After considering several options, university officials decided to support the creation of a not-for-profit corporation to be known as PrimeHealth. The main purpose of PrimeHealth was to assist USAMC in remaining financially viable and to provide the College of Medicine with needed referrals.[18] The hospital was facing a financial crisis and this solution was projected to allow it to remain fiscally secure and at the forefront of managed care in Mobile County.

Since its inception, PrimeHealth has gone on to achieve some impressive results. It was the first federally qualified HMO in the State of Alabama and has become the largest managed care company in Mobile County. Currently, PrimeHealth has a membership population of over 34,000 patients and a 7% market penetration in the city of Mobile and surrounding areas. It has also been a significant source of referrals for USAMC hospital and currently accounts for a significant portion of its outpatient services. Thus, by utilizing PrimeHealth and the University of South Alabama's hospital system, Mobile County Medicaid patients will be largely serviced by their traditional providers and university-qualified specialists. And because PrimeHealth is a staff model HMO, Medicaid officials maintain that it will be easier for them to control such aspects as patient utilization, pharmacy services, and general costs.

In overview, Alabama's Medicaid pilot project will not be a statewide effort, but rather encompass only the city of Mobile and its surrounding county area. Patients will be able to choose their primary care providers from a number of individuals who have historically provided care to Medicaid recipients. Participating doctors are employees of PrimeHealth and thus paid on a set salary level. This should help mitigate many of the perverse incentives that are often cited as contributing to the withholding of care. The project will also implement a freestanding Resource Center several months prior to demonstration project implementation. The purpose of this center is to help facilitate the transformation of the traditional Medicaid program over to the managed care plan. One of the primary functions of the center will be to help Medicaid recipients understand how the program works and provide instruction on accessing its services. The center will also act as a clearing house for a variety of ancillary services such as a patient education library and detailed information on how to select a primary care provider or file a complaint. In essence, the Resource Center is designed as a type of one-stop shopping for Medicaid patients to receive information on a variety of topics concerning Medicaid managed care, along with other ancillary services.

OUTCOMES AND CONCLUSION

This overview of the development of Alabama's current Medicaid reform plan is an important compendium in how state and federal events help to shape social programs and policy. The incremental nature of the state's Medicaid managed care movement has allowed it to establish a reasonable record of success and political acceptability. The 1988 Medicaid Waiver project has been the cornerstone of this process. The program has been instrumental in helping to reduce Alabama's infant mortality rate and in providing expectant mothers with a continuum of ongoing prenatal and postpartum care. 1994 figures indicate the women participating in the waiver program are reported to receive an average of nine prenatal visits as opposed to only three such visits prior to the program's implementation. Babies born to Maternity Waiver mothers also require fewer neonatal intensive care days, which results not only in healthier infants, but helps to reduce agency expenditures as well. The general success of the Medicaid Waiver Project has helped Medicaid officials take further steps toward developing comprehensive Medicaid managed care.[19]

The Mobile Medicaid Demonstration Project was implemented during the spring of 1996. After submitting its Medicaid Waiver application to the Health Care Finance Authority in September of 1995, the agency encountered several setbacks before obtaining approval. The majority of questions encompassed two main areas, the choice of using a single-source provider and specific details related to program operations and budget neutrality. A compromise was reached in which the Mobile pilot project proceeded with its decision to exclusively utilize PrimeHealth for the first three years and then send out for competitive bids for the remaining two years of operation. Operations began in the Mobile area and the waiver application was approved in 1997.

NOTES

1. See Anthony B. Kovner, *Health Care Delivery in the United States* (New York: Springer Publishing Company, 1990).

2. Most of this historical information was obtained from current and former Medicaid employees and an internal Medicaid report entitled ''A Historical Overview of the Alabama Medicaid Agency 1970–1995.''

3. See Alabama's Medicaid Agency Annual Report, 1995.

4. Ibid.

5. Ibid.

6. ''A Historical Overview of the Alabama Medicaid Agency 1970–1995.''

7. Ibid.

8. See Culley Scarborough, ''One Crisis After Another,'' in a local bi-monthly publication entitled *Health Care Alabama.*

9. Ibid.

10. Here I have been influenced by several reports and publications including the multi-article exposé on Florida Medicaid Fraud in the Florida Sun-Sentinel and David Osborne's chapter on the AHCCS program in *Laboratories of Democracy* (Boston: Harvard Business School Press, 1988).

11. Most of the information in this section was obtained from a copy of the Alabama's 1995 HCFA Medicaid Waiver application.

12. Ibid.

13. Ibid.

14. For an excellent overview of Medicaid managed care or just managed care in general, see Peter R. Kongstvedt, *Essentials of Managed Health Care* (Gaithersburg, Md.: Aspen Publishers, 1995).

15. I was influenced here by a study I did for the Alabama Department of Public Health in 1995. The project encompassed reviews of several state managed care systems, which included Minnesota, Maryland, Arizona, Tennessee, and Washington. Nearly all Medicaid officials expressed a preference for using health maintenance organizations with a mix of both commercial patients and Medicaid recipients.

16. State records show that as of January 1996, there are eleven HMOs licensed to do business within the state of Alabama.

17. Most of the information in this section was obtained from a copy of the Alabama's 1995 HCFA Medicaid Waiver application.

18. Ibid.

19. See Alabama's Medicaid Agency Annual Report, 1994.

3

Arizona Health Care Cost Containment System

MICHELLE A. SAINT-GERMAIN

With AHCCCS we are like Columbus: we don't know exactly where we are headed, and we don't know what we will find when we get there.
Arizona House Majority Leader Burton Barr, 1981

POLITICAL, HEALTH, AND ECONOMIC ENVIRONMENT PRE-ADOPTION

Arizona was the last of the 48 continental states to join the union, postponing statehood until 1912.[1] This frontier legacy still prevails to some extent in Arizona. Natives take pride in being self-reliant and maintaining as much independence as possible from the federal government. In a state legislature dominated by conservatives and Republicans, Medicaid was a dirty word, being associated with Democrats and liberals. There was little support for Medicaid from community groups and none from professionals. This feeling was so pervasive that, fifteen years after the enactment of Medicaid in 1965, Arizona was the only state without a functioning program. As theorized by Bachman,[2] it would take a substantial crisis for the state to reconsider its position.

Actually, a Medicaid program had been adopted by the Arizona state legislature in 1974 and signed by the governor. However, a key provision to allow the state to assess the counties for the local share of funds was ruled unconstitutional. Several influential legislators, fearful of open-ended budgets and the scandals that plagued the California Medicaid program, succeeded in killing any bill that would have appropriated enough state money to fund the program. This stalemate persisted for years. For example, in 1977, the legislature passed a bill to repeal the Medicaid program, but it was vetoed by the governor and the legislature was unable to override his veto. Thus the law was on the books but the program never functioned.

Another unique feature of Arizona is the large number of Native American residents. About 400,000 Native Americans live in Arizona, of whom about 170,000 live on 20 reservations scattered throughout the state. The Indian Health Service (IHS), funded entirely by the federal government, has traditionally provided health care to on-reservation Native Americans; the Bureau of Indian Affairs (BIA) has covered nursing home costs. Arizona legislators were fearful that if a Medicaid program was adopted, the federal government might discontinue funding the IHS and BIA programs, leaving the state to pick up the financing of health care for the Native American population in Arizona.[3] These fears were partially realized later on when Arizona sued the federal government to recoup $18.6 million in a dispute over which party was fiscally responsible when reservation residents were referred off-reservation for care.[4]

The Arizona State Constitution mandated that counties assume responsibility for indigent health care. Each county had its own program, eligibility requirements, services, and fee structure. Arizona counties had quite low eligibility ceilings, covering only about 40% of persons below the federal poverty level, compared to 60% in other states.[5] Counties with more generous benefits complained that people migrated in from other counties just to receive health care. There was little or no private sector involvement, although some nonprofit hospitals had traditionally provided care to the poor.

Years later, analysts were astounded at the numbers of people who participated in Arizona's Medicaid Waiver program. Their participation was much greater than could have been predicted by using county statistics on indigent care. The underserved population was grossly underestimated in Arizona because many people chose not to use county services. Some underuse was caused by adverse county requirements for eligibility. For example, some counties required applicants to make a public declaration of indigence in order to qualify for health care. Also, as programs migrate from the local to the state and national levels, eligibility requirements are often loosened. This prompts previous nonusers to take advantage of the program—a phenomenon termed the "woodwork effect."

There is evidence that Arizona had been thinking about managed care and cost containment even before the advent of its Medicaid Waiver program, the Arizona Health Care Cost Containment System, or AHCCCS (pronounced "access"). For example, in 1978 the state filed suit against two foundations for medical care organized by county medical societies. The foundations got competing physicians to agree to set rates to be charged to policy holders of certain health insurance companies. In 1982, the U.S. Supreme Court found that these arrangements violated anti-trust legislation but that HMOs did not. HMOs were different because they were agreements between noncompeting physicians and were conducive to cost containment.[6]

POLITICAL PROCESS OF POLICY FORMATION AND ADOPTION

How was this configuration of seemingly hostile factors overcome? The Arizona case provides a classic example of the Streams and Windows model of policy making described by John W. Kingdon.[7] Policy making is often described by others as a linear process consisting of several stages, such as problem definition, agenda setting, alternative generation, policy adoption, and implementation. Kingdon's model, however, is quite different.

There are three possible sources or streams of influence that affect policy making. First is the problem stream, which identifies potential agenda items by defining which things are problems. Not all situations or events are perceived as problems; rather, problems are conditions that we believe we should do something about.[8] Second is the policy stream, which identifies potential policy alternatives that reflect both advances in technical and scientific knowledge as well as basic consensus on specialists' values.[9] Third is the political stream, which contains events such as elections, changes in the political party in power, public opinion, and media campaigns that can influence what government does.

Kingdon's insight is that these three streams operate relatively independently of one another, each with their own forces, considerations, and styles.[10] That is, politicians may search around for a problem to solve, in order to win favor with their electorate. Policy specialists may develop solutions for which problems have not been formally acknowledged to exist. And a problem may exist that never gets onto the formal agenda, because no feasible solution exists or no politician is interested in it as it is defined.

Agenda and policy change occur when the three streams are joined in an opportunity called a "policy window."[11] Policy windows are not tightly scheduled, but are influenced by events mainly in the problems and politics streams, which can range from cyclical elections to unexpected dramatic events. None of these events will rigidly determine what must be done; what actually occurs is also influenced by the policy stream.[12] Often it takes a perceptive and persistent policy entrepreneur to sense that a window is opening and to seize the initiative of linking (or coupling) policy alternatives with problems and political events.[13]

The major concern in the problem stream in Arizona was not so much health as it was the dire fiscal condition of the counties. An analysis in 1982 stated that the two goals of AHCCCS were to alleviate the counties' financial burdens from providing indigent care, and "to implement price competition and deregulation in the health care market to control costs."[14] Arizona had passed a "Prop-13"-type measure that capped the amount of revenue that could be raised by property taxes. Revenues would increase only if there was economic growth, but the economy was in a downturn. In 1974 the counties spent $58.6 million on indigent care; by 1980 the cost was $122.6 million. Counties were spending up to 25% of their budgets to meet their constitutional mandate to provide health care for the indigent; one county attempted to declare bankruptcy. Swallowing their pride, the counties petitioned the state to either take over the health care program or bring in federal Medicaid dollars. It was estimated that Arizona would gain between $40 million and $60 million per year in Title XIX funds. However, the counties were under the mistaken notion that under the latter alternative they would receive and/or manage Medicaid funds directly.

At the same time, a group of grassroots activists began a statewide campaign for a traditional Medicaid program. A coalition began to emerge, consisting of county supervisors; legal aid and other indigent-related groups; Democratic state representatives from Tucson including Sister Claire Dunn, the AAUW, several Hispanic groups, and so forth. Pink-colored petitions were circulated throughout the state to put a Medicaid initiative on the fall ballot. In the summer, one Sunday was designated ''Medicaid Sunday.'' Tables were set up outside a great many churches to gather signatures. The actual number of signatures was never clear, but the event generated substantial publicity and put pressure on the state legislature to do something.

In the policy stream, a group of legislative staffers had been doing research on Medicaid alternatives. In 1981, Congress had adopted an act which allowed alternatives in delivery and financing for Medicaid and permitted program waivers to be issued.[15] The public was for Medicaid but the legislature was not. The staffers' idea was to get Medicaid dollars without the Medicaid program. Arizona was leery of the waste, fraud, abuse, and runaway budgets in states with traditional Medicaid programs. The staff investigated capitation projects, which had been tried on a limited basis in some states, such as Oregon. Debates about health care issues stormed in the Arizona House and Senate; interested parties ping-ponged back and forth across the courtyard separating the two chambers. Some legislators began to focus on the idea of an alternative to Medicaid—a clean slate. At that time it was still unusual to consider a managed care approach to a health program for the poor. Public hearings were proposed.

At the hearings, a wide variety of groups testified. A representative from the Arizona Hospital Association remarked that while there was room for improvement, it was something they could live with. An attorney for the Arizona Medical Association reported that the bill addressed most of their concerns. Qualified support was also expressed by such groups as the Arizona Academy of Family Physicians, the Governor's Council on Children, Youth, and Families, the Statewide Health Coordinating Council, the Governor's Advisory Council on Aging, the Arizona Association of Counties, the Director of the Arizona Department of Health Services, the Arizona Association of Home Health Agencies, the Arizona Optometric Association, and the Arizona Pharmacy Association.[16] Some Arizona physicians expressed concern about socialized medicine. Rural physicians, however, saw a chance to be reimbursed for services that they had been providing for free to the indigent, and in the end the medical establishment agreed not to oppose it. Interestingly, the state-supported medical school at the University of Arizona testified that it would not be impacted because it had nothing to do with indigent care—a far cry from its position years later when it lost its AHCCCS contract, its income fell by 25%, and several faculty physicians resigned.[17]

Community groups expressed concerns over services that were not to be covered (more than thirteen waivers were obtained) but also extended tentative support. These included the League of Women Voters of Arizona, the Arizona Ecumenical Council, the Grey Panthers, the President of Senior Now Generation, the American Association of University Women, Arizona Right to Life, Tucson Metropolitan Ministry, Jewish Family Services, the Medicaid Statewide Health Care Task Force, and the Arizona Community Action Association, and so on.

In the politics stream, recent electoral changes provided a policy window. The state governor, Bruce Babbitt, a neo-liberal or new Democrat, was looking for issues on which to exercise leadership. The new Republican president, Ronald Reagan, was a champion of market-based initiatives. Political appointees in the federal Health Care Financing Administration (HCFA) wanted a demonstration project; career bureaucrats wanted the chance to extend the Medicaid program to the last holdout among the 50 states.[18] In many ways, the Arizona case foreshadowed some of the principles of the reinventing government movement of the 1990s, such as injecting competition into service delivery.[19]

As described by Kingdon's model, Governor Babbitt emerged as the policy entrepreneur. Working with the Republican-controlled state legislature, grassroots activists, and the health care industry, Babbitt forged a consensus on a new type of health care program for the indigent that promised to keep the overall budget low. Babbitt made the program palatable to Republicans by promising that it would be run completely through contracts with the private sector, and would deregulate the provision of health care to the poor by obtaining waivers from Medicaid program requirements. It was acceptable to the poor because it promised to be better than what they had. It was acceptable to the medical establishment because it would bring new dollars into the health care industry. The counties did not like giving up program control but accepted it on the basis of fiscal relief. And finally, the Democrats had no choice politically but to support it.

The legislative staff realized that this was their window of opportunity. They drafted a proposal almost overnight, drawing on articles from the *New England Journal of Medicine* and other sources. They cobbled together a plan based upon the availability of votes for the various component parts. One observer likened it to six blind men and an elephant: it was different to each of them, but all could find something they liked about it.

An initial version of the Arizona alternative program was adopted by the legislature in May 1981, but was vetoed by the governor. Babbitt felt that it did not have the explicit go-ahead from HCFA, and that it would be foolish for the state to embark on such a program without a firm guarantee of federal funding. Legislative staffers began to meet with HCFA officials to negotiate waivers from the traditional Medicaid program. HCFA staff were apprehensive about the plan, because they would have to issue waivers that had never been approved before and a large number (13) of waivers.[20] Even the flexible waiver process had some limits, whether under a Republican or a Democratic administration. Little did they realize that Arizona's program would still officially be a "demonstration" project more than a dozen years later.[21] Arizona Republican state legislators who had contacts in the White House sent messages to HCFA that they wanted to work something out—and soon. Also, Arizona wanted assurances from the federal government that it would not withdraw Indian Health Service funding from Arizona if a Medicaid program was adopted.

Finally, the governor called a special session of the legislature and the program that had been reviewed by federal officials was passed in November 1981. An emergency clause stipulated that the program must be implemented before the next regular session of the legislature and also appropriated the necessary funds. This move ensured that funding would not be sabotaged by the following year's legislature, as had occurred with the 1974 bill. This proved to be a double-edged sword that on the one hand guaranteed that the program would go forward but on the other hand caused plenty of problems for program implementation.

TYPE OF SYSTEM ADOPTED

AHCCCS has been described in many ways, and the description has changed as the program has evolved over time. In 1981, several alternatives existed. These included a traditional Medicaid program; a state bailout of the counties; a statewide program for catastrophic expenses; or a Medicaid Waiver program.[22] Arizona opted for the last of these, adopting the Arizona Health Care Cost Containment Program, or AHCCCS. The legislation was deliberately adopted with few specifics. As is well-known in policy-making studies, it is often necessary for legislation to be rather vague in order to garner the votes necessary for passage; AHCCCS was no exception.

The purposes of the program were, first, to bring Medicaid dollars to Arizona. These dollars would benefit the fiscally strapped counties (and, by extension, the state, which would otherwise be forced into a financial bailout of the counties). Second, the purpose was to accept Medicaid dollars only in such a way as to deregulate them from federal control. Deregulation would allow market-based strategies of price competition to be applied to the delivery of health care to the indigent. Third, the purpose was to allow Arizona to control program costs. Waivers obtained from HCFA would allow Arizona to control costs mainly by limiting the amount and type of services that AHCCCS would be required to provide to program participants, and by limiting the number of the indigent who would be eligible for the program.

The legislation that established AHCCCS was not lengthy. Salient points are shown in Figure 3.1. These program features reflected the primary purposes of the program.

Figure 3.1
Features of the AHCCCS Program

1. The Arizona Health Care Cost Containment System (AHCCCS) was established as a unit within the State Department of Health Services, with a Director, and $20 million was appropriated for an operating budget.

2. County responsibility to provide medical care for the indigent was limited to that not covered by AHCCCS and the formula for county financial contributions to AHCCCS was determined at about half their previous health care budget.

3. The Director, through competitive bidding, would award a contract for the administration of AHCCCS to a private sector entity.

4. The Director, through competitive bidding, would award prepaid capitated service contracts to providers for inpatient and outpatient services.

5. The state would provide reinsurance against catastrophic costs to providers.

6. The state would define the type of services to be offered to participants by the providers.

7. The state defined eligibility for participation of indigents.

8. Nominal co-payments were required from some eligible participants.

9. State, county, and private sector employees were eligible to participate in AHCCCS with no public subsidy, as one of their health care plan options.

10. A Joint Legislative Health Care Cost Containment System Committee was established to oversee the development of the program and to conduct studies.

The first purpose was to bring federal Medicaid dollars to Arizona. Accordingly, authority to initiate AHCCCS was linked to the receipt of federal funds. The second purpose was to deregulate the provision of medical care to the indigent and to institute price competition. Therefore, implementation was contingent upon obtaining waivers from HCFA. These waivers would allow for substantial deregulation of not only the medical service provision portions of AHCCCS, but also its entire administration.

The third purpose was to control costs. Costs would be controlled, first, ostensibly through the competitive bid process from service providers. The state would establish the total budget to be expended on AHCCCS based on the projected number of enrolled members. The plans would then agree to provide specific health care services for a fixed fee per member per month, based on categories of eligibility and geographic location. But the state would also be partially "at-risk." Until 1991, HCFA provided money to Arizona based on capitation rates that were set at 95% of the estimated costs under traditional fee-for-service Medicaid plans. Since then, however, Arizona has received reimbursement on a cost basis identical to other states with traditional Medicaid programs.[23] In addition to capitation payments, the state is also responsible for fee-for-service payments, reinsurance, deferred liability claims, Medicare Part B premiums, disproportionate share hospital payments, third-party recoveries, and administrative costs.

Costs would be controlled, second, by limiting eligibility for participation. The upper limits were set at incomes of less than $2,500 per year and a net worth of less than $30,000 for individuals qualifying as medically indigent; limits for the medically needy were between $2,501 and $3,200 per year. The limits were increased by 33⅓% for a spouse and 17% for each additional dependent. Generally, only persons with incomes less than 40% of the federal poverty standard are eligible for AHCCCS. As the original limits were established by statute, they were difficult to change to keep up with inflation. In 1989, a family of four was limited to an income of $5,354 per year, compared to the federal poverty level of $12,700. In 1995, the Arizona limit was raised to $5,476, compared to the federal level of $14,800.[24] Furthermore, those determined medically needy were to pay a premium equal to 10% of the cost of their care. Nominal co-payments were also assessed for doctor visits and prescriptions, for elective surgery, and nonemergency use of emergency rooms.

Cost would be controlled, third, by limiting the services provided. Examples of excluded services were mental health, dental care, eyeglasses, family planning, home health care, long-term care, and liver, pancreas, lung, and bone-marrow transplants. Costs were also limited through the adoption of a managed care approach. While there is no universally accepted definition, managed care generally limits the choice of provider, limits patient utilization of services, and modifies the role of the primary care physician.[25] Each participant is assigned to a primary care provider (PCP). PCPs act as gatekeepers, holding down utilization to what is deemed to be necessary and appropriate services.

OUTPUTS, OUTCOMES, AND IMPACTS

The Arizona program can be evaluated from several aspects. First, has it met its own stated goals of bringing Medicaid dollars to Arizona, to alleviate the fiscal crisis of the counties? Second, has it developed an alternative delivery and payment system for providing health care services to the indigent, a system based on deregulation and price competition? And third, has it controlled costs? Additionally, we might also incidentally enquire as to whether it had any impact on the health of indigent Arizonans. Finally, we might ask, has it changed the health care sector in Arizona?

Bringing Medicaid Dollars to Arizona

Arizona has been successful at obtaining Medicaid funding (Table 3.1). Battles with the federal government over issues such as fiscal responsibility for off-reservation care for Native Americans, which once threatened funding for the entire AHCCCS program, have now been settled. Although AHCCCS is still technically a "demonstration project," its continued approval for funding is largely pro-forma. The total budget of the AHCCCS program has grown from

Table 3.1
Financing the Arizona Health Care Cost Containment System

YEAR	FEDERAL	STATE	COUNTY/ OTHER	TOTAL
1982-83	37,800,000	22,050,000	55,300,000	$ 115,150,000.00
1983-84	57,063,316	81,270,100	80,457,000	$ 218,790,416.00
1984-85	66,772,402	124,620,647	63,073,476	$ 254,466,525.00
1985-86	70,120,000	141,311,000	62,912,000	$ 274,343,000.00
1986-87	87,147,800	127,822,300	72,201,600	$ 287,171,700.00
1987-88	111,983,000	187,193,000	78,050,000	$ 377,226,000.00
1988-89	311,402,000	245,216,000	123,906,000	$ 680,524,000.00
1989-90	457,789,500	320,289,400	153,870,600	$ 931,949,500.00
1990-91	521,200,000	350,600,000	160,200,000	$ 1,032,000,000.00
1991-92	647,900,000	422,800,000	156,200,000	$ 1,226,900,000.00
1992-93	822,525,260	477,191,800	177,234,140	$ 1,476,951,200.00
1993-94	952,177,310	480,116,500	195,312,790	$ 1,627,606,600.00
1994-95	1,080,888,783	499,879,327	187,921,800	$ 1,768,689,910.00
1995-96	1,186,486,800	575,530,700	197,868,500	$ 1,959,886,000.00

Sources: AHCCCS Annual Reports.

$115 million in 1982–1983 to $1.9 billion in 1995–1996. The federal and state contributions did (at least at first) alleviate the fiscal stress of Arizona's counties for acute medical care for the indigent. With AHCCCS, counties contributed only about half the amount they had been spending for acute indigent care before. County contributions did eventually increase, but only after the incorporation of a long-term care component into AHCCCS with its own cost-sharing formula that required additional county contributions beyond the acute care contribution.

By avoiding the need to bail out the counties financially in the short run, however, the state may have gotten itself into an even more unfavorable situation in the long run. The state portion of the AHCCCS bill has grown from $22 million to $575 million. The federal share has grown most of all, from $37 million to nearly $1.2 billion, as shown in Table 3.1.

Developing an Alternative System

There were really two different parts to the alternative system: one, the contracting out of program administration; and two, the contracting out of service provision. The first was a complete failure; the second has been more of a qualified success.

The AHCCCS Administrator

Since nearly every facet of program administration was to be contracted out, the legislature would approve the creation of only a handful of new state employee positions (estimates varied between six and thirty). These employees would be responsible for "policy and regulations, research and planning, financial management, and public relations."[26] The point was stressed that this was not to become a new mega-agency. The state would exercise only an oversight role and would not have its own eligibility workers, providers, and so on. A joint legislative committee would also exercise control.

The governor pushed for early implementation in order to get federal dollars flowing into Arizona. There was talk in Congress of turning Medicaid into a block grant, where state allocations would be based on past Medicaid dollars spent in each state. This would leave Arizona out completely. There was clearly pressure to make things happen, which left little time for pilot projects. Not doing pilots was an administrative gamble, because this approach had never before been tried on a statewide basis. But doing pilots was politically risky, since if something went wrong the whole program would be in jeopardy. In Arizona, the "can-do" approach prevailed. It was decided to forge ahead in the present and to tidy up afterward.

Another unique characteristic of the Arizona experience is that there was no preexisting Medicaid program. On the one hand, there was no entrenched bureaucracy to deal with or organized power base to overcome; on the other hand, there was no history of experience in the state on which to draw. Not only was there no experience, there was no organized state Medicaid agency, health plan, eligibility process, or service provider network.

The Arizona Department of Insurance and Department of Health Services were given oversight responsibility, but they had no experience in managed care. No state had ever contracted out the entire program administration.[27] HCFA officials had no such experience, either. Also, some HCFA officials were apprehensive about the implications for Medicaid in the other 49 states, should the Arizona experiment succeed.

The Request for Proposals were sent out to select a program administrator. A number of bids were received. Allegedly, Ross Perot's EDS bid but lost, sued, and settled out of court. The contract was awarded to McAuto Systems Group, Inc., or MSGI, part of McDonnell Douglas in St. Louis, Missouri. It was later discovered that McAuto had formerly been doing business as Bradford National Corporation, which had been convicted of defrauding the federal government on a defense-related computer contract. McDonnell Douglas bought the computer services group for $11.5 million.[28] Also, there was speculation that McDonnell Douglas might withdraw a planned helicopter manufacturing plant from Arizona if it did not win the contract.[29]

The contract was originally awarded for $8.2 million for 40 months, and later raised without rebidding to more than $11.4 million to cover unexpected administrative costs. By 1984, however, MSGI had submitted claims for more than $42 million. The state terminated the contract in 1984. MSGI sued for $16.2 million, while Arizona countersued for $18.6 million. Eventually, Arizona was paid $3.5 million to settle the lawsuit.

The state took back responsibility for program administration, and retains it to this day, having established a quasi-independent administrative entity for AHCCCS. With regard to developing an alternative administrative system, one article concluded that "AHCCCS is a managerial success because it has survived."[30] There were many setbacks in the first few years, and at times the program's future looked very tenuous. An early report by the General Accounting Office (GAO) raked the implementation process over the coals.[31] Newspapers did not hesitate to publicize potential scandals. Continuous shortfalls made the program a favorite whipping post for legislators at budget time. But AHCCCS has not only survived, it has become the largest single government program in Arizona, with more than 1,000 full-time staff and a total annual budget approaching $2 billion.

Service Delivery

Arizona was the first state to attempt to implement statewide "a system of comprehensive, prepaid capitation contracts awarded to providers using a competitive bidding process."[32] When the timetable for drafting rules and regulations was announced, many groups demanded to be included as a reward for their silence or tacit approval during the legislative process. Governor Babbitt included not only health care providers but also advocates and activists in the drafting committees. This astute move gave everyone a stake in seeing the program succeed and effectively bought off any potential opposition.

To take full advantage of deregulation and price competition, the bidding process set almost no barriers to entry to potential bidders. It had been expected that existing private sector HMOs would become involved in AHCCCS. But there were only six in the entire state (two in Phoenix and four in Tucson), and, being staff models, they had limited facilities and no easy way to expand rapidly. AHCCCS did result in the formation of six new HMOs using the alternative independent physician association (IPA) model. However, none had previous private sector managed care experience. Only three plans survived and the market share of this type of plan is only about 22%.[33] Of eighteen contracting providers in the first year, only two had prior prepayment experience; in the second year, only one of nineteen had pre-AHCCCS prepayment experience.[34]

Demolishing barriers to entry brought out not only the naiveté but also the "greed and apparent corruption among some providers."[35] There was considerable movement of plans into and out of the market, due to financial losses, mismanagement, and fraud.[36] Of course, the federal agency charged with oversight, HCFA, did not have much experience in this area either and so could offer little guidance.[37] This resulted in wholesale disruption of continuity of care to thousands of AHCCCS participants who had to be shifted to new plans when their assigned providers went bankrupt or lost their AHCCCS contracts.

Congressional Rep. Henry Waxman (D-Calif.) held hearings in 1984 on the management of the Arizona Medicaid Waiver by HCFA. Waxman had experience with the Medicaid scandals of California, where he found that: "The strong economic incentive to under-serve that is inherent in prepayment, combined with the lack of effective State monitoring of the contracting providers, led to frequent denials of care and extensive profiteering."[38] He further went on to state his concerns about the AHCCCS program: "AHCCCS may . . . prove to be a system that offers high-quality care to the poor in a cost-effective manner, or it may . . . offer nothing more than a second-class medical care for the poor and offer opportunities for exorbitant financial gain for providers."[39]

The GAO testified that HCFA requirements for written quality assurance plans from the providers that explain how health services are monitored and corrected, for collection of utilization data by the state, for medical audits by the state, and for the establishment of grievance procedures, had not been fully implemented. However, steps were being taken by HCFA and the state to work toward compliance with these requirements. A GAO auditor reported that: "It is clear that the program started before it was ready. When AHCCCS began, eligibility and enrollment systems weren't fully ready. Policies, rules, and regulations weren't finalized. Quality assurance requirements such as management information systems, grievance procedures, and the encounter data requirements weren't specifically communicated to the providers."[40]

After a rocky start, AHCCCS did eventually iron out these problems. Quality assurance measures adopted included performance standards in six areas: administration, subcontracting, organization, program service, program operation, and finances. There is multi-factor rating of bids on the basis not only of price but also adequate financial resources; an adequate health care network to provide services; acceptable accounting standards and practices; an adequate quality assurance program; adequate management organization; an adequate management information system; an adequate capitation proposal. The state conducts reviews of performance standards and makes frequent site visits throughout the term of the contract. Annual medical audits are conducted by the AHCCCS Medical Director and outside evaluators selected through competitive bidding. All utilization of health care services by eligible participants must be documented (called encounter data) so that a determination can be made whether participants are being denied access to services. An office of client advocacy helps members resolve problems with their plans, and investigators deal with charges of fraud or abuse. And quarterly and annual financial statements and certified annual financial audits must be submitted by all plans.

Despite the fact that Arizona's AHCCCS program is still operating as a "demonstration project" under HCFA waivers, it is commonly accepted as an established, ongoing program. A report prepared for HCFA in 1996 identified a number of areas that anyone attempting a similar program should take seriously. These include comprehensive administrative structures, strategies for setting capitation rates, quick eligibility and enrollment systems, wide-ranging fiscal and medical audits, and, above all, an adequate management information system.[41] A GAO report found common problems in all the states with Medicaid managed care approaches, including implementation planning, attracting commercial HMO participation, and participant education.[42]

Cost Containment

There have been a number of reports that AHCCCS medical care does not cost as much as a traditional Medicaid program.[43] However, others have charged that there are significant problems with the methodology employed to calculate the cost savings. The difficulty is that there is not now, and never was, a concurrent traditional Medicaid program in Arizona with which to compare AHCCCS. Thus cost-saving calculations must be based on comparisons with the private sector or with Medicaid in other states. Furthermore, even these limited comparisons have not demonstrated remarkable cost savings, never even approaching 10%. And the rate of growth of costs in Arizona was 9.1% per year compared to 10.3% per year in traditional Medicaid programs.[44]

In addition, it is not possible to point to any single aspect of the Arizona program as the major cause of the savings, or to assign a proportion of savings to each of its aspects. That is, it is not possible to untangle the effects of competitive bidding from the effects of the gatekeeper model or the other facets of the Arizona program. Perhaps with the increase in the number of Medicaid alternative models, some comparison will be possible that can isolate (statistically speaking) the contribution to cost containment of each of the various strategies or specific combinations of them.

Moreover, AHCCCS administrative costs seem to be at least twice as high as those of traditional Medicaid programs (for the acute care program only; the long-term care program is not considered here). From 1983–1984 to 1988–1989, AHCCCS administrative costs rose from $10 million to $56 million, nearly twice the rate of health care costs, which rose from $219 to $643 million.[45] These higher administrative costs are due to the management of the bidding process, the oversight of quality of care, contract enforcement, and the monitoring of plan financial integrity. Major programs such as AHCCCS may entail "high start-up costs associated with developing an appropriate infrastructure (for example, management information systems, provider networks, and bidding processes)."[46] Recently, AHCCCS changed from a one-year contract cycle to two and now three-year cycles, to cut down on the expenses associated with the bidding process.

The competitive bidding process that eventually emerged in Arizona did not completely fulfill expectations for cost control.[47] As there was only very general guidance in the enabling legislation, it is not unusual that the process evolved in response to market forces. Bidders faced considerable uncertainty because of downturns in local economic conditions, recent U.S. Supreme Court decisions about the provision of services to undocumented immigrants, a rocky administrative start (poor agency coordination and multiple decision makers), and a lack of historical data on utilization trends and costs.[48] In the early stages, program officials were under pressure to demonstrate that the alternative delivery system could work as well as be cost-effective.[49]

Besides political factors, other nonmarket forces also constrained competition in the Arizona case. For one, the desire for universal access to and availability of care caused AHCCCS officials to want to implement the program throughout the state, even though some areas would not be as cost-efficient as others. For another, the state felt it had a vested interest in protecting some existing health care providers to the poor, such as county hospitals, which had significant investments in infrastructure, personnel, and ties to the community.[50]

Program officials were pleasantly surprised at the large number of bidders who competed in the first round of RFPs. It may be that providers saw AHCCCS as an attractive alternative to regulation.[51] As a whole, however, the bids were far above the amount the state had budgeted for the project. Program officials wanted to spread the AHCCCS dollars as widely throughout the state as possible but still keep total expenditures under budget. This resulted, on the one hand, in awards being made to multiple bidders in each county (rather than a single contract, franchise arrangement) and, on the other hand, a pseudo-negotiation process where the state requested—and got—voluntary price reductions from bidders whose offers were judged too expensive by the state.[52]

The multiple winning bidder strategy results in weak incentives to keep prices low because economies of scale are reduced when the total volume of participants is divided among several plans. But by the same token plans have little incentive to keep bids low, since the chances of winning at least a partial contract are high. The pseudo-negotiation process also produces strong incentives for gaming. Plans may bid at a level above their actual costs but below other plans' bids, or they may try to make up losses from one category of participant with higher profits on other categories.[53]

Another danger inherent in competitive bidding is that over time the administration may come to resemble a regulatory agency as it fulfills its enforcement responsibilities, with the bidding process becoming "regulation-driven rather than market driven."[54] Similarly, as the program may come to depend, over time, on the same group of providers, it may be "captured" by its clients,[55] with the result that both prices and costs may rise over time.[56] Providers have several times resorted to filing suit to force AHCCCS to reveal the data it uses to set rates and the formulas it uses to make award decisions, when they felt they did not get their "fair share" of the patient pie.[57]

One example of AHCCCS regulatory initiatives is the ongoing medical audits of primary care physicians in outpatient settings. The audits have been carried out by AHCCCS staff in conjunction with contracts to the Accreditation Association for Ambulatory Health Care (AAAHC). An unanticipated finding was that the majority of offices visited were not in compliance with state fire marshall fire safety codes. Other regulatory moves have included the implementation of grievance procedures at both the plan and state levels; client advocacy at the state level; and the investigation of cases that fall below statistically expected norms of service.[58] In fee-for-service programs, these concerns are often left to the private sector.

There are several instances of how AHCCCS works to countermand the "at risk" status of contracting providers. There is constant turnover in the patient base. In response, all state-funded participants are certified as eligible for at least six months (federally funded participants are eligible for twelve months). Further, participants may only change plans once per year, during a limited open enrollment period. This guarantees providers a stable cash flow.[59] Also, the state limits risk by providing reinsurance for catastrophic costs [60]; and the reinsurance threshold may not be set at the optimum level to keep bids low. Finally, plans are judged on several criteria, not just the amount of the bid. Thus, plans do not have to have the lowest bid in order to win a contract.

Another strategy to contain costs was to limit the number of indigents who are eligible to participate in AHCCCS. This strategy is still being pursued, although at times it seems counterintuitive. Arizona still does not participate fully in Medicaid. That is, by raising its limits on eligibility to stipulated federal levels, additional categories of indigents could be covered and more federal funding could be received. However, the state chooses not to do so, despite arguments that the state would actually save money in the process, because more of those now funded fully by state dollars would be shifted to categories with federal financial participation as well.

The persisting AHCCCS eligibility process has also confounded attempts to control costs. While low ceilings attempt to hold down the total number of eligibles, people may be eligible under a number of different criteria, as shown in Table 3.2.

These criteria are linked to different social welfare programs and the funding source of the programs. For example, persons who receive Aid to Families with Dependent Children (AFDC) are certified as eligible by county welfare department workers. Persons receiving social security have their eligibility certified by federal Social Security Administration workers. Persons receiving unemployment compensation are certified by state Department of Economic Security workers. None of these workers is under the supervision of AHCCCS. One audit found that some counties were making mistakes in 16.7% of eligibility determinations.[61] In addition to the problems occasioned by multiple agencies being involved, their computer systems have been found to be incompatible. Thus, inconsistencies in the records of other agencies compared to AHCCCS records cannot be rectified electronically. Other audits have routinely turned up capitation payments being made for dead or ineligible recipients.[62]

Table 3.2
History of Enrollment in the Arizona Health Care Cost Containment System

YEAR	TOTAL	AFDC	SSI	MI/MN	CHILD	CMP	SOBRA	SES	FES	ALTCS
1982	89,683	53,195	28,322	8,166						
1983	147,124	66,520	29,506	51,098						
1984	185,409	74,898	30,582	79,929						
1985	144,450	71,948	32,340	40,162						
1986	151,140	74,043	34,869	42,234						
1987	192,305	88,059	36,949	47,003	20,294					
1988	216,425	100,014	38,760	47,680	24,138		5,833			
1989	278,099	118,989	36,698	44,626	39,648		28,830			9,308
1990	318,383	143,480	38,828	40,176	29,244		54,275			12,380
1991	377,208	178,112	43,692	40,347	27,264		73,774			14,019
1992	439,405	209,472	49,726	48,787	27,006		88,344			16,070
1993	467,659	217,845	56,055	49,201	10,467	14,127	102,404			17,560
1994	463,340	220,568	61,316	31,314	2,312	14,108	111,201	276	3,437	18,808
1995	451,587	208,325	66,006	30,179	2,444	9,410	110,227	283	4,352	20,361

Source: Overview of the Arizona Health Care Cost Containment System (Phoenix: AHCCCS, June 1996, Appendix I).

Other cost control measures have been similarly frustrated. The initial legislation envisioned a small co-payment for some services (e.g., $0.50 for prescriptions), for some AHCCCS participants. However, this feature proved extremely cumbersome to enforce, and in practice participants were not denied services for lack of ability to pay. Eventually, these cost containment measures were dropped.

While AHCCCS has endured, it continues to be the target for many investigations and accusations. One investigation by the Office of Inspector General of the U.S. Department of Health and Human Services, concerning the oversight of AHCCCS administration by the HCFA, has dragged on for more than eighteen months. As the largest program in Arizona, it is not unusual for rumors to swirl about. Many former AHCCCS officials have been recruited by provider organizations as consultants or executives to help them prepare winning bids. Charges of wrongdoing have been leveled against program officials but none have been found to have merit.[63] As with the beginning of AHCCCS, there may be many groups which are not completely satisfied with the program, but none wants to see the program shut down.

Impact on the Health of Indigents

Measures of the impact of the AHCCCS program are largely absent. A common failing of evaluations of public programs is to report how many units of output were produced, for example, numbers of participants enrolled, dollars spent, and volume of services provided, but not to report whether these outputs had any significant impact on their presumed target—the health of the indigent. Perhaps this only reinforces the point that the main purpose of the AHCCCS program is to demonstrate that a market model can be applied to the delivery of health care services to the indigent.

As no specific goals with regard to the health of the indigent population were part of the original program, very little data was collected on this subject. While Arizona registered the largest increase (161%) in per capita spending on health care from 1980 to 1990 ($848 to $2,211)—undoubtedly partially a function of Medicaid dollars flowing into the state—statewide rates for some health indicators had not improved.[64] Infant mortality rates eased from 12.4 (per 1,000 live births) in 1980 to 8.8 in 1990 and 8.4 in 1992.[65] But low birth weights increased as a percentage of all births from 6.03% to 6.51% over the same period.[66] Among unmarried women, low birth weights climbed from 18.7% of all births in 1980 to 32.7% in 1990.[67]

A Flinn Foundation report noted that Arizonans were sicker but received less medical care than other U.S. citizens. Despite high rates of teen suicides, alcohol abuse, and mental illness, Arizona had obtained a waiver from HCFA's requirement to provide mental health services. It ranked tenth lowest in 1990 on mental health expenditures per capita, spending only $10 in 1981, $12 in 1985, and

$27 in 1990 (when services for children were phased in), compared to U.S. averages of $27, $35, and $48.[68] In 1989, 25% of Arizonans had no regular source of care compared to 18% of all Americans; and 13% of Arizonans reported they didn't get needed care in the past year. The percentage of persons without health care coverage in Arizona increased from 15.5 in 1990 to 20.2 in 1994,[69] compared to U.S. averages of 13.9 and 15.2 in the same years. In Arizona, one-third of the poor and one-quarter of Hispanics, Blacks, and American Indians had no health insurance. From 1980 to 1994, Arizona fell from 27th to 37th in terms of disposable personal income per capita.[70] The report concluded that there were two Arizonas: one whose citizens had health insurance and were healthy, and one whose citizens did not and were not.[71]

An early evaluation of AHCCCS reported that the percentage of poor children seeing a doctor increased from 58.8% in 1982 to 75% in 1984, and the percentage of the poor with no regular source of care decreased from 15.3% in 1982 to 5.2% in 1984.[72] Another study documented a decrease in premature births among AHCCCS participants from 7% to 4% of all births.[73] More recent data show increases in the percentage of women between 1989 and 1995 who received cervical and breast cancer screening, family planning services, and blood pressure screening under AHCCCS. With regard to children aged 0–2, some progress was made in the percentage receiving measles immunizations and TB tests, but the rates fell for other measures, such as DPT and polio immunizations, physical exams, and hearing and vision tests. The rates of coverage for AHCCCS children for these services are generally lower than for children in employer-sponsored HMOs, but generally higher than for uninsured children.[74] While it would be difficult to ascribe changes in the health status of the poor solely to the presence or absence of AHCCCS, much more attention needs to be paid to the impact of AHCCCS on the health status of the Arizona population.

However, there are complications with attempting to measure impacts. For one, the AHCCCS population is generally in poorer health than persons with private insurance, and sees doctors more often.[75] The AHCCCS population also differs in other important ways from the private sector HMO population. Thus studies of the health care impact of AHCCCS must be investigated on different categories of the indigent (those who are participants and those who are not), as well as the nonindigent with and without health care coverage.

At the individual level, a few studies have explored participant access to care, with mixed findings. One report found that, overall, AHCCCS participants have comparable or better access to health care services and better quality of care for children than comparable groups in New Mexico's Medicaid program. However, some areas of concern were raised by the evaluation, including lower quality indicators for nursing home care and prenatal care.[76] New Mexico, while contiguous to Arizona geographically, is rather different in terms of the mix and distribution of its population, and is consistently at the bottom of the states in terms of disposable income. These factors make it a questionable comparison program; or, put another way, to say Arizona's program did only as well as New Mexico's is faint praise.

Additionally, at least one early study[77] found evidence that overall refusal-of-care rates had increased from 5.4% in 1982 to 6.9% in 1984, and that denial-of-care rates were higher among those enrolled in AHCCCS (8.4%) than for those not enrolled (4.7%). Some explanations may be that as expectations were raised, people became more aware of not obtaining needed services. Also, in the early years of AHCCCS, there was some confusion among participants about which providers they were allowed to visit. Participants who claimed to be denied care may either have not been eligible to be seen by that provider, or have lost their eligibility for AHCCCS altogether.[78] This issue is important because a goal of AHCCCS was to mainstream the indigent into private sector health care. AHCCCS literature boasts that nearly all hospitals and the vast majority of physicians in the state participate in AHCCCS. Nevertheless, there were many charges that AHCCCS contractors were grouping their indigent patients into only a few facilities, to minimize contact with and possible inconvenience to their private pay or privately insured patients.[79]

What few gains there are for the indigent in Arizona seem to have been achieved at the expense of the poor who do not qualify for AHCCCS. For them, both access to care and satisfaction with care have declined. Competitive bidding, cost containment, and other state controls put contracting providers under extreme financial pressures. Those in the system have better access to a comprehensive set of services and are generally more satisfied. Those not in the system, however, are more completely without medical care, as excess or marginal capacity is taken up by the low capitation rates of the AHCCCS system.[80] Arizona was tenth highest in the percentage of persons with no health insurance coverage in 1989, when one in five was not covered. The Arizona Hospital Association reported that its members wrote off more than $211 million in care to charity or bad debt in 1988 treating the noncovered poor. This resulted in cost-shifting to private pay or insured patients.[81] The percentage of persons using hospital emergency rooms as their usual source of care declined among AHCCCS enrollees from 17.8% in 1989 to 6.2% in 1995, but increased among the uninsured from 13.7% to 14.2% over the same period.[82] Among current AHCCCS participants, those who had no usual source of care before joining increased from 43% in 1989 to 60% in 1995,[83] reflecting the increasingly desperate situation of the poor in Arizona.

It is important to pay attention to health impacts because prepaid capitation gives providers many incentives to limit participant access to and utilization of care. And while the managed care principle works in theory to counteract those incentives, the finding that 62% of AHCCCS enrollees stay in a plan less than twelve months diminishes the theoretical benefits of managed care. The reasoning is that with managed care, the indigent will have increased access to a regular source of care. This will decrease inappropriate utilization of medical services, such as emergency room visits for routine care or minor acute illnesses that could be easily handled on an outpatient basis. Also, having access to a stable source of care would improve the health of the indigent through better continuity of care and the application of preventive as well as curative medicine. However, the benefits of preventive care are realized over the long run. This lessens the incentive of each provider plan to administer preventive measures (e.g., immunizations) because the odds are that the participant will be in another plan when the preventable illness manifests itself. Nor is there any incentive to restore the AHCCCS population to or maintain them at the highest levels of health since most are presumed to not be in the paid labor force.

In fiscal year 1994–1995, the AHCCCS program did begin to develop health indicators for acute care, long-term care, developmentally disabled, and behavioral health care. It also developed indicators for contracting provider financial health, as well as a member survey. In subsequent years, data will be presented on such things as the childhood immunization rate, the low birth weight rate, prenatal care utilization, mammography screening, and so forth. Finally, while most studies of satisfaction with care among AHCCCS participants have indicated that respondents are mostly satisfied, participants still remain largely uninformed about their rights to legislatively mandated transportation to health care sites, how to file a grievance, and other rights.

Impacts on the Health Care Market in Arizona

One of the hopes for the AHCCCS program was that it would stimulate the entry of new health care providers into the market. In 1989, one report lamented the lack of new plans.[84] In 1994, however, a significant new development was noted: the entry of some "heavyweights" into the bidding process. More than twice the number of bids was received than in the previous round.[85] These more established providers had followed a three-stage strategy over the twelve years of the program's existence: no participation, participation as subcontractor, participation as primary contractors. Finally, the goal of mainstreaming AHCCCS patients seemed about to be realized. But the entry of these giants pushed out several of the smaller plans that had been awarded AHCCCS contracts for years.

The more established providers gave several reasons for their entry: they wanted to diversify; they wanted access to a large and new patient base; they were facing increased demands from private sector insurers to cut costs; and they wanted to become players in the government contracts market—a safe alternative to the open market. They also wanted to position themselves should the long-delayed provisions for including public sector employees in AHCCCS be implemented.[86] They could not have helped but notice, in addition, that AHCCCS providers had reported $44 million in profits in the previous year, a 44% increase over the previous year and the largest ever. Profit margins for AHCCCS providers averaged 4.1% compared to 3.5% for other health maintenance organizations in the state.[87]

Another remarkable feature of the Arizona case is the entry of county-sponsored plans. Much of the market-centered rhetoric of the original legislation was aimed at getting health care out of the hands of public bureaucracies (associated with high costs and inefficiency) into the hands of the private sector. Counties, traditional providers of care for the poor in Arizona, were alarmed by this aspect of the AHCCCS program, since it could steer the indigent into managed care plans that used other facilities.[88] This represented a potential loss to counties with large investments in infrastructure. For them, AHCCCS represented a new source of revenue for previously unreimbursed care. However, if indigent patients were enrolled in other AHCCCS plans, this would reduce the use of county facilities by patients whose care was reimbursed, and it would increase the use of county facilities by those who were not eligible for AHCCCS, as they were turned away from other facilities. This would have a significant negative impact on county facilities in terms of reduced potential revenues from AHCCCS coupled with a need for more support from county revenues to deal with a larger burden from the uninsured "notch group."[89] It would shift the burden back to the counties in the continuing intergovernmental game of fiscal musical chairs.[90]

At first, some counties underestimated their actual costs and while successful at obtaining contracts, lost money with each additional patient they were awarded. Eventually, however, the county plans were able to compete successfully with the other providers. County-sponsored plans now enroll about 25% of eligibles to provide a continued flow of patients to county-owned hospitals. These hospitals suffered from lower occupancy rates and shorter average stays with the implementation of AHCCCS. There were also some bailouts, as when Maricopa County lost its contract and was later awarded a partial contract. This attempt to introduce competition into the public sector again anticipated the reinvention movement by several years.[91]

While none of the preexisting private sector HMOs became directly involved in AHCCCS in the early years, the program did affect the private health care market in Arizona indirectly. Thirteen new private sector HMOs arose in Arizona, resulting in a two-tiered market (one for the indigent and the other not) which was not the intent of the original legislation.[92] In general, the use of managed care has increased in the private sector in Arizona as well as in the public sector.

The original AHCCCS legislation envisioned a system where public sector employees would also be enrolled, allowing state and local governments to participate in the cost savings derived from a managed care program. Small businesses were also to be allowed to buy into AHCCCS to procure health care insurance for their employees at a reasonable cost. More than 66,000 Arizona small businesses with 25 or fewer employees would be eligible. The public sector program was never implemented, due to vigorous protests by public employees' unions; the small business provision was implemented but has very few participants. Some plans, which were formed specifically to bid on

AHCCCS contracts, no doubt thought that they would be able eventually to add the more lucrative public employee and private business employer contracts. They would use AHCCCS to capitalize and then quit the AHCCCS program to focus on the healthier working population of public sector and small business employees. This may have contributed to the demise of some of the early plans. Still, AHCCCS is credited with sparking the development of managed care plans in Arizona to serve the non-AHCCCS employed population.[93]

Nonprofit hospitals assumed a much greater role in AHCCCS than originally predicted; they now have about a 50% market share. They changed from a wait-and-see position to that of subcontractors, to primary contractors. One reason was that the bankruptcy and volatility among plans left the subcontracted hospitals often unreimbursed in the early days of the program. Another reason was that the market was changing, with the introduction of such cost control measures as diagnostic related groups (DRGs) and HMOs in the private sector as well. Finally, the hospitals realized that, as primary contractors, the reimbursement rates from AHCCCS would be greater than their marginal costs from treating new indigent patients. These organizations have better financial stability, more sophisticated management information systems, and greater experience with utilization review and quality assurance initiatives.[94]

Other potential impacts on the health care system in Arizona include the number of practicing physicians per 10,000 population in patient care. After increasing steadily until 1985, the rate of increase slowed and then fell in 1994. In comparison, the U.S. average continued to rise over the same period.[95] The number of hospital beds per 1,000 population showed an even more dramatic decline. After rising steadily in Arizona from 1940 and peaking in 1970, it fell substantially until 1992. Arizona, at 2.5, was a full bed lower than the U.S. average of 3.6 beds in 1992.[96] Arizona hospital occupancy rates, at 57.1%, are similarly lower than the U.S. average of 64.5% in 1992.[97] The number of nursing homes and nursing home beds increased in Arizona after long-term care was incorporated into AHCCCS in 1989. However, the number of beds per 1,000 persons aged 85 and older is substantially lower in Arizona than the U.S. average. At the same time, the number of full-time equivalent employees per 100 daily hospital patients has increased at an astounding rate. Arizona, at 720, is far above the U.S. average of 635 in 1993. Table 3.3 displays physician and hospital bed data.

CONCLUSIONS

Since the installation of the Clinton administration, federal evaluations of AHCCCS seem much more positive than before. Arizona appears to be compiling impressive achievements. Increases in the average annual per capita costs of AHCCCS reportedly averaged 6.8% in Arizona from 1983 through 1991, compared to 9.9% for a traditional Medicaid program. Administrative expenses

Table 3.3
Health Care System Indicators in Arizona

Mds per 10,000 patients	1975	1985	1990	1994				
AZ	14.1	17.1	18.4	17.9				
US	13.5	18.0	19.5	20.7				

Beds per 1,000 pop	1940	1950	1960	1970	1980	1990	1992	1993
AZ	3.4	4.0	3.0	4.1	3.6	2.7	2.5	2.5
US	3.2	3.3	3.6	4.3	4.5	3.8	3.6	3.6

Hospital Occupancy %	1940	1960	1970	1980	1990	1992	1993
AZ	61.2	74.2	73.3	74.2	62.4	60.2	57.1
US	69.9	74.7	77.3	75.2	66.7	65.7	64.5

Nursing Homes (N)	1975	1985	1990
AZ	70	107	112

Nursing Home Beds	1975	1985	1990
AZ	5884	11250	13265

Beds per 1,000 over 85 yrs.	1975	1985	1990
AZ	406.2	374.7	329.3
US	685.3	542.1	494.5

Employees per 100 patients	1960	1970	1980	1990	1992	1993
AZ	222	327	455	590	683	720
US	226	302	394	563	610	635

Sources: Charity Ann Dorgan, ed., Statistical Record of Health and Medicine (Detroit, Mich: Gale Research, 1995); Health United States 1995 (Washington, D.C.: U.S. Department of Health and Human Services, Public Health Service, Centers for Disease Control, National Center for Health Statistics, May 1996); Statistical Abstract of the United States 1995 (Washington, D.C.: U.S. Department of Commerce, September 1995).

appear to be coming down in Arizona from twice that of other programs, to about 7% of total expenditures, compared to 4% or 5% in other states. AHCCCS providers began to turn a profit in 1990 (0.29%) and the margin has increased steadily. Finally, AHCCCS capitation rates fell by an average of about 11% from 1994 to 1995, while national averages were projected to rise.[98]

However, Arizona's success is mixed at best. First, it has attracted Medicaid dollars. Second, it has backed away from an entirely deregulated system for the provision of medical care to the indigent. And third, there is little evidence that Arizona has been able to control program costs other than by limiting eligibility and services. Finally, it has not provided any evidence that the health of the indigent population in Arizona has been improved by AHCCCS.

Furthermore, a 1993 GAO report noted that while states are moving to managed care Medicaid systems to control costs while improving services, most are not moving to Arizona's capitated prepayment system. Although there is a wide range of possible variants, most states seem to be adopting a Primary Care Case Manager (PCCM) system.[99] The PCCM system pays a capitation fee to a primary care provider to become a case manager for each participant enrolled, but reimburses provided services on a fee-for-service basis. Fully capitated managed care programs such as Arizona's appear to work fairly well at controlling the costs of medical services,[100] but not so well at controlling administrative costs, both of which are crucial for holding down overall costs. Thus, there seems to be little evidence for the GAO's rather cheery 1995 conclusion that Arizona can serve as a model for other states.[101]

NOTES

1. This case study of the Arizona Medicaid-waiver program (AHCCCS) was undertaken in the summer of 1996. It is based on research conducted in Arizona with legislative and other records, as well as interviews with some of the key personnel involved in the early days of the AHCCCS program. It also made extensive use of published and unpublished materials made available by some of the authors cited in the references. The author wishes to especially thank the Center for Health Services Administration at Arizona State University. Of course, the author alone remains responsible for any errors or omissions in this study.

2. Sara S. Bachman, Stuart H. Altman, and Dennis F. Beatrice, "What Influences a State's Approach to Medicaid Reform?" *Inquiry* 25 (Summer 1988): 243–250.

3. "AHCCCS Wins Federal 5-Year Extension; Long-Term Care for Handicapped Also Authorized." *Arizona Republic* (December 2, 1988): A1.

4. "Indian Health Care Job of Feds, Judge Decides." *Arizona Business Gazette* (February 2, 1990): 28.

5. Howard E. Freeman and Bradford Kirkman-Liff, "Health Care Under AHCCCS: An Examination of Arizona's Alternative to Medicaid," *Health Services Research* 20, no. 3 (August 1985): 245–266.

6. Eric L. Richards, "Anti-Trust and the Future of Cost Containment Efforts in the Health Profession," *Nebraska Law Review* 62, no. 1 (1983): 49–85.

7. John W. Kingdon, *Agendas, Alternatives, and Public Policies* (New York: HarperCollins, 1984).

8. Ibid., 115.

9. Ibid., 140.

10. Ibid., 93.

11. Ibid., 94.

12. Ibid., 177.

13. Ibid., 188.

14. Frank G. Williams, "The Political Impact of the Arizona Health Care Cost Containment System" (Tempe: Arizona Center for Health Services Administration, Arizona State University), 1.

15. Deborah A. Freund and Edward Neuschler, "Overview of Medicaid Capitation and Case-Management Initiatives," *Health Care Financing Review* (Annual Supplement, 1986): 21.

16. Transcript of Public Hearings, Arizona State Senate, Health Welfare and Aging Committee (Phoenix, November 15 and 16, 1981).

17. "AHCCCS Loss Costly for UA's Medical School; Income Dips, Staffers Quit." *Arizona Republic* (November 21, 1994): B10.

18. Charles Breacher, "Medicaid Comes to Arizona: A First Year Report on AHCCCS," *Journal of Health Politics, Policy and Law* 9, no. 3 (Fall 1984): 411–425.

19. David Osborne and Ted Gaebler, *Reinventing Government* (Reading, Mass.: Addison-Wesley, 1992).

20. Chris Ferrara and Doug Bandow, "Finding an Alternative to Medicaid," *Journal of the Institute for Socioeconomic Studies* 9, no. 3 (Autumn 1984): 34–42.

21. Rhona S. Fisher, "Medicaid Managed Care: The Next Generation?" *Academic Medicine* 69, no. 5 (May 1994): 319.

22. "Background on the Implementation of AHCCCS and Summary of Activities for Years One Through Five," n.d. (Xerox), 52.

23. Nelda C. McCall, William Wrightson, Lynn Parringer, and Gordon Trapnell, "Managed Medicaid Cost Savings: The Arizona Experience," *Health Affairs* 13, no. 2 (Spring 1994): 235.

24. "Health Care for the Poor: Expand AHCCCS Coverage," *Arizona Republic* (April 7, 1995): B6.

25. Deborah A. Freund, "Competitive Health Plans and Alternative Payment Arrangements for Physicians in the United States, Public Sector Examples," *Health Policy* 7 (1987): 165.

26. Nelda McCall, Douglas Henton, Michael Crane, Susan Haber, Deborah Freund, and William Wrightson, "Evaluation of the Arizona Health Care Cost Containment System," *Health Care Financing Review* 7, no. 2 (Winter 1985): 78.

27. Ibid.

28. "State Gets AHCCCS Settlement; McDonnell Douglas Yields $3.5 Million," *Arizona Republic* (October 24, 1987): A1.

29. Bradford L. Kirkman-Liff, Frank G. Williams, and L. A. Wilson II, "Medical and Capitated Competitive Contracting: The Arizona Experiment," *New England Journal of Human Services* (Summer 1985): 33.

30. Bruce Babbitt and Jonathan Rose, "Building a Better Mousetrap: Health Care Reform and the Arizona Program," *Yale Journal on Regulation* 3, no. 2 (Spring 1986): 275.

31. "Curing AHCCCS," *Phoenix Gazette* (April 17, 1987): A14.

32. Jon B. Christianson, Diane G. Hillman, and Kenneth R. Smith, "The Arizona Experiment: Competitive Bidding for Indigent Medical Care," *Health Affairs* (Fall 1983): 88.

33. Bradford L. Kirkman-Liff, Jon B. Christianson, and Tracy Kirkman-Liff, "The Evolution of Arizona's Indigent Care System," *Health Affairs* 6, no. 4 (Winter 1987): 51.

34. "Medicaid Issues": Hearings of the Subcommittee on Health and the Environment of the Committee on Energy and Commerce of the U.S. House of Representatives (June 15, 1984): 208.

35. Frank G. Williams, David Phoenix, and Bradford L. Kirkman-Liff, "The Prospects for Pre-Paid Long Term Care: The Arizona Medicaid Experiment," *Journal of Health Politics, Policy and Law* 14, no. 3 (Fall 1989): 562.

36. "Fourth-Largest AHCCCS Provider Will Drop Plan; Was Losing Money," *Arizona Republic* (August 5, 1987): B4; "Three Indicted in Fraud Against AHCCCS." *Arizona Republic* (March 10, 1989): A1.

37. Elizabeth Andersen, "Administering Health Care: Lessons from the Health Care Financing Administration's Waiver Policy-Making," *Journal of Law and Politics* 10, no. 2 (Winter 1994): 215–262.

38. "Medicaid Issues": Hearings, 158.

39. Ibid., 159.

40. Ibid., 203.

41. Nelda McCall, "The Arizona Health Care Cost Containment System: Thirteen Years of Managed Care in Arizona" (San Francisco: Henry J. Kaiser Family Foundation, 1996).

42. General Accounting Office, "Medicaid: States Turn to Managed Care to Improve Access and Control Costs" (Washington, D.C.: United States General Accounting Office, Number GAO/HRD-93-46, March 1993).

43. Arizona Health Care Cost Containment System Administration, *AHCCCS Overview* (Phoenix, January 2, 1989, Arizona Health Care Cost Containment System Administration, 1989); David Azevedo, "No Kidding—There's a State where Doctors Like Medicaid," *Medical Economics* 69, no. 24 (December 21, 1992): 126–135; Chris Ferrara and Doug Bandow, "Finding an Alternative to Medicaid," *Journal of the Institute for Socioeconomic Studies* 9, no. 3 (Autumn 1984): 34–42; John K. Inglehart, "Health Policy Report: Medicaid and Managed Care," *New England Journal of Medicine* 332, no. 25 (June 22, 1995): 1727–1731; McCall, "The Arizona Health"; SRI International, "Evaluation of the Arizona Health Care Cost Containment System: Final Report" (SRI International, January 1989, HCFA #500-83-0027).

44. McCall, "The Arizona Health."

45. "Probe of AHCCCS Dropped After Complaints." *Phoenix Gazette* (September 1, 1988): D1.

46. McCall et al., "Managed Medicaid," 244.

47. Diane G. Hillman and Jon B. Christianson, "Competitive Bidding as a Cost-Containment Strategy for Indigent Medical Care: The Implementation Experience in Arizona," *Journal of Health Polities, Policy and Law* 9, no. 3 (Fall 1984): 446.

48. Christianson et al., "The Arizona Experiment," 97; Hillman and Christianson, "Competitive Bidding," 436.

49. Hillman and Christianson, "Competitive Bidding," 437.

50. Arizona Department of Health Services, Division of Health Resources, "Health Care Cost Containment Issue Paper" (September 1, 1982), in "Skyrocketing Health Care Costs—Causes and Solutions: Phoenix, Arizona," Hearings of the Subcommittee on Health and Long Term Care, Select Committee on Aging, U.S. House of Representatives, June 10, 1993.

51. Frank G. Williams, "The Political Impact of the Arizona Health Care Cost Containment System" (Tempe: Arizona State University, Center for Health Services

Administration, 1982), 14; Arizona Hospital Association, "Critique of Reporting Requirements for Arizona Health Care Cost Containment System (AHCCCS)" (Santa Rosa, Calif.: Jurgovian and Blair April 6, 1993), 6.

52. Hillman and Christianson, "Competitive Bidding," 432.

53. Jeffrey S. McCombs and Jon B. Christianson, "Applying Competitive Bidding to Health Care," *Journal of Health Politics, Policy and Law* 12, no. 4 (Winter 1987): 703–722.

54. "Objective AHCCCS Study Needed," *Phoenix Gazette* (March 23, 1989): A14.

55. McCombs and Christianson, "Applying Competitive Bidding."

56. Lynn Parringer and Nelda McCall, "How Competitive Is Competitive Bidding?" *Health Affairs* 10, no. 4 (Winter 1991): 229.

57. "AHCCCS Providers Suing for Rate Data: It's 'Inside Information,' Officer Says," *Phoenix Gazette* (February 19, 1988): E8.

58. Donald F. Schaller, Albert W. Bostrom, Jr., and John Rafferty, "Quality of Care Review: Recent Experience in Arizona," *Health Care Financing Review* (Annual Supplement, 1986): 66.

59. Arizona Hospital Association, "Critique of Reporting Requirements for Arizona Health Care Cost Containment System (AHCCCS)" (Santa Rosa, Calif.: Jurgovian and Blair, April 6, 1983), 10.

60. Williams, "The Political Impact."

61. "$3.3 Million in Fines Threatened for AHCCCS Errors," *Arizona Republic* (January 7, 1987): B1.

62. "Health Plan Has Survived Stormy Times," *Arizona Republic* (April 5, 1987): 12; Bill Muller and Pat Flannery, "AHCCCS Head Quits, Denies U.S. Probe a Factor," *Arizona Republic* (February 28, 1996): A1.

63. Bill Muller, "AHCCCS Web Tangles Program: Former Officials, Critics Charge Favoritism," *Arizona Republic* (April 21, 1996): A1.

64. Guy Webster, "State Health Costs Soaring, Study Says, Yet Spending Still Is Below U.S. Average," *Arizona Republic* (November 7, 1990): B1.

65. *Statistical Abstract of the United States 1995* (Washington, D.C.: U.S. Department of Commerce, Economics and Statistics Administration, Bureau of the Census, September 1995), 91.

66. *Health United States 1995* (Washington, D.C.: U.S. Department of Health and Human Services, Public Health Service, Centers for Disease Control, National Center for Health Statistics, May 1996, DHHS Publication No. (PHS) 96–1232), 92, 103.

67. Charity Ann Dorgan, (ed.), *Statistical Record of Health and Medicine* (Detroit, Mich.: Gale Research, 1995), 115–116.

68. *Health United States 1995*, 273.

69. Ibid., 274.

70. *Statistical Abstract of the United States 1995*, 462.

71. "Arizonans Ill More But Receive Care Less; State Gets 'Failing Grade,' Study Says," *Arizona Republic* (November 28, 1989): A1.

72. Babbitt and Rose, "Building a Better Mousetrap."

73. Azevedo, "No Kidding."

74. Bradford L. Kirkman-Liff, "AHCCCS in 1989 and 1995: A Detailed Comparative Analysis" (Phoenix: Arizona State University, School of Health Administration and Policy, 1995): 39.

75. Flinn Foundation, "AHCCCS in 1989: A Progress Report" (Phoenix: Flinn Foundation).

76. McCall, "The Arizona Health."

77. Bradford L. Kirkman-Liff, "Refusal of Care: Evidence from Arizona," *Health Affairs* 4, no. 4 (Winter 1985): 18.

78. Ibid.

79. Breacher, "Medicaid Comes to Arizona."

80. Williams, Phoenix, and Kirkman-Liff, "The Prospects."

81. "Group's Goal: Aid Uninsured; 20% Lack Health Coverage." *Arizona Republic* (October 13, 1989): B1.

82. Kirkman-Liff, "Refusal of Care," 10.

83. Ibid., 15

84. "Objective AHCCCS Study Needed." *Phoenix Gazette* (March 23, 1989): A14.

85. Guy Webster, "Some AHCCCS Patients Adrift on Health Plans; State Making Big Changes in Care Providers." *Arizona Republic* (August 16, 1994): B1.

86. John DeWitt, "State Health Plan Suddenly Popular." *Arizona Business Gazette* (June 30, 1994): 1; Jodie Snyder, "New Providers Get Big Portion of AHCCCS; Huge Profits Lure Bidders," *Phoenix Gazette* (July 15, 1994): B1.

87. Jane Erikson, "HMO's Earn $44 Million Caring for State Indigents." *Arizona Daily Star* (May 5, 1994): 1.

88. Inglehart, "Health Policy Report."

89. Howard E. Freeman and Bradford Kirkman-Liff, "Health Care Under AHCCCS: An Examination of Arizona's Alternative to Medicaid," *Health Services Research* 20, no. 3 (August 1985): 248.

90. Steve Yozwiak, "Plan Would Cut Health Aid to 30,000; Symington Seeks to Save $80 Million," *Arizona Republic* (January 14, 1992): B1.

91. Kirkman-Liff, Christianson, and Kirkman-Liff, "The Evolution"; Christianson et al., "The Arizona Experiment," 97.

92. Kirkman-Liff, Christianson, and Kirkman-Liff, "The Evolution," 57.

93. McCall, Henton et al., "Evaluation," 84.

94. Kirkman-Liff, Christianson, and Kirkman-Liff, "The Evolution"; Jon. B. Christianson, Bradford L. Kirkman-Liff, Teddylen A. Guffey, and James R. Beeler, "Nonprofit Hospitals in a Competitive Environment: Behavior in the Arizona Indigent Care Experiment," *Hospital and Health Services Administration* (November 1987): 483, 484.

95. *Health United States 1995*: 235.

96. Ibid.

97. Ibid.

98. General Accounting Office, "Arizona Medicaid: Competition Among Managed Care Plans Lowers Program Costs" (Washington D.C.: United States General Accounting Office, Number GAO/HEHS-96-2, October 1995), 5.

99. Robert E. Hurley, and Deborah A. Freund, "A Typology of Medicaid Managed Care." *Medical Care* 26, no. 8 (August 1988): 764–774.

100. General Accounting Office, "Medicaid: States."

101. General Accounting Office, "Arizona Medicaid: Competition Among Managed Care Plans Lowers Program Costs" (Washington D.C.: United States General Accounting Office, Number GAO/HEHS-96-2, October 1995), 19.

4

Managed Health Care in California: The Economic and Political Issues and the Strategic Plan

PATRICIA A. WILSON

INTRODUCTION

California's "Health Care Reforms" occurred in the 1970s and again in the 1990s. The purpose of this chapter is to discuss "Medi-Cal Reform" in California. Section one will begin with background information about the Medi-Cal Program and the 1970s reform. Section two will present a chronology of economic issues which led to reform. Also included in section two will be a discussion of events relating to goals, structures, controls, and standardization processes, and so on, of the Medi-Cal program. Finally, recent political demands and their impact on California's strategies and designs for the 1990s health care reform will be presented in section three.

BACKGROUND

The California Medical Assistance Program (Medi-Cal) was the result of Chapter 4, Statutes of 1965, by the Secondary Extraordinary Session of the California Legislature. The program had two major purposes: (1) to provide "basic and extended health care and related remedial or preventive services to recipients of public assistance and to medically needy aged and other persons, including such related social services as are necessary;" (2) to establish a system whereby medical care could be "mainstreamed." Prior to Medi-Cal many public assistance and medically needy persons relied primarily on county hospitals and/ or other charitable institutions for their medical care. Mainstreaming health care meant that the needy would have access to medical care that was comparable to that purchased "out of pocket" or through private insurance.[1]

March 1, 1966 was the federal implementation date for Medi-Cal, which extended coverage to 1.3 million people. The Office of Health Care Services, Health and Welfare Agency, had responsibility for policy determination, fiscal management control, program planning and review, training assistance, and federal program relations. In 1978, however, the Medi-Cal program became one of the major divisions of the Department of Health.

Prior to Medi-Cal, public assistance recipients (welfare recipients) relied on the Public Assistance Medical Care (PAMC) program or the Medical Assistance for the Aged (MAA) program. The PAMC was the main medical program; however, it had major exclusions. For example, "Aid For Dependent Children" (AFCD) adults were not covered except for dental care and out-patient rehabilitation services. Also, acute hospital care was provided only for the blind; medical attention for other beneficiaries was provided by the County Hospital. Except for former MAA beneficiaries, the medically needy were also not covered. Medi-Cal, however, required that certain basic services be made available to all beneficiaries.[2]

Medi-Cal was a very comprehensive medical program. Public assistance recipients were offered a wide range of medical services, such as inpatient and outpatient hospital services, physician services, laboratory and x-ray, nursing home care, prescription drugs, and ambulance services. The program also covered hearing aids and other medical services such as chiropractic, podiatry, dentistry, and home health care, organized outpatient mental health programs, birth control devices and drugs, and rehabilitation center services.

The Medi-Cal recipients were classified into two groups: Group I eligibles, and Group II eligibles. Group I recipients could receive all of the above benefits. Group II recipients were defined as persons who had income and/or property in excess of the public assistance limitations. This group was extended care but not to the extent of that provided for Group I. By 1970, however, Medi-Cal had contracted to pay for Medicare Part B premiums, which included coverage of physician and outpatient services, for both Groups I and II.[3]

FINANCIAL CUTBACKS: THE ECONOMIC ISSUES AND REFORM

There were two major program cutbacks in 1967 and 1970, respectively. In 1967, emergency administrative regulations were designed to curtail expenditures for fear a potential overexpenditure of $210 million would happen before June 30, 1968. Medi-Cal, therefore, eliminated coverage for the following medical services: chiropractors, freestanding clinics, special duty nurses, psychiatrists, audiologists. Additionally, dental care, prescription drugs, certain physician services, hospital services, optometrists, and so on, were greatly reduced. In 1970, a second state of emergency was declared and "Cost-Trim" regulations were put in place because it was again feared that the Medi-Cal program would exceed the budget—this time by $140 million.

As a result of the "Cost-Trim" regulations, several restrictions and cuts were imposed. For example, the amount providers received for services was reduced by 10%; physician office services and home visits were limited to two per month without prior authorization; prior authorization requirements became stricter for other providers; specific medical procedures were defined as "elective," which meant that such services could be postponed 90 days or more without causing significant disability or death; new and stricter drug rules were established, including additional wholesale price ceilings and minimum quantities for prescriptions for patients with chronic conditions. These emergency regulations remained in effect until June 30, 1971, although numerous lawsuits against the Department were filed because of them.[4]

MEDI-CAL REFORM

The Medi-Cal Reform Act of 1971, which represented a compromise of views of the Republican administration, the Democratic legislature, county governments, welfare organizations, and provider groups, attempted to make major changes in the scope and direction of Medi-Cal. It changed the program in the following five ways.

First, program benefits were divided into a basic schedule of benefits and a supplemental schedule. The basic schedule covered the same services previously available under the Program, but limitations were placed on the number of times the services could be used without authorization. Under the basic schedule, outpatient services were limited to two visits per month without prior authorization. Unused visits for one month only could be carried over to the next month for physician services. Prescription drugs also had the two-per-month limitation. These provisions were enforced by having special labels on each beneficiary's Medi-Cal card: if labels were gone, the provider knew he had to get authorization or postpone the services until the next month. Emergency services did not require authorization. The supplemental schedule covered outpatient physician services, inpatient hospital care, and prescription drugs in excess of coverage provided under the basic schedule. Treatment for elective services was not covered, and all care under this schedule was subject to utilization controls.

Second, medically indigent persons were extended Medi-Cal program coverage. This coverage extended to certain children not otherwise eligible for assistance, and to adults under 65 who were neither blind, totally disabled, nor heads of household with deprived children (according to welfare standards). These persons have been referred to as the "working poor," unable to obtain care except through the county hospitals. It was estimated, and included in the legislation, that county hospital systems were treating 800,000 persons per year who would be picked up under this category. State and some federal funds would then be available to help pay for care of these persons. The monthly number of medically indigent has never totaled over 450,000 persons. Since each person was not given a unique identification number to use throughout the state during the course of the year, it was not known exactly how many persons are annually eligible for this program.

Third, prepaid health plan development was encouraged by provisions that eased certain technical legal requirements and also by an aggressive program to establish such plans. Desirability of such an approach to the provision of health care had long been indicated. The original Medi-Cal law stated: After December 31, 1966, such care shall, to the extent feasible, be provided through a prepaid health care system or contracts with carriers. Up until this time, however, the program had only experimented with relatively limited pilot projects. For example, the San Joaquin Foundation (SJF) Pilot Project, established in February 1968, was the first prepayment agreement entered into by the Medi-Cal program. The original agreement was from physician services to public assistance cash grant beneficiaries who were residents of the four counties of San Joaquin, Amador, Calaveras, and Tuolumne. The Department of Health Care Services entered into a prepaid capitation agreement which was a pilot program with the Family Health Program of Southern California that purchased medical care from a medical practice group, composed of salaried physicians. Also, in October 1969 the Sonoma Foundation for Medical Care entered into a capitated prepaid pilot project with Medi-Cal. The project covered all public assistance and medically needy eligibles in Lake, Mendocino, and Sonoma counties, and the first contracts were signed in 1972.

Fourth, co-payment experiment started. The program obtained a waiver from the Secretary of the Department of Health, Education, and Welfare to perform a statewide experiment with co-payment. Essentially, the beneficiary had to pay $1 per outpatient medical visit for each of the first two visits and $0.50 for each of the first two prescriptions per month under the basic benefit schedule. Co-payment was scheduled to run from January 1, 1972 through June 30, 1973. A household survey of beneficiaries was completed in late 1971 in order to collect data on socioeconomic, health, and medical experience prior to implementation of co-payment. Approximately one-third of the eligible beneficiaries had sufficient income or resources to be on co-payment status.

Fifth, county option financial provisions were eliminated.[5] In January 1972, the co-payment experiment was started. There were 471,381 persons who received Medi-Cal cards indicating that they had to co-pay. The highest number of those who were involved in co-payment occurred in May 1972, when 833,066 of 2,258,048 persons were required to co-pay. The experiment ended on June 30, 1983. In April 1972, as a result of an amendment to the Social Security Act, intermediate care services became a Medi-Cal program benefit. However, prior authorization by a Medi-Cal consultant was required for admission to an intermediate care facility.

The first prepaid health plan contract with Innovative Health Systems in the Anaheim area became effective on May 1, 1972. By December, 5.8% (128,631 out of 2,235,945 persons) of Medi-Cal beneficiaries were enrolled in prepaid health plans. Major hospital billing modifications were instituted in June 1972. As a result of the 1970–1971 cutbacks and the 1971 Reform, many county hospitals were administratively overburdened. The billing process required hospitals to submit an estimated billing to the Department for payment, but this billing was to be substantiated and adjusted by regular individual claims submitted to the program's fiscal intermediaries. These billing processes were a "nightmare" for hospitals. Consequently, the counties sought legislative relief from Medi-Cal administrative requirements. The relief that they obtained eliminated the requirement for county hospitals and teaching hospitals operated by the University of California to present individual bills for each person treated during 1971–1972 before being paid. Alternatively, these hospitals were allowed to submit directly to the Department a quarterly statement which indicated a little more than the amount due them by the Medi-Cal program.

In July 1972 a "reimbursable cost list price (RCLP)" for pharmaceuticals was established. The RCLP established wholesale cost price ceilings for 196 multi-source generic drug types and medical supplies. It was replaced by the "Maximum Allowable Ingredient Cost (MAIC) program for pharmaceuticals in December 1973. The MAIC provided new procedures for establishing drug price ceilings in accordance with the Administrative Procedure Act.

Several other changes and/or services were added to the Medi-Cal program in 1974, including dental and dialysis services, and the Vietnamese and Indochinese Refugee program. The program entered into an agreement with the California Dental Service (CDS) to provide dental care through a prepaid statewide dental pilot program. Approximately 12,000 or 95% of all dental practitioners in California participated in the program. All Medi-Cal beneficiaries could receive these services.

Additionally, Medi-Cal coverage was extended for dialysis and related services to persons not otherwise eligible for Medi-Cal. Each beneficiary had to pay 1% of the cost of his dialysis and related services for each $5,000 of his annual net worth. This was increased to 2% in January 1980.

The Vietnamese and Indochinese Refuge Assistance Program, implemented in April 1975, covered 16,400 refugees. The federal government provided for 100% federal reimbursement for Medi-Cal assistance to these people.

Also in September 1975, Senate Bill 970, which established a single schedule of benefits under the Medi-Cal program, was signed into law. The benefits provided by this law included all the previously discussed benefits; additionally, beneficiaries could obtain an unrestricted number of physician outpatient services and Medi-Cal formulary prescription drugs without prior authorization. Beneficiaries were allowed, also without prior authorization, to have two outpatient visits per month from the following categories: optometrists, chiropractors, psychologists, audiologists, Christian Science practitioners, and occupational and speech therapists. Rehabilitative services were also added as a benefit for patients in intermediate care and skilled nursing facilities.[6]

CONTROL AND STANDARDIZATION

Control of Medi-Cal fraud and abuse was very important in the mid-1970s. The "Professional Standards Review Organizations" (PSRO) was established as a result of Federal Public Law 92–603. These organizations, composed of physician groups who would contract with the federal government, provided utilization control over Medicare and Medicaid inpatient stays. Physicians began forming these organizations, and because they were empowered by the law, their control decisions were binding. The PSRO ensured that the Medi-Cal program was not adversely affected.

More pharmaceutical drug utilization controls and programs were also instituted in January 1976; for example, minimum dispensing quantity requirements for certain drugs used on a long-term basis, and the establishment of onsite audits of pharmacy providers. Other examples of controls include changes, for example, in the number of visits to psychiatrists. Psychiatric services were changed to eight visits per 120 days without prior authorization.

During 1976 there were also attempts at simplifying the Medi-Cal eligibility requirements. Inequities between groups of Medi-Cal applicants, who were in similar circumstances but who were treated differently, were corrected. For example, the application and redetermination procedures for the medically needy and medically indigent persons were standardized. These changes were designed to simplify the county's administrative responsibilities relating to the Medi-Cal program and to provide more accurate eligibility determinations throughout the state. In January 1977, Medi-Cal eligibility regulations were completely rewritten to become a comprehensive set of instructions for patient/client determinations, case management, and general county administration. A Medi-Cal eligibility manual was published.

Other procedures aimed at standardization were implemented with regards to the statewide fee schedule for physician services. A uniform statewide schedule of maximum reimbursement replaced the physician profile reimbursement system. There was an overall rate increase for physician services, in general, of 9.5%. Maternal care, primary care, and anesthesia services increased by 30%, 20%, and 65%, respectively. A major change in the funding of the Medi-Cal program was made in July 1978. The 1978–1979 Budget Act, which eliminated county sharing in funding of the program, was in response to the passage of Proposition 13. This act placed a limitation on funds the counties could collect through property taxes.[7]

Although funding for the Medi-Cal program was becoming more and more of a problem, the number of Medi-Cal enrollees was increasing with great rapidity. For example, the federal government mandates the provision of emergency health care of illegal immigrants through the Medi-Cal program. Joining this political bandwagon, California legislation enacted in 1988 (SB 175) added prenatal care services to the scope of benefits provided to illegal immigrants. "From 1989–90 to 1995–96, the demand for prenatal services by illegal immigrants drove state program expenditures from $17.7 millon to $79.4 million, a 350 percent increase in just six years."[8]

To reiterate a growing problem, the number of enrollees in the Medi-Cal program was greatly increasing, which in turn was causing skyrocketing costs. The program "provides health care coverage to more than 5 million women, children, and aged or disabled people in California. Between 1980 and 1992, enrollment in Medi-Cal climbed to 79 percent, while the cost of the program tripled."[9]

Ironically, however, although the number of enrollees and costs were greatly increasing, patients were not receiving quality care. The system in which the care services were being provided was less than efficient and/or adequate. The Department of Health Services addressed such inadequacies:

The care [that] patients were receiving was fragmented, patchwork and out-dated. Instead of being cared for in a doctor's office or a clinic, . . . patients [would] wind up waiting hours in emergency rooms for simple problems like a child's ear infection. Thousands of Medi-Cal beneficiaries are hospitalized each year for service health conditions that could have been prevented by primary care—an ordinary doctor visit by preventive tactics like immunizations and early detection of disease through pap smears and mammograms.[10]

THE POLITICAL ISSUES AND CALIFORNIA'S STRATEGIC PLAN

There were two political demands on the Medi-Cal program: (1) constraining the above-mentioned costs and achieving the best value in services and quality on limited funds, and (2) "support for the continued existence of a safety net for the care of the medically indigent, with protections for the continuation of existing relationships between clinical providers and the patients they care for."[11]

Although, since the early 1970s, the State of California had operated a program of managed care contracting for Medi-Cal beneficiaries, its effort to respond to these conflicting and competing goals was manifested in legislation—Chapter 95, Statutes of 1991 (AB 336) and Charter 722, Statutes of 1992 (SB 485) "which require[d] the Medi-Cal Program to place an . . . emphasis on efforts to arrange and encourage access to health care through enrollment in organized, managed care plans of the type available to the general public, and which authorize[d] the Department of Health Services to accelerate the transition of Medi-Cal beneficiaries into managed care plans."[12]

Managed care is a comprehensive approach to health care provision. It refers to an organized and coordinated system of individual health care providers—a system with emphasis on primary and preventive health care. Under managed care, a health plan is paid a fixed rate, as opposed to a fee-for-service in which a provider bills for every visit.

Managed care's emphasis on access to primary care is intended to increase utilization of clinical preventive services and thus reduce the unnecessary use of emergency rooms for ambulatory care and to eliminate preventable hospitalizations. In addition, quality care can better be assured in managed care systems than in "fee-for-service" (FFS). Unlike FFS, providers operating in a managed care environment are formally and systematically linked in a manner that allows quality of care to be rationally assessed and accountability for care to be established and monitored.[13]

Major opposition to the Department of Health Services (DHS) came from traditional and safety net providers. Traditional providers were "those which historically have delivered services to Medi-Cal beneficiaries," for example, medical and hospital providers only, either profit or nonprofit entities, publicly owned and operated. Many have been Medi-Cal providers for more than 20 years and have consistently maintained a substantial Medi-Cal portion of their practice.

Safety net providers were clinical providers that provided comprehensive primary care and/or hospitals providing acute inpatient services to the medically indigent and special needs segments of the state's population. They were the providers of charity care. Typically, they receive charitable or public grants and contributions for the purpose of providing indigent health care. Most safety net providers also provided services to Medi-Cal beneficiaries. For example, safety net providers could include: governmentally operated health systems; community health centers, rural and Indian health services centers; and disproportionate share hospitals, public and university hospitals, and rural and children's hospitals.[14]

To many traditional and safety net providers a conversion from the FFS to a managed care system was tantamount to a "financial death." In many cases, since Medi-Cal patients were their best, and in some cases only, paying patients, losing Medi-Cal revenues would seriously erode the ability of many such providers to continue to operate. For this reason, the traditional and safety net providers generated major opposition to such a conversion.[15] As a result of such opposition, in November 1992 a moratorium was placed on further expansion until the development of a strategic plan.

Governor Wilson's administration and legislature (SB 845), however, recognized the obstacles that Medi-Cal's traditional "fee-for-service" system imposed on such goals as: adequate and appropriate access to care, quality service, and cost-effectiveness. As a result of their economic and political analyses, the administration embarked on an initative to move approximately 3.2 million Medi-Cal recipients into "managed care" plans by the end of 1996–1997. This initiative was designed for long-term advantages; it was not intended to produce budget savings in the short term. Its emphasis was on primary and preventive services, which in turn was believed to reduce "costly interventions and associated hospital inpatient costs."[16]

On January 13, 1993, the Director of the Department of Health Services released the Draft Strategic Plan for the expansion of efforts to transpose Medi-Cal to managed care. At the time of the Plan there were already "over 600,000 Medi-Cal beneficiaries in 20 counties covered by Medi-Cal managed care arrangements." As part of the political process involved in this transition, however, the DHS mailed 1,500 copies of the Draft Plan to "provider associations, organizations concerned with health care, Medi-Cal providers, State and local governmental and elected officials, and other interested persons." Those who received the letter were asked to submit written comments, concerns, and recommendations. Additionally, interested and concerned persons were invited to speak and/or present testimony at public forums concerning the transition.[17] The Plan replaced the moratorium discussed above.

The Two-Plan Model is California's principal model for the expansion of managed care. DHS will contract with two managed care plans: one locally developed, comprehensive managed care system (the Local Initiative), and the other a commercial plan (nongovernmental-operated Health Maintenance Organization or HMO), referred to as the mainstream option.

DHS gave the County Board of Supervisors the first opportunity to initiate the development of the local initiative. If the Board was not interested in such development, the Department would review proposals from other local stakeholders. Under the Mainstream Plan, the DHS would select a single HMO for each region through a competitive "invitation for bid" process. The local initiative, on the other hand, could have taken any of the following forms: (1) a health care consortium, in which local stakeholders share governance of an organization that is responsible for administering Medi-Cal managed care; (2) a County Organized Health System (COHS) "Look-A-Like," in which the County Board of Supervisors establishes an entity for purposes of administering the local initiatives as one of two full-risk plans in a region; and (3), any alternative system developed by local stakeholders that meets the requirements of state and federal law, and the criteria described in the Department's Plan.[18]

In addition to fiscal management concerns, the continued involvement of traditional safety net providers in the care of Medi-Cal patients was another important political goal. To accomplish this, the DHS made certain assurances to these providers. First, the state would provide technical assistance which would include suggestions for developing or obtaining access to management information systems, expanding or developing provider networks, understanding and complying with Medi-Cal managed care program requirements, and assistance in forming relationships with existing managed care organizations which can provide ongoing training and support. Second, the local initiative would be required to include all safety net providers that agree to provide services in accord with the same terms and conditions that the plan requires of any other similar provider that affiliates with the plan, and would be required to submit to the Department its participation standards for including traditional providers. Third, in securing contracts for mainstream plans, DHS would publicize the favorable weighting it would assign to bids and proposals which provide the inclusion of traditional and safety net providers within the service delivery networks.[19]

CONCLUSION

In conclusion, the above discussion demonstrates how the economic and political environments of an organization or system can determine the need for structural change and/or reform. The declining economic conditions in California, and the growing number of Medi-Cal enrollees caused the DHS to necessarily investigate new health care structures, hence the managed care movement. In some ways California may be a leader in "Health Care Reform." Its managed care model provides a design for prudent fiscal management, as well as a strategy for the continuance of traditional and safety net providers in health care, that is, a plan for the accomplishment of two conflicting political goals. What is needed now is sufficient time after implementation to evaluate the impact that such reform has had upon the plight of traditional providers and upon access, quality, and cost of health care in the Medi-Cal program.

NOTES

1. "The Medi-Cal Program—A Brief Summary of Major Events," Medical Care Statistics Section, Department of Health Services (Sacramento, California, March 1990), 1.
   2. Ibid., 2–3.
   3. Ibid., 2–4.
   4. Ibid., 4–10.
   5. Ibid., 11–12.
   6. Ibid., 13–20
   7. Ibid., 20–25.
   8. "Governor's 1996–97 Budget Highlights," California Department of Health Services (Sacramento, California, January 1996), 10.
   9. Letter from Dr. Molly Joel Coye, Director, "Expanding Medi-Cal Managed Care," California Department of Health Services (Sacramento, California, March 31, 1993), 1.
   10. Ibid., 1.
   11. Ibid., 1–2.
   12. "Expanding Medi-Cal Managed Care," Executive Summary, California Department of Health Services (Sacramento, California, March 1993), i.
   13. Ibid.
   14. Ibid., 23.
   15. Ibid.
   16. "Governor's 1996–97 Budget Highlights," California Department of Health Services (Sacramento, California, January 1996), 8.
   17. "Expanding Medi-Cal Managed Care, California Department of Health Services (Sacramento, California, March 1993), 2–4.
   18. Ibid., ii.
   19. Ibid., 24.

5

The Diamond State Health Plan: Delaware's Experience with Medicaid Managed Care

ERIC D. JACOBSON AND AMY B. DROSKOSKI

INTRODUCTION

Effective January 1, 1996, the State of Delaware implemented a statewide Medicaid managed care program known as the Diamond State Health Plan (DSHP). The state sought to achieve three major goals: (1) improve and expand access to health care for more adults and children throughout the state, including all uninsured adults below 100% of the federal poverty level; (2) expand access to care for the Medicaid population using a managed care delivery system; and (3) control the growth of health care expenditures for the Medicaid population. In order to implement this program, the state submitted and obtained approval from the Health Care Financing Administration (HCFA) for a Section 1115 Demonstration Waiver to introduce a new health care delivery program to serve roughly 63,000 eligible individuals, including approximately 9,000 previously uninsured. The state submitted the proposal in July 1994 and received approval ten months later (May 1995). Delaware was the seventh state to receive HCFA approval for this type of waiver and one of the first states to implement a statewide, fully capitated managed care plan. The program is built on the principles of managed care and strong quality assurance. Program eligibles are enrolled into comprehensive, prepaid health plans that contract with the state to provide a specified scope of benefits to each eligible in return for a capitated payment made on a per member per month basis.

Despite some early implementation problems, the plan is generally considered a success. In a lead editorial, Delaware's most widely read newspaper, the *Wilmington News Journal*, announced "Managed care is best for Medicaid despite the initial difficulties."[1] The program has received strong support from Delaware's Democratic and Republican state leaders. Democratic Governor Thomas

R. Carper trumpeted "the [DSHP] waiver approval is an important part of our ongoing effort to reduce the number of uninsured throughout Delaware ... vaulting Delaware to the forefront of the nation with regard to provision of health insurance for low income families."[2] Senate Minority (Republican) Leader Myrna L. Bair expressed similar enthusiasm: "I am very supportive of the new Medicaid managed care program. Not only will it help to contain costs ... but it will go a long way to increasing availability to a population that is very under served medically."[3] Representatives from HCFA's Office of State Health Reform Demonstrations told us that the implementation of Delaware's Medicaid managed care program was "much smoother" than the experiences of other states that had received 1115 Waivers. This case study will help the reader to gain a better understanding of Delaware's experience and lessons that might be learned about how to make the transition from a traditional Medicaid program.

METHODOLOGY

Information for the report was obtained primarily through detailed onsite and phone interviews conducted by the authors during the second quarter of 1996, supplemented by a review of newspaper articles, documents, and related written materials. We talked with policymakers, providers, health plans/insurers, consumers, and advocacy groups. To begin the interview process, we generally mailed or faxed a preliminary set of open-ended questions. As issues and themes began to emerge in each interview, additional questions were added to clarify interview content gained from the structured interview questions. A variety of interests were represented in our survey panel, including private practicing physicians and safety net providers such as hospital emergency departments and community health centers.

We also attended two public hearings in May 1996 conducted by the Delaware Health Care Commission. During these hearings on the transition to managed care, more than 60 speakers testified on subjects ranging from HMO profit motives to lack of understanding by managed care organizations about the special needs of disabled enrollees. To gain additional insights about the new Medicaid managed care program, we interviewed selected speakers following their formal presentations.

Several documents given to us by the State Medicaid Office and the Delaware Health Care Commission provided very helpful information about the DSHP and recent developments in Delaware's health system. We also used an insightful 1996 report, *The Community Snapshot Project*,[4] published by the Robert Wood Johnson Foundation. This report, which included a chapter describing the Wilmington, Delaware market, offered new and interesting perspectives on the state's health care environment. Its content also seemed to be reflected in many of the responses we obtained during our interviews.

LIMITATIONS

There are five limitations to our study that should be noted. To begin with, this case study should be considered a preliminary investigation, and therefore it is limited in scope. Observations and opinions are based on only six months of experience with the new DSHP. Second, our findings are not based on quantitative analysis of large administrative data sets, chart reviews, or satisfaction surveys of consumers or providers. Third, many of our findings are based on the opinions and insights of our survey panel. Frequently, the responses of different groups were at odds, and our attempt to understand the "complete picture" was difficult. The fourth limitation is a common criticism of most opinion surveys: We quickly discovered that some opinions were not based on solid factual foundations. Several respondents, for example, admitted that their opinions were based on what they had heard about experiences in other states—situations that obviously did not apply to Delaware. Finally, we also suspect that many critics tended to present the saddest and most serious cases (such as disabled children) as representative of the entire class of enrollees seeking treatment. We tried to piece together key issues and present an analysis based on reliable observations and viewpoints. To correct factual inaccuracies, we sent a draft of this case to key state officials and other key stakeholders for review. The case has been revised on the basis of their comments.

The main body of this study is divided into three parts. Part I describes the context of reform. It presents four forces that encouraged the adoption of Medicaid reform in the state. Part II contains a detailed description and analysis of the key components of the DSHP and experience to date. Part III discusses key issues faced by the state; the three sections address implementation issues, the number of Delawareans without health insurance, and an innovative pre-DSHP program that improved access to primary care.

Before proceeding to the next section, we will provide some basic background information about Delaware. When traveling outside the Mid-Atlantic region, Delawareans frequently are asked: "By the way, where is Delaware?" Delaware, the second smallest state, is located in the Boston–Washington, D.C., urban corridor. The state's population, like its industry, is concentrated in the north around its largest city, Wilmington. Two-thirds of the state's 715,000 population lives in northernmost New Castle County. The state often is described as being dominated by the business community, especially by the DuPont Company and financial service corporations such as MBNA America Bank. The state also is home to thousands of very small employers—close to two-thirds of the state's 22,000 business establishments employ less than five people. The central and southern counties, Kent and Sussex, are mostly rural and have economies that feature agriculture, government (the state capital and the Dover Air Force Base are located in Kent County), tourism, and manufacturing sectors.

THE CONTEXT OF REFORM

There were many different economic, political, and health care related forces that led to Medicaid reform in Delaware. In this section, we describe four: improving access, restructuring work–welfare choices, meeting Delaware's health care needs, and responding to public and business community support for Medicaid managed care.

Improving Access

The DSHP initiative seeks to increase the number of insured individuals by implementing a more cost-effective delivery system. Unlike other states such as Hawaii, that focused on slowing down hemorrhaging health care costs, Delaware's primary intention was to improve access—a long-recognized need throughout the state. In a 1990 report to former governor Michael Castle, the Indigent Health Care Task Force emphasized the severity and urgency of the problem. "The [task force] report represents a unanimous view by the task force that the problems associated with the lack of health care are manifested in both social and economic ways throughout Delaware, and that the burden of dealing with this issue and the affordability of health care is becoming a serious problem."[5] The task force report presented 1988 and 1989 Census Bureau data showing that 12% of nonelderly Delawareans were without health insurance. In recognition of this problem, the Delaware Health Care Commission was created in 1990. The mission of the commission was "to provide basic, affordable, equal quality, accessible health care to all Delawareans."[6]

In 1996, the Commission supported a comprehensive study of the demographics of the uninsured. The study, conducted by Edward Ratledge of the University of Delaware's College of Urban Affairs and Public Policy, generated estimates for 1995 indicating that 13.6% of the state's nonelderly population did not have health insurance, a rate roughly equivalent to the 13.5% uninsurance rate in the region which includes Maryland, Pennsylvania, New Jersey, and New York.[7]

In a separate 1996 report to the Health Care Commission, two Duke University consultants, Christopher Conover and Frank Sloan, warned Delaware's leaders of a projected secular decline in employer-based coverage.[8] Most troubling is that Delaware's overall uninsurance rates could increase in spite of the aggressive Medicaid improvements. This prognosis should be sobering news to state officials committed to improving access to health insurance. Given the importance of the Conover and Sloan argument, we will discuss its logic and the recent experience in a later section.

Restructuring Work-Welfare Choices

Governor Thomas Carper has received national attention for the fundamental changes Delaware is making to its welfare program. The new program, which will be phased in over four years beginning in 1995, is built on five key principles: (1) work should pay more than welfare; (2) welfare recipients must exercise personal responsibility in exchange for benefits (for example, by participating in job training and accepting a job if offered); (3) welfare should be transitional, not a way of life (i.e., two-year time limits for benefits); (4) both parents should help support their children; and (5) the formation and maintenance of two-parent families should be encouraged, and teenage pregnancy should be strongly discouraged.

The new welfare program enables recipients to take jobs while continuing to be eligible for a portion of their welfare grants. It also encourages work by allowing welfare recipients to take a job without losing their eligibility for coverage under the Diamond State Health Plan. This new Medicaid program extends health coverage to all adults—with or without jobs—up to 100% of the poverty level. The program also allows welfare recipients to keep their Medicaid coverage for 24 months if they obtain jobs that raise their incomes above the poverty level. These provisions eliminate the difficult choice faced by an unemployed welfare recipient who must decide whether to accept a low-paying job that does not provide health coverage or forego the job to keep health insurance.

The Carper administration's decision to take a leading role in reforming the nation's welfare programs added fuel to Delaware's Medicaid reform engine. Many health care observers in the state told us that they supported the Medicaid initiative, but wondered why the state created "unnecessary stress and hardships" by rushing implementation, particularly during the enrollment phase. (This problem is described later.) One reason suggested to us was the linkage between the Welfare and Medicaid reforms. To "make work pay" effective January 1, 1996, required the DSHP to be up and running by the same date.

Meeting Delaware's Health Care Needs

While Delaware takes pride in having been the first state to ratify the constitution, it's not even close in health status statistics. A leader in the state's provider community argues that the state's public health status statistics are "woeful." The Robert Wood Johnson Foundation's *Community Snapshot Project* claims that "the health of people in Wilmington compares unfavorably with that in other areas."[9] Based on a composite of 23 factors, Morgan Quintno's *1994 Health Care State Rankings* places Delaware fifth from the bottom, up from next-to-last in 1993.[10] Northwestern National Life conducts an annual analysis of seventeen indicators, including access to health care, disabilities, disease, and mortality, and in 1992 ranked Delaware as the 26th healthiest state. The state's infant mortality rate is more than two times the national average. In terms of new cancer cases, Delaware consistently is one of the ten unhealthiest states.[11] (Pennsylvania and New Jersey, two of Delaware's three neighboring states, also have very high rates of new cancer cases.)

The State Division of Public Health reports there are insufficient primary care providers to meet the needs of Delawareans. "Analyzing the primary care needs by county shows that all three counties have unmet needs for primary care providers." New Castle County (a primary urban area that contains the city of Wilmington) has small, underserved areas characterized by high poverty rates. Sussex County is a federally designated underserved area and Kent County has a similar primary care provider shortage.[12] (Kent and Sussex counties are mostly rural regions with agriculture-based economies.)

By increasing insurance coverage, improving access to primary care, and expanding managed care networks, the state expects the expanded Medicaid program to improve the health status of Delaware's poor.

Responding to Public and Business Community Support for Medicaid Managed Care

A 1995 public opinion survey, conducted by the University of Delaware's College of Urban Affairs and Public Policy, indicates a high level of support for Medicaid managed care.[13] Delawareans expressed a strong desire to increase access without an increase in costs—the fundamental principle of the Diamond State Health Plan. The survey asked people to select the most important priority for statewide health care reform. The most popular choice, chosen by 37% of the respondents, was making health care more affordable for people and their families. Selected by almost as many respondents (34%) was ensuring universal coverage for all Delawareans. Furthermore, more than 80% of respondents agreed that all citizens of Delaware should be entitled to the same right to necessary medical care whether or not they can pay for the care.

The survey also revealed that most Delawareans do not see a great difference between the quality of care offered by health maintenance organizations and traditional fee-for-service health plans; 64% said that HMOs offered at least the same quality of care as fee-for service plans. When asked to identify specific concerns about managed care, a majority of the respondents questioned the difficulty of appealing an HMOs decision about denial of coverage, the amount of money HMOs spend on administration and advertising, physician disenrollment, and financial rewards given to providers when patients use fewer services.

The survey included specific questions about both Medicaid and Medicare managed care. Encouraging Medicaid patients to receive health services from HMOs in order to save money was supported by 72% of Delawareans. Encouraging Medicare patients to receive health services from HMOs received slightly less support; nevertheless, 67% were in favor of this proposal.[14]

One can look at the recent experience of Delaware's largest employer, the DuPont Company, to find strong support for a managed care delivery system. DuPont's is viewed as a market leader whose decisions about health benefits have a direct effect on the state's health care system. In 1993, the company surprised the health care community by moving to create managed care options for its employees. Corporate response has been very positive. At a May 1996 public hearing on the topic of managed care, Robert F. Miller, DuPont's Health Care Program Manager, talked about the company's very positive experience:

We acknowledge that managed care is a change from the traditional fee-for-service plans which many employers, including DuPont, offered before rapidly rising health care costs made them prohibitive. The cost trend had to be reversed and managed care was the free market system's response—and I will add the only solution that exists! I recognize that managed care adds "tension" to the delivery of health care. Our 1995 survey of our employees/retirees, however, reflects a 78 percent satisfaction rating among DuPont employees with our managed care plans. . . . We cannot retreat to the good old days and still afford to provide quality health care plans to our employees.[15]

In all probability, the state would not have the Diamond State Health Plan if DuPont had not moved to managed care. There are two reasons for this. To begin with, DuPont's decision, which has been followed by other businesses, drove the health care and insurance communities to reposition themselves to meet the changing demands. This created the necessary managed care infrastructure for the new Medicaid delivery system. A second important reason reflects Delaware's political culture which has been described by political observers as a "consciously cultivated, a probusiness climate that is carefully sustained."[16] This view suggests that business opinion and experience are of major importance for the determination of state policy. So, support from the business community likely was a necessary prerequisite for the state's aggressive action on Medicaid reform.

KEY COMPONENTS OF THE INITIATIVE AND EXPERIENCE TO DATE

The DSHP marks a fundamental shift in the state's health care program, both in terms of how clients seek and receive care and the manner in which providers are paid. Before describing the plan in more detail, it will be helpful to summarize the pre-reform Medicaid environment. Delaware received (and continues to receive) 50% matching funds from the federal government for the Medicaid program. In state fiscal year 1995, total expenditures equaled $352 million with approximately 66,000 average monthly eligibles. Although three-quarters of the eligible persons were children, their mothers, and other younger adults, expenditures were approximately the reverse; 73% was spent on the aged and disabled recipients and the remaining 27% went to all other recipients.

Prior to the 1996 DSHP reforms, the state had done little to fill gaps in coverage for adults. Other than pregnant women, very few adults were eligible for Delaware's Medicaid program; the pre-reform program covered welfare recipients who had incomes only up to about 35% of the poverty level (and certain two-parent families when the chief salary earner was unemployed). Moreover, the state's funding for adults fell significantly below national averages. In 1993, the state spent $1,502 per nonelderly adult enrollee, just 87% of the national average.

By opening the Medicaid program to adults with incomes between 35 and 100% of the poverty level, the state expects to add 9,000 beneficiaries to the Medicaid program. For these new enrollees and the 56,000 participants who were previously eligible, the DSHP offers a basic benefit package including medical and mental health services. Examples of covered services include the following: inpatient, outpatient, and ambulatory medical and surgical services; gynecological, obstetric, and family planning services; rehabilitation services such as physical therapy, emergency transportation, limited mental health and substance abuse services; as well as a variety of other services. Several "wrap-around" services are not included in the managed care package but continue to be provided on a fee-for-service basis. These include pharmacy, nonemergency transportation, extended mental health and substance abuse benefits, and some other services such as private duty nursing and prescribed pediatric extended care.

The state does not require beneficiaries to pay premiums, deductibles, or co-payments. At first glance this decision seems to be fundamentally different from the pricing policies established by the six states (Arizona, Tennessee, Oregon, Hawaii, Rhode Island, and Minnesota) that implemented Section 1115 Demonstration Medicaid Managed Care programs before Delaware. All of these states require some form of participant cost-sharing. Closer examination of the fee schedules, however, shows that most of these states tie fees to income levels and exempt individuals with incomes at or below 100% of the poverty level. Since Delaware's program covers adults only up to this income level, a no-fee program seems to fit the established pricing practices. By offering all services for free, the state avoids addressing several very difficult questions: Should participants be denied coverage if they don't pay? Should the state invest its limited resources in collecting unpaid balances from low-income families facing difficult financial pressures? Does the state want to face the possibility that fees will reduce use and have an adverse effect on health outcomes?

Health Benefits Manager and the Enrollment Process

Delaware has contracted with a health benefits manager (HBM) to facilitate and monitor member enrollment in managed care plans. The HBM was selected to provide outreach, education, and enrollment services for the Medicaid managed care program. The national firm, which previously processed Delaware's Medicaid claims, was selected in a competitive process during which state officials and community representatives evaluated and reviewed bids. The contract requires the HBM to help former Medicaid eligibles and new clients select a health plan, educate them about the new health care system and importance of primary care, and assist them in resolving any problems with the managed care organizations that they select.

Many questions have been raised about the quality of the services provided by the HBM and the overall education and enrollment process. At this point, it will be helpful to briefly present the major steps in the enrollment process. At least 30 days prior to the start of the plan year, the HBM mailed an enrollment packet to each eligible individual or family. This package contained a personalized enrollment form, general information about DSHP, brochures and provider directories from the three managed care organizations serving the county of residence. Enrollees were encouraged to attend in-person meetings, health fairs, and individual counseling sessions organized by the HBM. Individuals or families who did not enroll within 30 days were automatically assigned (autoassigned) to the default plan selected for them by the state's Medicaid management information system and printed on their enrollment form. Indicating the default plan on the enrollment form caused confusion for the state, the HBM, health plans, and health providers: a nonreturned form could indicate either that the enrollee was satisfied with the default selection or that the enrollee did not receive, read, or understand the enrollment materials.

Organization of Health Services Delivery

Managed Care Organizations

All health services under DSHP are delivered through fully capitated managed care health plans. To increase the managed care infrastructure in underserved subcounty areas, the state required bidding managed care organizations to submit proposals covering at least one of Delaware's three counties. Health plans showed a high level of interest in obtaining DSHP contracts. The state decided to contract with four managed care plans/organizations: AmeriHealth First, Blue Cross/Blue Shield of Delaware, First State Health Plan, and DelawareCare. AmeriHealth and DelawareCare were awarded statewide contracts. Blue Cross and Blue Shield was selected to serve Kent and Sussex counties (mostly rural areas). The First State Health Plan was awarded a contract for one county, New Castle County (mostly urban area that accounts for nearly two-thirds of the state's population).

At this point, it will be helpful to describe the process of change in Delaware's HMO and insurance markets and to examine the impact of that change on the development of the DSHP. Blue Cross and Blue Shield, which has dominated the local health insurance market, has a history of offering generous payments to providers and imposing minimal prior authorization requirements. More aggressive HMOs—ones that try to reduce costs by implementing strict physician oversight mechanisms and sharply discounted payment rates—have received frequent criticism from Delaware's physician community and until recently have not been well received by the state's business community. One health care leader we interviewed pointed out that the strong loyalty to Blue Cross/Blue Shield of Delaware (a "buy Delaware" attitude) has been extremely expensive for consumers and taxpayers. Employer and consumer concerns about the unrelenting rise of health care costs attracted commercial insurance companies to compete with Blue Cross/Blue Shield for customers.

The DelawareCare Medicaid managed care plan started as a joint venture between Principal Health Care of Delaware and Mercy Health Plan, a large Medicaid plan based in Philadelphia.[17] Principal Health Care entered the market relatively early and followed Blue Cross/Blue Shield's practice of being physician friendly. Consumers seemed very willing to switch from Blue Cross and Blue Shield. By 1993, for example, more than half of Delawareans enrolled in HMOs were covered by Principal. Costs seem to have been a major driving force. To keep costs low and attract a larger market share, Principal started implementing stricter managed care practices and restructuring fee schedules to drive down costs. Even though these practices are commonly used in other states, Delaware's provider community has been very critical. Several physicians we interviewed told us that due to these concerns, DelawareCare had difficulty recruiting physicians. DelawareCare's enrollment rates have lagged behind those of the three other health plans. If strict managed care requirements have been a major influence on physician participation and client enrollments, then DelawareCare (and the three other managed care organizations) might be forced to reexamine these requirements and become more physician and consumer friendly. Without managed care organizations applying stringent rules, the state—in the long run—may not realize the full per enrollee cost savings it anticipates.

The Medical Center of Delaware, which provides care to nearly 60 percent of all inpatients admitted statewide, recently decided to compete with insurers by establishing a physician-hospital organization (PHO). In April 1995, the Center obtained an insurance license and began operating the PHO called Mid-Atlantic Health Systems, Inc., and formed a Medicaid health plan called the First State Health Plan. (Many consumers had difficulty differentiating this plan name from the overall state Medicaid managed care plan name. We were told of a Medicaid client who asked "If I'm already part of the Diamond State Health Plan, why do I need to enroll in the First State Health Plan?") Physicians we spoke to rated the First State Health Plan as the best of the plans. This is not surprising since it's the only plan that pays providers on a fee-for-service basis, and it has the most flexible preauthorization requirements. The plan also has introduced innovations to Delaware's Medicaid managed care market. Two of these innovations include electronic mail authorizations for specialist referrals and "fast track" primary care in the Medical Center's emergency departments. Clients needing emergency or nonemergency medical attention can continue to receive treatment from the Medical Center's Emergency Department. Unlike the procedures required by the state's other Medicaid health plans, First State's enrollees do not face the frustration of being turned away from the health provider with whom they're most familiar. The "fast track" program also helps to cut the number of disputes over denial of claims for emergency medical services.

Consolidation has occurred in the Delaware market at an increasing pace. AmeriHealth was formed when three HMOs—Delaware Valley HMO, Healthcare Delaware, and Keystone—merged into one. To benefit from greater economies of scale and secure a stronger funding base, Blue Cross and Blue Shield of Delaware recently announced its intention to merge with two larger organizations: Blue Cross and Blue Shield of New Jersey, and Anthem, Inc., an Indianapolis-based Fortune 500 insurance company conducting business in all 50 states. Under this proposed agreement, Blue Cross/Blue Shield of Delaware will be part of a national company with $9 billion in consolidated revenues and six million members (nearly nine times the entire population of the State of Delaware). In exchange for the right to convert to for-profit status, the new Blue Cross and Blue Shield organization will create a $103 million investment fund to establish the Center for HealthCare Economics. This nonstock research organization will collect health care information and use it to provide "Consumer Report" format health care report cards providing information on health plans, hospitals, and physicians. The transformation of Blue Cross /Blue Shield to a for-profit status along with the increased availability of comparative health care information could have a major impact on the state's employers and the state government as a purchaser for low-income health consumers. Larger insurers, for example, might have the leverage to force Delaware's physicians to accept deeper discounts and more aggressive managed care arrangements.

The health plans see both short- and long-term gains from participating in the state's Medicaid Managed Care plan. The immediate benefit will be increased demand for their products and expanded HMO networks. Without obtaining a Medicaid contract, Blue Cross/Blue Shield would have experienced a deepening erosion of its market share. The newly formed First State Health Plan desired to establish a presence in the state's insurance industry. The First State Health Plan and AmeriHealth, the two of the four Medicaid plans that currently do not have contracts for state employees, also recognize the importance of enhancing their relationships with the state. According to a *Wilmington News Journal* article, the general manager of AmeriHealth's Delaware operations said he also has his sights on the more than 27,000 Delaware state employees whose health care contract is up for bids in 1997.[18]

Alfred I. DuPont Institute

One unique aspect of Delaware's current health care system is a public–private partnership set up between the state and the Nemours Foundation to provide health care for the majority of Medicaid and uninsured children in the state without a medical home. This program was designed to determine if a financially secure, nonprofit entity, the Alfred I. DuPont Institute of the Nemours Foundation, could increase access to Delaware Medicaid children under a managed care approach with risk-based capitation. The Institute, located just outside Wilmington, is a pediatric acute care hospital that has evolved during the past decade from an orthopedic hospital. To set up this managed care system for children, the state received a Section 1115 Waiver from HCFA in 1992. Under this arrangement, the Alfred I. DuPont Institute planned to expand medical care by opening thirteen new satellite children's clinics throughout the state. Under this agreement, seven clinics will be located in New Castle County and the remaining six will be in southern Delaware, three each in Kent and Sussex counties. The Institute agreed to accept a capitated rate that was substantially lower than the average cost per child for an equivalent package of services under the Medicaid fee-for-service program. In 1995, approximately 15% of the Institute's funding came from the Nemours Foundation. The Nemours contributions allowed the Institute to keep fees low, and it provided the hospital with additional financial resources to purchase state-of-the-art technology and maintain strong hospital capacity.

By 1995, the year prior to implementation of the Diamond State Health Care Plan, nearly one-third of the state's Medicaid eligible children had become members of the Institute's network. Realizing the significant role the Institute plays in health care delivery, the state wanted to continue its partnership in the new Medicaid managed care program. The state encouraged the four plans to include Institute primary care physicians and specialists in their provider networks, and all of the plans have done so. Under this arrangement, the plans have been able to offer comprehensive pediatric provider networks. The adult speciality networks provided by the four plans have been criticized for having obvious gaps with respect to specialists. Due to low fee schedules, for example, very few orthopedic surgeons are available to adults enrolled in any of the plans.

The implementation of the DSHP has not significantly impacted the Institute's ability to provide quality care to the state's Medicaid children. Even though complete data is not available, Institute officials do not expect to find significant changes in enrollment trends. By the end of 1995, the Institute had opened nine of the planned thirteen satellite clinics. The tenth will open during the summer of 1996; the implementation of the DSHP has not affected this decision. The Institute has been recognized by peer organizations for the strong commitment it has made to improving the health of Delaware's underserved children. In 1995, the Health Strategy Network awarded the Institute its third annual ''Award in Recognition of Significant Contribution to Health Care in the Delaware Valley.''

Community Health Centers

Delaware has three community health centers (CHCs) that historically have provided primary and preventive care to the very poor in their geographic areas. The Henrietta Johnson Medical Center and Westside Health Service, two federally qualified health centers (FQHCs), operate in New Castle County. Henrietta Johnson, the larger of the two, serves a predominantly African-American patient population. Westside has a predominantly minority patient base, but has twice as many Hispanic as African-American patients and employs a bilingual medical staff. Delmarva Rural Ministries, a rural health clinic, operates a clinic in Kent County and a Match Van that delivers health services to Sussex County. The clinic has been recognized for the care it provides for farm workers, including a large number of migrants.

To learn how the new Medicaid program might impact Medicaid and non-Medicaid populations, we interviewed directors of two centers and a senior-level representative of the third. Given DSHP's primary goal of improving access and the CHCs' important role in providing health services in underserved areas, the state encouraged all health plans to contract with the CHCs. This goal has not been achieved. In New Castle County, one center has contracted with only two of the three health plans. Sussex and Kent counties, which are medically underserved areas, have been served by only one CHC, Delmarva Rural Ministries. Because Delmarva Rural Ministries does not have a primary care physician, it cannot be reimbursed for any services provided by its nurse and nurse practitioner staff. (Nurse practitioners, under state law, must practice under the general supervision of a physician.) Therefore, it currently does not have a contract with any of the three health plans. Even though 20% of its patients are Medicaid eligible, Delmarva Rural Ministries does not receive any fees for treating these patients. To improve its services and funding base, Delmarva Rural Ministries plans to recruit for a staff physician by the end of 1996; however, the health center likely may not have the financial resources to attract a primary care provider to practice in a rural and underserved area. The growing number of A.I. Institute satellite clinics has helped to improve the physician network in southern Delaware, but Delmarva Rural Ministries programs remain essential for the two underserved counties.

The situation is much better in New Castle County. The CHCs have physicians on staff and therefore can contract with the health plans. However, one health plan has not contracted with the Henrietta Johnson Center. According to the center director this has created a significant problem. Many former patients were auto-assigned to this noncontracting health plan and either had to select another health care provider or had to work through the DSHP transfer procedure. This resulted in patient and provider confusion, loss of reimbursement for the center, and the use of many staff hours to correct the related problems.

How will the Medicaid reforms impact the Community Health Centers? In the Robert Wood Johnson Community Snapshot Study of Wilmington, the authors provide a very insightful observation: "The CHCs seem less worried about their fate under the DSHP than they are about the operational consequences of moving to capitation. These issues can be a major challenge to health centers lacking the financial and administrative resources for restructuring their information systems and rethinking patient care delivery."[19]

During our interviews, the CHCs offered several examples and suggestions that seemed to support this observation. First, the CHCs reported that the new plan has placed a financial burden on their organizations. At a minimum, increased administrative requirements have raised the average cost of providing services. One center reported that the change from fee-for-service along with delays in payments from the health plans have caused their cash flow to drop by 30%, even though their patient flow has not declined. Second, unlike many private practices that have experience working with managed care organizations, the CHCs expressed concern that they lacked the necessary financial and administrative expertise needed to move to a managed care environment. One CHC informed the health plans that it refused to accept capitated payments and negotiated a fee-for-service payment schedule similar to the one used under the former Medicaid system. Another CHC, which accepts capitated payments, suggested that transition would have been much easier if the state or the Health Benefits Manager had expanded the DSHP education program by offering provider orientation sessions. Third, one CHC expressed concern about the structure of the new "safety net" service delivery mechanism. Prior to the start of the DSHP, the CHC considered the state to be an experienced and caring partner in providing health care to the underserved population. Now, CHCs feel they've lost an ally and, according to one representative, are required to "go through a third party [a managed care organization] that seems to lack experience in providing health care to members of low income communities."

Based on admittedly early and incomplete evidence, the CHCs generally remain optimistic that the DSHP should improve access, particularly for the 9,000 uninsured being picked up by the state's new Medicaid program. Moreover, there seems to be an expectation that the CHCs, at least in the short run, will continue to serve as safety net providers to more than 60% of their clients who remain without health insurance after reform.

HCFA has contracted with an outside organization to conduct an evaluation of the DSHP. (HCFA requires comprehensive evaluations of all Section 1115 Demonstration Waivers.) One of the questions likely to be examined will be whether the health plans had sufficient experience working with low-income, Medicaid patients. We did not explore this question in sufficient depth to comment. One should note, however, that experience serving a Medicaid population was one of the criteria used to select health plans. Before we move on to a more thorough discussion of several key policy and management issues, it seems appropriate to briefly present the reporting and monitoring requirements that HCFA and the state developed for the Diamond State Health Care Plan. Even though the quality assurance plan seems similar to the ones developed for other Section 1115 Waiver programs, we found that many "knowledgeable" individuals, including providers, advocates, and consumers, seemed totally unaware of the quality assurance process.

Quality Assurance

Delaware has devised a quality assurance plan based on the HCFA Quality Assurance Reform Initiative guidelines for Medicaid managed care plans.[20] The federal government has delegated the responsibility for administering the Medicaid program to states. In its Section 1115 Waiver application, the state committed to monitor the four health plans for compliance with the contract through at least five mechanisms:

1. *Contractor reporting.* Managed care organizations will report information such as utilization by category of service, analysis of provider networks, enrollee complaint and grievance reports, and financial statements.

2. *Onsite reviews and medical audits.* As part of this review, an external quality review contractor will assess whether the health plans meet the current standards of medical care. The medical audits will focus on questions such as whether all necessary care was provided, whether discharges from the inpatient settings were appropriately timed and executed, and whether outreach and education of clients was adequately performed.

3. *Beneficiary surveys.* Satisfaction surveys will be conducted at several times during the plan year to address issues such as accessibility (travel time, waiting times for scheduling appointments, availability of medical advice by telephone), satisfaction with the quality of medical treatment, satisfaction with education on plan rules and how to use a health plan, and satisfaction with health plan rules and procedures.

4. *Provider surveys.* Mail surveys will be conducted once a year to assess the level of network provider satisfaction with the managed care program in general and with the health plan(s) to which they belong. Specifically, the following issues will be addressed: satisfaction with provider/patient relationship, satisfaction with health plan and related rules and procedures, ability of providers to satisfactorily deliver services, and accessibility to information regarding the eligibility of clients.

5. *Analysis of internal data and reports.* On an ongoing basis, the Medicaid Office will track disenrollment surveys, letters, phone calls, physician and hospital appeals, and requests for enrollment termination. This information will help state and federal administrators to identify problems related to referral procedures, payment mechanisms, quality of care, access to care, and the education and enrollment process.

Based on our investigation, we suspect that the quality assurance study will raise at least five major questions: (1) could the state and health benefits manager have improved the quality of the marketing, education, and enrollment phases? (2) did the state rush implementation? (3) how do safety net providers fare in the long run? (4) does the DSHP underserve the disabled? (5) does medicaid managed care provide adequate access to behavioral health services?

In the next section, we will address the first two questions. It is too early to comment about the third question. We would have liked to provide more insight and tentative answers to the last two questions, particularly because they have received a great deal of attention in the press and by critics of the DSHP. It is important to note that the majority of comments we heard about these two issues were very critical. Here are two examples of the criticisms: Parents of disabled children claimed the health plans were denying health care services that they had been allowed under the traditional Medicaid program; and, advocates from the mental health provider community told us that the mentally ill and substance abusers were experiencing great difficulties obtaining needed care. A representative from HCFA pointed out that, unlike many other Section 1115 Waiver programs, Delaware's Medicaid officials have been very responsive to the special needs of the disabled. For example, the state started to hold monthly meetings with a group representing families of children with disabilities.

Even though we received a great deal of input about disability and behavioral health-related issues, much of this information seemed to be incomplete, contradictory, and/or based on questionable evidence. A more extensive investigation backed by quantitative data, nevertheless, might indicate severe problems here. Experience from other states indicates that the beneficiaries that have fared the worst under managed care initiatives are the mentally ill, the substance abusers, and the disabled. We do not have enough solid evidence to determine if this also is true in Delaware.

KEY ISSUES AND DISCUSSION

Implementation Issues

Nearly every person we interviewed for this case study expressed significant concerns about the DSHP's implementation. Other states have faced similar problems. In a spring 1995 *Health Affairs* article, John Holahan and his colleagues at the Urban Institute describe the experience of the first five states to implement Medicaid managed care programs using HCFA Section 1115 Waivers. The authors emphasize that states will face many obstacles when they decide to implement Medicaid managed care programs.[21] Delaware, the seventh state to implement, encountered many of these same obstacles. Rather than echo the contents of the Holahan article, we will just point out several of the more severe problems from the Delaware experience.

Enrollment

Rapid enrollment in managed care has not been easy. Previously eligible Medicaid clients became eligible for the DSHP either on January 1 or February 1, 1996. Eligibles were assigned on a random basis to one of two groups defined by the eligibility dates. The health benefits manager mailed enrollment materials to the first group during the third week of November 1995. Several problems quickly became apparent. Introductory letters to all recipients were sent bulk mail. Incorrectly addressed bulk mail is not returned to the sender. As a result, the health benefits manager lost the opportunity check recipient addresses before sending out personalized enrollment kits. Enrollment kits were mailed in envelopes showing the health benefits manager as the sender. Many clients did

not recognize the company name, assumed the package was nothing more than
"junk mail," and threw it away. The enrollment kits arrived immediately before
Thanksgiving; clients were asked to complete the enrollment process during the
Thanksgiving-Christmas-New Year holiday season. Scheduling the enrollment
process during the holiday season resulted in many eligible beneficiaries failing
to select their own health plan and consequently being auto-assigned by the
health benefits manager.

According to Mary Kenesson, a consultant studying Medicaid enrollment and
the role of health benefits managers, a high voluntary enrollment rate and a low
rate of auto-assignment "is in everyone's best interests." Those auto-assigned
often don't understand managed care, often do not like the "idea of managed
care," are likely to file complaints and grievances, do not provide a current
address and phone number for the state and health plans, and generally "put
dust in the air."[22]

Delaware's voluntary enrollment rate has been close to the target level of
60+% set for the health benefits manager. Recent experiences in Missouri and
New Jersey, which have achieved rates better than 80%, indicate that this target
might have been set below what might be feasible through intensive outreach
efforts and three-month enrollment periods.

In addition to stronger marketing and advertising strategies, representatives
from two health plans suggested that a more aggressive follow-up system would
have helped to raise the voluntary enrollment rate and helped the plans to ease
the transition to the mandatory managed care system. When the health benefits
manager discovered that a client had not enrolled, the company was required to
contact the client "at least via mail" to remind them about the pending enrollment choice. The plan representatives told us they received an "excessive number" of incorrect enrollee addresses from the health benefits manager, and felt
this problem was symptomatic of a weak follow-up system. The state could
have achieved a higher voluntary enrollment rate by requiring the health benefits
manager to use the Missouri model where a minimum of *five* contacts were
attempted by mail and by phone.[23]

State officials told us that splitting the previously insured Medicaid population
into two enrollment groups unnecessarily complicated the enrollment process.
Many clients assigned to the second enrollment group (February enrollees) experienced a great deal of anxiety when they did not receive an enrollment during
the first mailing cycle; many of these individuals contacted the health benefits
manager or the state to find out why they hadn't received enrollment materials
or whether they had been dropped from the new Medicaid plan.

Communication and Education

During our interviews we asked respondents to tell us about the weakest or
most negative aspect of the DSHP. In terms of frequency of response and depth
of negative feelings, the communication and education components clearly were
the weakest components. Overall, there seemed to be a strong consensus among

the individuals we interviewed that the health benefits manager (HBM) did a poor job of helping enrollees (and their physicians) understand the myriad of issues that can confront any health care consumer. There also seemed to be serious concern that in comparison to the nation's two leading firms in this field, the HBM selected by Delaware lacked sufficient experience to effectively deal with the socioeconomic pressures common to Medicaid consumers.

Before describing specific concerns, it's important to point out that the health benefits manager faced several obstacles outside the company's control. First, the tight implementation schedule established by the state required the health benefits manager to use one-month enrollment periods rather than two- or three-month periods successfully used in other states such as Missouri. Second, the state's schedule required that enrollments occur during the Thanksgiving and Christmas holiday seasons when beneficiaries face numerous outside pressures. The state, unfortunately, was hit by a major snow storm during the enrollment period. This in effect decreased the number of days available for educational sessions and health fairs offered by the health benefits manager. Third, the state paid the health benefits manager a lower rate than other contracts around the country. These savings might have encouraged the company to "cut corners" and may not have been a "sound investment" for the state.

In spite of these constraints, many legitimate concerns were raised about the quality of the consulting services provided by the HBM. Among the list of specific concerns are the following abbreviated items. The enrollment materials developed by the health benefits manager were criticized for being much too complicated and confusing for the target audience to understand. Interestingly, in the Request for Proposal the state required that all materials be understandable at a sixth-grade reading level. Based on the feedback we received, the materials did not pass the "ease of understanding" test. One health care provider said that a person would need a college degree to work through the materials. A former benefits manager for a major corporation said his former employer would never accept such "poorly written and poorly designed" materials. Several physicians told us that the materials were so difficult to understand that they decided to send informational letters to their Medicaid patients. To help us learn more about innovative communication and education strategies, we interviewed a benefits communications consultant who has extensive experience working with Medicaid managed care plans. The consultant sent us material suggesting that the health benefits manager had not employed "state-of-the-art" oral or visual communication strategies such as increased use of billboards, bus posters, and radio announcements.

The health benefits manager hired 35 specially trained temporary workers, many of whom were Medicaid enrollees themselves, to answer phone inquiries about the DSHP, and speak with Medicaid clients at neighborhood centers, clinics, and health fairs. Many people we interviewed questioned the quality of the training received by these temporary workers. The director of one health plan told us that the health benefit's enrollment counselors frequently called his plan's staff to ask "very basic" questions about managed care and the Diamond State Health Plan! Another director told us that "the health benefits manager staff was not hired or trained in a timely fashion which had a negative impact on our plan." The director of one community health center complained that his staff "ended up doing a lot of the work that others [the health benefits manager] had been paid to do." The benefits consultant we spoke to suggested an interesting solution: The consultant's firm has demonstrated that all phone counselors do not have to be located in the client state (e.g., Delaware) to deliver "culturally appropriate and operationally effective" services. By tapping a health benefits manager's capacity and human capital in other Medicaid managed care states, Delaware might have been able to save money and expand the expertise of its toll-free Medicaid support.

The first few months of enrollment and implementation left many enrollees and providers confused. The headline to a *Wilmington News Journal* article read, "Managed-care program confusing doctors, patients: Medicaid experiment plan raises coverage, continuity of care issues."[24] Problems were particularly difficult for practices that had less experience with managed care and less experience with Medicaid patients. The Federally Qualified Health Clinics (FQHCs) had little experience with managed care and therefore had a particularly difficult time learning (and accepting) the new administrative requirements and administrative constraints. A physician in Sussex County, a medically underserved area, told us that overall he has been pleased with the DSHP, but early confusion caused two of his office assistants to quit. When Oregon introduced its Medicaid managed care plan, the health benefits manager conducted 65 well-attended provider information sessions across the state. Similar types of sessions organized and conducted by senior benefit consultants likely would have helped to lower the level of anxiety and confusion experienced by Delaware's provider community.[25]

The state's health providers suggested they could have been encouraged to play a more active role in educating their patients about the new Medicaid program. Provider information sessions would have helped to ensure that the Medicaid patients received accurate information from their physicians. Most physicians we spoke to felt that the health benefits manager should have marketed in providers' offices and health centers and should have supplied educational materials for distribution in the offices of physicians and other health care providers that interact with Medicaid patients.

Several providers suggested that the HBM and the state should have encouraged physicians and other health providers to help their Medicaid patients select the "best" health plan. Even though informal counseling certainly occurs in physicians' offices, there are two serious conflicts of interest here. First, there is a risk-selection problem: physicians who are compensated on a capitated basis will have a financial incentive to encourage their healthy (low-cost/low-risk) patients to remain with their practices while steering unhealthy (high cost/high risk) patients away. Second, physicians will encourage their patients to select the health plan that pays physicians the highest fees and has the least stringent managed care requirements. (The state's primary care providers typically affiliate with several health plans.) This advice will benefit providers, but in the long run it will limit the savings that can be generated from managed care—savings that the state is using to finance expanded Medicaid coverage.

We would like to conclude this section by addressing the question of whether the state rushed implementation. Based on the above discussion, one could easily conclude by answering "yes." We would like to present the case that the better answer is "no." We would agree that enrollees and providers faced serious problems during the enrollment periods and the first few months of the DSHP. (This seems to be a common problem faced by many states implementing Section 1115 Waiver programs.) Many—but certainly not all—of these problems could have been alleviated by making two fundamental changes in the DSHP. First, many enrollment-related problems seem like the result of the health benefit manager's lack of experience with a statewide Medicaid managed care program. Two firms with much more experience decided not to bid for the state contract. We suspect that these firms would have expressed much more interest if the state had been willing to pay higher fees for the HBM contract. The second change would have eliminated the staggered enrollment periods for previously eligible Medicaid clients. By using two one-month enrollment periods, the state spread the administrative burden over two months. But if the state had gone with one two-month enrollment period, there would have been less enrollee confusion about arbitrary assignments to the two groups. Moreover, auto-assignment rates likely would have dropped if eligibles were given two months to enroll.

The Number of Delawareans without Health Insurance

Improving access to health care is a primary goal of the Diamond State Health Plan. Access to health care has several dimensions, but the one most immediately impacted by the DSHP is the availability of health insurance coverage for the estimated 9,000 new Medicaid eligibles. Those with health insurance typically enjoy greater access to health care providers than those who don't have any.

Given that Delaware's Medicaid Waiver will expand Medicaid coverage, it seems reasonable to expect a significant drop in the number of uninsured residents. This conclusion is questioned in a 1996 report of Delaware's Cost Containment Committee. The Cost Containment Committee was created by an act of the Delaware General Assembly in 1992 for the purpose of recommending measures by which hospital and other health care costs could be contained. During its deliberations, the Committee discussed several interrelated issues that went beyond the scope of their work, but were thought to be important enough to include in their final report, *Evaluation of Certificate of Needs and Other*

Health Planning Mechanisms. One of these issues was the possible increase in the number of uninsured. The report indicates that even after accounting for increased Medicaid coverage, "the state can expect to see its uninsured population rise by 10,000 to 21,000 during the next six years."[26]

The Cost Containment Committee based its pessimistic projections on several national studies. These studies show that there has been a steady growth in the uninsured during the 1990s, largely attributable to an erosion in employer-based coverage. More workers reported securing health insurance coverage from their own jobs, but this gain was more than offset by a drop of dependents from employer-based plans. These dependents include secondary family workers without employer-based coverage on their own jobs, and nonworking adults and children. The Committee's report also sites a Tulane University study that estimates that if the loss of employer-based coverage continues at the current rate, holding Medicaid enrollments constant, the number of uninsured nationally will increase by approximately 67% by the year 2002. Recognizing that the erosion in employer-based coverage is likely to slow, the Tulane study lowers these national projections to a loss in the range of 25–40%. In Delaware, this level of change would translate into 22,000 to 33,000 additional uninsured. However, due to the "strength and unique characteristics of Delaware's economy," the Committee agreed that it should lower these estimates. On balance, after adjusting for the new Medicaid eligibles, the Committee reports that "the state can expect to see its uninsured population rise by 10,000 to 21,000 during the next six years."[27] Interestingly, very few of the people we interviewed for this study seemed aware of the nationwide erosion in employer-based coverage or the increased number of uninsured projected by the Cost Containment Committee. To better understand the nature of the uninsured problem, Delaware health care officials likely will be confronted with these key trends.

The Cost Containment Committee released its report in May 1996. One month later, Edward Ratledge of the University of Delaware completed the demographic study of the state's uninsured. Ratledge's report, "Delawareans without Health Insurance: A Demographic Overview," presents time series data indicating that, unlike overall U.S. trends, the number of Delawareans with health insurance has increased during the 1990s. From 1990 to 1995, the estimated number of individuals without health insurance dropped from 101,000 to 96,000 and the uninsurance rate dropped from 14.8 to 13.6%. During this same period, the uninsurance rate in the region (Maryland, Pennsylvania, New Jersey, and New York) increased from 10.4 to 13.5%. Ratledge attributes the increased rate of coverage to Delaware's strong economy, "a job creation machine that was even able to absorb the impact of major job cuts from the state's larger employers." He also credits the rapid employment growth in Delaware's FIRE (finance, insurance, and real estate) sector which has an extremely low uninsurance rate. In 1994, for example, the state's FIRE sector's uninsurance rate was 2.8%, compared to rates ranging from 8.8 to 31.4% in the manufacturing, trade, service, and construction sectors.[28]

Ratledge's work suggests that researchers need to be very careful when they apply national trends to the specific situations in individual states. U.S. data may reflect a continuing trend, but the numbers do not tell such a consistent story in every state. The Cost Containment Committee bases its gloomy insurance forecasts on nationwide trends. One might challenge whether this methodological approach works for Delaware.

The Voluntary Initiative Program

In 1993, Delaware established an innovative program to improve access to primary care for its Medicaid population. What is noteworthy about this program, known as the Voluntary Initiative Program (VIP), is that it aimed to reduce hospital emergency department use before the state had received a federal waiver. At the time, the state also lacked an adequate provider network to operate a statewide managed care program for Medicaid patients.

The VIP was a joint program between the Delaware Medical Society and the State of Delaware, where Medicaid patients without a regular source of care were referred to primary care physicians who agreed to become their primary care physicians. The intention was to establish a medical home for Medicaid recipients, thereby improving the quality of care for these patients and reducing the need for the use of emergency departments and hospitalizations. Clients and physicians participated on a voluntary basis. All state Medicaid clients were invited to initiate the referral process by calling the VIP referral number. The only managed care component was the expectation that the primary care physicians would remain the regular source of care for patients who were referred to them. By the end of the second year of the program, 3,000 referrals were made to 200 physicians. To add some perspective, Delaware has approximately 70,000 Medicaid clients and 1,000 primary care physicians.

Dr. James Gill (M.D.) and Dr. James Diamond (Ph.D.) examined the impact of the VIP. Using claims data for a study group (VIP patients) and a comparison group (non-VIP patients), the researchers sought to determine whether the program was successful in decreasing use of hospital emergency departments and in increasing use of office-based physicians during the first six months of operation. Both the study and comparison groups were primarily female and non-white, and about half were children under age fifteen. For each person in the study group and comparison group, Gill and Diamond calculated the rate of use of hospital emergency departments and the rate of physician office visits before and after referral. (For the comparison group, individuals were assigned artificial "referral dates.")

Gill's and Diamond's study demonstrates a positive effect of the VIP. After referral, emergency department use decreased 24% for the study group as compared to 4% for the comparison group. This occurred without requiring physicians to take on the role of gatekeeper. Physician office visits increased 50%

for the study group but decreased 13% for the comparison group. These results provide support for Delaware and other states' public officials who have built new managed care programs on the assumption of lower emergency room utilization and resulting budget savings. "These findings confirm the importance of primary care in improving the efficiency of health care delivery for the Medicaid population."[29] The Gill and Diamond study also suggests that referral to a primary care physician can have benefits even without managed care programs. The VIP could serve as a model for health care leaders in areas that have not developed large managed care programs or are waiting for federal waivers or greater support at the local level. The program could serve as an incremental program encouraging Medicaid recipients to obtain care from primary care physicians, thereby easing the transition to the full requirements of a managed care delivery system.

CONCLUSION

Despite early implementation problems, the Diamond State Health Plan on balance is considered a success. Unlike many other states that focused on slowing down hemorrhaging health care costs, Delaware's primary intention was to improve access—a long-recognized need throughout the state. By opening the Medicaid program to adults with incomes between 35 and 100% of the poverty level, the state expects to add 9,000 beneficiaries to the Medicaid program. For these new enrollees and the 56,000 participants who were previously eligible, the Diamond State Health Plan offers a basic benefit package including medical and mental health services. By increasing insurance coverage, improving access to primary care, and expanding managed care networks, the state expects the new Medicaid program to improve the health status for Delaware's poor. A public opinion survey and testimony of business leaders indicates a high level of support for Medicaid managed care. Governor Thomas Carper's decision to take a leading role in reforming the nation's welfare program added fuel to Delaware's Medicaid reform engine.

The Delaware experience suggests several important findings that states might want to consider in developing effective health care programs for low-income beneficiaries. First, the success of a program depends on the program design, leadership, and an external environment that reinforces the development and implementation of Medicaid reform. There is no question that Delaware's leaders made a strong commitment to meet a set of realistic goals. In all probability, though, the state would not have a statewide Medicaid managed care plan if the Alfred I. DuPont Institute had not worked to improve the distribution of providers in the state or if the state's largest employer, the DuPont Company, had not moved to managed care in 1993. DuPont's decision helped to create the necessary managed care infrastructure and demonstrated the business community's support in a state which sustains a probusiness political culture.

Second, moving the Medicaid population from traditional programs to managed care requires states to develop effective enrollment procedures and education programs—for both enrollees and providers. This issue has been a recurring thorn in the sides of most—if not all—state initiatives that preceded Delaware's. The communication and education components clearly were the weak links in Delaware's new Medicaid program. State officials with support from a health benefits manager developed written materials aimed at a low-income population, established a toll-free help line, and offered independent group and individual counseling sessions. Nevertheless, there seemed to be a clear consensus that the health benefits manager selected by the state made critical enrollment mistakes and did a poor job of helping beneficiaries and their physicians understand the myriad of issues that can arise during transition to a new Medicaid program. The Delaware experience demonstrates that states deciding to contract for enrollment and education services should pay close attention to the adequacy of funding levels and develop mechanisms to clearly monitor the performance of outside contractors. The problems associated with the health benefits manager shows that contracting out (government privatization) is not always a panacea. There is no question that privatization strategies can, in many instances, enhance productivity and enable Medicaid programs to accomplish more with fewer resources (such as full-time staff). A case in point is the partnership set up between the state and the Alfred I. DuPont Institute that offers Medicaid children a comprehensive specialist network and satellite primary care clinics in medically underserved areas of the state.

The third lesson is that states should pay special attention to meeting the needs of existing safety net providers and the difficulties of moving to a capitated payment system. One of Delaware's three community health centers, located in a medically underserved region, does not have a physician on staff and therefore could not be reimbursed for the care provided by its nurse and nurse practitioner staff. Another community health center expressed concern that it lacked the necessary financial and administrative resources needed to understand and meet the requirements of the new managed care delivery system.

Fourth, states looking to Medicaid managed care programs to expand coverage might be "swimming against a very strong tide." National trends suggest a continued erosion of employer-based coverage, particularly for dependents of employees. There is reason to suspect this trend to be strong enough to more than offset coverage gains of the Medicaid population. A study conducted for the State of Delaware indicates that even after adjusting for the new Medicaid eligibles, the state can expect to see an increase of 10,000 to 21,000 in its uninsured population during the next six years. What should be troubling to health care leaders across the country is that this trend is occurring in Delaware, a state with a strong economy which has been characterized as a "job creation machine."

Finally, Delaware's Voluntary Initiative Program demonstrates that by establishing a medical home for low-income persons—even without a full managed care program in place—low-income persons can be encouraged to seek treatment outside of hospital emergency departments. This program can serve as a model for health care leaders in areas that have not developed statewide Medicaid managed care programs; it also can serve as an intermediate step to ease the transition to a full-scale managed care program.

ACKNOWLEDGMENTS

Many people helped bring this case study to fruition. Among them are numerous individuals in Delaware including Delaware state officials, plan representatives, advocates, analysts, and consumers, who generously contributed their time, granting interviews and furnishing written materials. Kay Holmes, Paula Roy, and Philip Soule deserve special recognition for their exceptional commitments of energy to the Diamond State Health Plan and to their high level of support for this study.

We also are deeply grateful to a group of national experts who generously offered background materials, time, and overall guidance. This group includes Alisa Adamo, Lisa Adatto, Marsha Gold, Mary Kenesson, and Joseph Newhouse. Their input was extraordinarily helpful.

NOTES

1. Editorial, *Wilmington News Journal* (February 2, 1996).

2. Office of the Governor News Release, "Feds Approve Carper's Medicaid Waiver Extending Health Care Coverage to 9,000 Working Poor" (May 17, 1995).

3. Myrna L. Bair, interview by author, Newark, Delaware (May 20, 1996).

4. Kathryn D. Duke, Helene L. Lipton, and Karen C. Hertz, "Wilmington, Delaware Site Visit Report," in Paul B. Ginsburg and Nancy J. Fasciano, eds., *The Community Snapshots Project: Capturing Health System Change* (Princeton: The Robert Wood Johnson Foundation, 1996).

5. State of Delaware Indigent Health Care Task Force, cover letter to "Access to Health Care in Delaware: Recommendations by the Delaware Indigent Health Care Task Force" (Dover, Delaware, May 1990).

6. The Commission's mission was amended in 1995 to recognize that the Commission itself is not the provider of care. The new mission is "to promote basic, affordable, equal quality, accessible health care to all Delawareans."

7. Edward C. Ratledge, "Delawareans without Health Insurance: A Demographic Overview" (Newark: University of Delaware College of Urban Affairs and Public Policy, June 1966, draft).

8. Delaware Health Care Commission, *Evaluation of Certificate of Need and Other Health Planning Mechanisms* (Dover, Delaware, May 1996), 101–102.

9. *Community Snapshots Project*, 1996, 2.

10. Kathleen O'Leary Morgan, Scott Morgan, and Neal Quitno (eds)., Preface to *Health Care State Rankings, 1994* (Lawrence, Kans.: Morgan Quitno Corporation, 1994).

11. Northwestern National Life, *The NWNL Health Rankings* (Minneapolis, Minn.:

Northwestern National Life, 1992), in Victoria Van Son, *State Fact Finder: Rankings Across America* (Washington, D.C.: Congressional Quarterly, Inc., 1993).

12. Delaware Health Care Commission, *Primary Care Committee DIMER Review Project: Report and Recommendations* (Dover, Delaware, January 1996), 4.

13. The College of Urban Affairs and Public Policy developed the survey instrument in conjunction with the State of Delaware Developmental Disabilities Planning Council and Robert Griss, a consultant to the Council from the Center on Disability and Health. The sample size was 442 respondents, randomly selected from each of Delaware's three counties proportionally to the total population of that county within the state. Sampling error in a population of this size is +/−5% at the 95% confidence level.

14. Amy B. Droskoski, Eric D. Jacobson, and Jeffrey Raffel, *Health Care Reform for Delaware: Issues and Options* (Newark: University of Delaware College of Urban Affairs and Public Policy, 1996).

15. Robert F. Miller, Health Care Program Manager at the DuPont Company, testimony at the Delaware Health Care Commission's Public Hearing on Managed Care, May 30, 1996.

16. Janet B. Johnson and Joseph A. Pika, "Delaware: Friends and Neighbors Politics," in Ronald J. Hrebenar and Clive S. Thomas, eds., *Interest Group Politics in the Northeastern States* (University Park: Pennsylvania State University, 1993), 71.

17. Effective September 1, 1996, Mercy Health Plan is no longer a partner in the DelawareCare plan. A representative from HCFA questioned whether Principle Health Care of Delaware has sufficient experience working with the Medicaid population.

18. Eve Tahmincioglu, "Medicaid: Loss Leader for Del. Insurers?" *Wilmington News Journal* (November 24, 1995, Business section): 10.

19. *Community Snapshots Project*, 1996, 17.

20. U.S. Department of Health and Human Services, Health Care Financing Administration, Medicaid Bureau, *A Health Care Quality Improvement System for Medicaid Managed Care* (Washington, D.C., 1993).

21. John Holahan et al., "Insuring the Poor through Section 1115 Medicaid Waivers," *Health Affairs* (Spring 1995): 199–216.

22. Mary Kenesson interviewed in "N.J., Mo. Log Impressive Voluntary Enrollment Rates," *State Health Watch* (May 1996): 2.

23. "N. J., Mo. Log Impressive Voluntary Enrollment Rates," *State Health Watch* (May 1996): 2.

24. Eve Tahmincioglu, *Wilmington News Journal* (February 6, 1996, Business section): 3.

25. State officials held numerous informational/educational sessions for providers and provider organizations. Provider comments suggested that these should have been supplemented by sessions conducted by the health benefits manager.

26. *Evaluation of Certificate of Need and Other Health Planning Mechanisms*, 1996, 102.

27. Ibid., 101.

28. Ratledge, "Delawareans without Health Insurance: A Demographic Overview."

29. James M. Gill and James J. Diamond, "Effect of Primary Care Referral on Emergency Department Use: Evaluation of a Statewide Medicaid Program," *Family Medicine* (March 1996): 1.

6

Medicaid in a Managed Care Environment: The Florida Experience

KHI V. THAI AND MARY ANN FELDHEIM

INTRODUCTION

Florida is America's fourth largest state with the fourth highest number of Medicaid recipients in the country.[1] The large number of Medicaid recipients in Florida has meant that Medicaid spending and reform have been public policy issues for the last two decades. Indeed, several incremental strategies were utilized to address the issue of providing Medicaid coverage prior to major health care reform in 1992.

In the early 1980s, business coalitions and the organized elderly petitioned the legislature for reform that addressed hospital spending, because for-profit hospitals were finding ways to avoid contributing to the state's burden of uncompensated care. The Health Care Access Act of 1984 created a Public Medical Assistance Trust Fund to expand and improve Medicaid and to enhance primary care. The trust fund was sustained by a tax of 1% of net hospital operating revenues, rising to 1.5% in subsequent years.[2]

Tax increases were also implemented by the Florida legislature to address the increased Medicaid spending that the state was experiencing. A politically popular "sin tax" on cigarettes was utilized to generate revenue earmarked for health care coverage, including Medicaid. Reflecting the political antipathy in Florida toward broad tax increases, the legislature also enacted specific tax increases, linked to programs that aided poor mothers and children.[3] Other methods to address Medicaid spending, without affecting the programs' structure, eligibility, or services, were utilized, including: a fee reduction (30% average) in the reimbursement level for physicians; small reductions in nursing home payment levels; the use of generic drugs and co-payments; and modifications in the utilization control programs that were targeted to reduce costs.[4] These measures, however, were scattered, stop-gap measures intended to help curb the growth of the Medicaid expenditures. By the early 1990s, a perceived health care crisis existed in Florida that precipitated major health care reform whose goal was to provide access to health care coverage for all citizens within the state. Medicaid in Florida has been inextricably linked with the overall Florida health policy reform.

This chapter will examine health care reforms in Florida in the early 1990s and the factors that led to these reforms. Organizational studies offer a model of the "emotional cycle of change" that explains significant emotional shifts which affect people and policy when change occurs. Florida's health care reform effort, which focused on many aspects of Medicaid, is reflected in this model. By studying Florida's response to change, other states can predict and prepare for responses to policy changes.

FACTORS LEADING TO HEALTH CARE REFORMS IN FLORIDA

The health care reform movement in Florida was set into motion by three key factors: the perception of a health care crisis, an activist governor, and an activist health care network. These three factors came together in the early 1990s.

Health Care Crisis

The public's perception of a health care crisis in Florida came to the forefront in the early 1990s. Four broad classes of conditions that impact the health care policy area have been identified: access to care, health care costs, the allocation of resources, and the administrative burden imposed on providers and patients.[5] The primary conditions that were present in Florida to stimulate health care reform were limited access to care and escalating health care costs for which the state was responsible.

As a precipitating condition to health care reform, access to care refers to the numbers of people without either private insurance coverage or eligibility for government programs such as Medicare or Medicaid.[6] Florida in 1991 ranked fifth in the nation in the percentage of nonelderly citizens without health care coverage. It was estimated that 2.5 million people in Florida were uninsured and another 2.5 million people were underinsured.[7] The fact that an estimated 5 million Floridians had limited access to health care in 1991 contributed to the development of a health care crisis in the state. In Florida access to care was perceived as a major condition in the health care reform process.

Coupled with the problem of access to health care, the cost of health care in Florida had become a major concern. Although the recession of the early 1980s reduced inflationary pressure on the economy, medical inflation continued to rise.[8] Moreover, federally mandated expansions of Medicaid[9] and large numbers of immigrants[10] were also responsible for the dramatic growth of Medicaid in Florida. Indeed, between 1980 and 1992 health care expenditures in Florida increased from $9.2 million to $30 million a year, with a Medicaid enrollment of more than twice the national average and an annual growth rate of 18.3%.[11] Without reform of the health care system in Florida the cost was projected to increase to $90 million by the year 2000.[12]

Of the identified conditions that impact health care policy, cost has become the primary focus in policy debates. The reason for this is that cost affects access, resource allocation, and administrative burden. However, the above conditions alone did not create enough impetus for health care reform in Florida; a change in the views of the public was required. In the early 1990s, the public's attitudes regarding expansion of the role of government in addressing access to care and to control the rising cost of health care became increasingly favorable.[13]

An Activist Health Care Policy Network and an Activist Governor

The values articulated by a society in the political process are manifested in the distribution of resources among society's members. Because the availability of resources does not remain static, the political process is a dynamic interaction that responds to changing conditions. This constantly changing interaction is between those who advocate the current system of distribution (stake-holders) and those who advocate change (stake-challengers).[14] The conditions of the 1980s and early 1990s made the stake-holders increasingly competitive and increased the numbers of stake-challenger groups in the health representational community, creating a heterogeneous representational network. This network replaced the autonomous policy community, or iron triangle, built on close relations between private interests, predominantly medicine, and legislators. The dynamic nature of the new heterogeneous health policy network constantly responding to environmental changes makes it more amendable to change and reform than the iron triangle it replaced.[15]

The health care policy network that formed in Florida was unique to the state's varied population. It was influenced by: (1) support for governmental activism by the state's numerous liberal senior citizens; (2) a split between voluntary and public hospitals and the for-profit sector of health care providers; (3) a group of seasoned legislators and staff committed to health care reform; and (4) a governor willing to take the lead in promising state health care reform.[16]

The issue of health care reform in Florida was at a political stalemate until the election of Governor Lawton Chiles in 1990.[17] Chiles's initial proposal, the ''Florida Health Plan,'' has been credited as being the catalyst that brought the players in the health care arena together in a serious effort to expand health care access through the political process.[18] In heterogeneous policy networks the key to policy change focuses on the role of major political leaders with the resources and influence to mobilize the broad coalitions necessary to enact legislation.[19] In Florida several factors came together in the early 1990s to precipitate health care reform. The factors of importance are: (1) the public's perception of a health care crisis; (2) the election of Governor Lawton Chiles; (3) and the coalescing of an activist health care policy network.

Political strategies—clubs, commissions, and consensus—have been utilized over the last decade to impact the passage of health care policy in Florida. The health care reform process of the 1990s began with the use of a health policy "club," a political strategy for dramatic policy change that constituents find threatening and undesirable. This strategy improves the appeal and eventual acceptance of moderate reforms.[20]

The use of the "club" strategy led to the passage in 1991 of a limited health care reform bill, that created a 21-member advisory council to canvas reform alternatives, including a single-payer system. This bill created momentum in moving health care reform in Florida forward.[21] The advisory council, a form of "commission" strategy, was created to study the Florida health care system and to make recommendations for reform to the legislature and the governor.[22] Moreover, the council provided a public forum to discuss and debate the issues.[23] This strategy has been used extensively in Florida health care reform to build consensus in creating legislation that honors the top priorities of each group.[24]

Also in 1991, prior to major health care reform, Florida began a pilot program (in four counties) for Medicaid recipients of primary care case-management utilizing a fee-for-service structure. The state-managed pilot program was called MediPass. MediPass was created as a managed care "overlay" to the Medicaid program. The philosophy of the MediPass program was that the patient/physician relationship is critical for quality, cost-effective health care. In the MediPass program the Medicaid-eligible recipient enrolls with an individual physician, who has been approved as a Medicaid provider. The physician provides to the recipient direct services for a fee, authorization for other services he/she is unable to provide, and 24-hour access availability to deal with emergency situations.[25] The MediPass pilot program was added to the traditional fee-for-service Medicaid and the increasing use of HMOs to provide health care to Medicaid recipients. These changes were small, however, compared to the health care policy reform the state was contemplating in 1992.

Early in 1992, the advisory council made recommendations to address Florida's health care crisis. The focus of the recommendations was to increase Floridians' access to the health care system. The key recommendations included: (1) the creation of a single state agency to coordinate and regulate the state's health care program; (2) the establishment of a public and private partnership utilizing the managed competition model; and (3) a focus on wellness and health promotion.[26]

The 1992 legislative session faced clashes over taxation and reapportionment.

The taxation problem and the health care crisis were very visible in the budget submitted to the legislature by Governor Chiles. The projected budget indicated that the normal growth in Florida's tax revenue for the coming year would be consumed by state health care costs with 43% of the budget going toward human services.[27] The liaison between a reform-minded Chiles and the conservative Associated Industries of Florida (AIF), a broad-based business association, was a powerful force in moving the state toward health care reform. Other factors that aided in the passage of reform were the distractions created by the redistricting and tax battles, and the polls in Florida which indicated that the public was demanding better care at an affordable price.[28]

Public leaders and private groups, except physicians, were accepting of a new public sector entity with the capacity to diagnose the workings and failings of the system and to consider the practical implications of change. Consensus was achieved by Representative Bloom, a skilled legislator, who crafted a bill that attempted to meet the most important needs of all the interested parties. The bill passed the House, but had difficulty in the Senate where the creation of a new public agency and public sector reorganization had not even been considered. Supporters of the bill, whom Bloom and others had accommodated, were contacted to lobby for passage. This in addition to strong lobbying by the governor created a broad consensus in the shifting health policy network, and the Health Care Reform Act of 1992 was passed.[29] Consensus-building from divergent interest groups has allowed Florida to enact sweeping health care reform, but the reform has been vague, idealistic, and unwieldy policy that is exceedingly difficult to implement, causing dramatic swings in public opinion.

HEALTH CARE REFORMS IN FLORIDA: AN EMOTIONAL CYCLE ANALYSIS

Florida experienced an ambitious reform effort with the goal of providing health care access to all Floridians, including Medicaid recipients. This reform effort fits very well the emotional cycle of change, a model in organization studies. The emotional cycle, which addresses the feelings and attitudes of individuals in response to organizational change, consists of five stages: uninformed optimism, informed pessimism, hopeful realism, informed optimism, and rewarding completion.[30] Thus, this model, modified by expanding the focus, from the individual in an organization to the public's response to health care reform changes and policy implementation, is used to analyze Florida health care reform and policy change.

Uninformed Optimism Stage of Health Care Reform: The Health Care Reform Act of 1992

The first stage in the emotional cycle of change is "uninformed optimism." The assumption that forms the basis of this stage is that the level of positive feeling (optimism) regarding a change is related to the expectations of what will be involved. This is a honeymoon period with high hopes and high morale because the major obstacles are identified on the basis of raw data.[31] This unrealistic optimism was seen in Florida with the 1992 and 1993 legislation and in the Health Security Plan.

The Florida experience with the emotional cycle of change began with the passage of the Health Care Reform Act of 1992, when the legislature, in a bold move, overwhelmingly passed legislation creating the first comprehensive Florida commitment to ensuring access to basic health care for every citizen. The law utilized a multi-strategy approach to reform the health care system, with Medicaid being part of the comprehensive reform. The Health Care Reform Act of 1992 embodied the recommendations of the advisory council and the basic components of Chiles's "Florida Health Plan."[32] The primary thrust of this reform was administrative reorganization through the creation of the Agency for Health Care Administration (AHCA).[33] The focus of the AHCA was to consolidate health care financing, purchasing, planning and health facility regulatory functions, health policy development and planning, and to coordinate the Medicaid program. A secondary component of the 1992 legislation was to give the AHCA the responsibility to establish a managed competition model for the provision of health care insurance using a public sponsor to guarantee access to health care insurance coverage for small businesses and the state's employees and Medicaid recipients.[34]

The legislation was extremely ambitious, attempting to achieve universal coverage and reasonable costs by 1995, but there were inherent obstacles. First, severe fiscal constraints arose because Florida is a high growth, small business, and low-tax state, making the generation of revenues a major obstacle in all legislation. Second, parts of the legislation required federal waivers and legislative approval for implementation, which could impact significant sections of the legislation. Third, health insurance regulation was under the purview of the state insurance commission, a cabinet-level partisan position, creating the potential of fragmentation of effort. Fourth, the AHCA reports to the governor, but legislative approval was, and continues to be, required for adoption of health policy plans. The legislature in Florida is in continual flux and subject to partisan rivalry. Lastly, the AHCA was given an extensive agenda that must address many of the tough questions that consensus was unable to solve. Florida put its faith in reorganization. The hypothesis was that reorganization of the public structures and processes that govern health care financing and regulation would provide a way for the state to achieve major health care policy reform.[35]

The 1992 legislation provided through the policy process an opportunity for businesses, insurance companies, and other health care interests to pursue a market-based solution to ensuring basic access to health care for all Floridians. This stimulated extensive private sector meetings and a state initiative labeled Healthy Paradigms.[36]

The newly created AHCA orchestrated the Health Paradigms project using a series of one-day workshops and a two-day health care summit as a "commission" to solicit ideas and suggestions to achieve the goals established in the 1992 legislation. The staff of AHCA examined successful pioneer health reform programs at the state, national, and international levels. The focus of the data collection was on local solutions over state solutions, echoing the Chiles gubernatorial campaign. The outcome of the project was a "Blueprint for Health Security," with the centerpiece of the package being the creation of eleven regional community health purchasing alliances (CHPAs).[37]

The "Blueprint for Health Security" became the basis for the Health Care and Insurance Reform Act of 1993. This legislation included the following: (1) a mandate requiring all Medicaid recipients to be enrolled in a managed care program to the maximum extent practicable and permitted by federal law; (2) evaluation of the MediPass program of primary care case management for Medicaid recipients and expansion of the program to the state by 1996, after application for a federal freedom-of-choice waiver; (3) the creation of a managed competition model for health care access utilizing state-chartered, nonprofit private purchasing alliances called Community Health Purchasing Alliances (CHPAs); and (4) the creation of the Med/Access program to expand Medicaid coverage to Floridians with incomes up to 250% of the federal poverty level after the required federal waiver was secured.[38]

The emotional stage of uniformed optimism regarding health care policy was at its peak in this extremely ambitious and optimistic legislation. This law exemplifies the limits of state health policy reform primarily because of its inability to finance broadened coverage.[39] The euphoria of the health care reform movement in Florida was captured in the 1992 and 1993 legislation and presented to Floridians in "The Florida Health Security Plan: Healthy Homes 1994," published by the AHCA. This publication was an extremely optimistic and detailed report on health care reform in Florida, and it marks the end of the period of extreme optimism regarding the state's health care reform efforts.

Informed Pessimism Stage of Health Care Reform: Emerging Problems in the Reform

The second stage of the emotional cycle of change is labeled "informed pessimism," when unplanned events and problems begin to surface. The underlying assumption for this stage is that the more that is learned about what is involved in the policy change the more pessimistic the expectations become. One of the elements in this stage is that there is a lack of needed personnel, the project is viewed as unattainable, morale drops, there is resistance to the changes, and a process of "checking out" begins. The result is an attitude of extreme caution and concern in advancing the change reflecting the reality of implementation.[40]

By the end of 1993, Florida moved into the "informed pessimism" stage of emotional change as several problems surfaced. The first problem of the ambitious health care reform process arose when the Florida legislature attempted to reduce Medicaid spending by eliminating the Medically Needy Program. The Medically Needy Program provides catastrophic health insurance for the working poor.[41] Eliminating this program violated the goal of health care reform, that was to provide health care access to all Floridians. The legislature contemplated a bill to eliminate the program, but this gave rise to significant public outcry from advocacy groups representing the disabled and the elderly. In response to public concern, this bill was never enacted.[42] The public was effective in this instance in setting the parameters for Medicaid reform in Florida, and the political realities were being felt by those attempting health care reform. This incident reflected a dilemma of health care access and cost control.

The second setback to the Florida health care reform process came when the legislature did not pass legislation creating the proposed Med/Access program, which was to expand Medicaid coverage to Floridians with incomes up to 250% of the federal poverty level. The Med/Access program during the reform process was merged with the Florida Health Security Plan and relabelled the Medicaid Buy-In plan, which required two important steps before implementation (1) a federal waiver and (2) legislative approval.[43]

The Med/Access program attempted to circumvent the two major constraints to health care reform at the state level—political opposition to employer mandates and tax increases. To circumvent these constraints, Florida looked to Medicaid expansion as a way of covering more of the uninsured. Medicaid was an attractive solution, since the federal government would pay 50–83% of the costs of a state's Medicaid program. Eligibility for Medicaid could be expanded in two ways: by utilizing the 1902 (r)(2) provisions of the Social Security Act to expand coverage to pregnant women, children under the age of nineteen, and qualified Medicare beneficiaries, which was self-limiting,[44] and by expanding Medicaid eligibility by utilizing Section 1115 of the Social Security Act to provide for research and demonstration using a waiver.

The federal government might waive select Medicaid rules if the research was "budget-neutral," with the project maintaining costs to the pre-waiver status. The waiver requirement to remain budget-neutral was addressed by Florida with creative financing, which proposed to use existing dollars more efficiently to pay for the expansion, using savings from managed care and managed competition to expand coverage to more people.[45]

Florida did receive the waiver that would have allowed new eligibility categories and income limits for Medicaid recipients, but political changes in Washington and in the Florida legislature that were against additional governmental subsidies destabilized the Florida health policy network. The new political conditions left Governor Chiles as the main proponent of the Med/Access program, and he was unable to garner enough support to have the enabling legislation passed.[46] The pessimism regarding health care reform was becoming stronger, and the Med/Access or Medicaid Buy-In program became the first victim of the increased skepticism regarding universal access and sweeping health care reform.

A third setback in the implementation of health care reform in Florida came from problems in the utilization of managed competition to reduce Medicaid costs. The objective of managed competition is to provide increased access to health care coverage through the buying power of a public sponsor. The plan is based on the economists' paradigm of a competitive market, where there are multiple producers and well-informed consumers. The competitive market approach should result in increased enrollment in health plans that offer high-quality care at low costs, while high-priced plans would lose enrollment.[47] Individuals covered under the new Medicaid Waiver eligibility categories were intended to have a choice of plans offered by the Community Health Purchasing Alliances (CHPAs), either HMOs, indemnity, or PPO plans.[48] However, this large block of beneficiaries has not been included in the purchasing alliances. This has been an administrative decision by the Agency for Health Care Administration,[49] so at this time the relationship between Medicaid recipients in managed care programs and the managed competition model does not exist and cannot be extrapolated.

The three major setbacks to initial legislation of 1992 and 1993—the controversy in a legislative attempt to eliminate the Medically Needy Program, the failure to enact the Med/Access program, and failure to utilize managed competition for Medicaid access to care—created a situation where the broad goal of universal access for all Floridians became unattainable. As the realities of policy implementation began to be felt, the state relied more and more on managed care to provide health care service for Medicaid recipients and to reduce health care costs.

Managed care is a broad term used to describe a variety of existing and developing health plans that integrate the delivery and financing of health care services. Organizations that provide managed care utilize a variety of techniques such as utilization review, quality assurance programs, and preadmission certification to control utilization and cost, while delivering quality care.[50]

Nationwide there has been an evolution in the use of managed care by states implementing Medicaid. Managed care plans offer Medicaid beneficiaries coordinated forms of care, and typically a primary care physician acts as gatekeeper and coordinator of care. States believe that managed care plans save money and make the future growth of Medicaid more predictable.[51] The Omnibus Budget Reconciliation Act of 1981 promoted state-level experimentation in alternative forms of medical service delivery. Florida was slow in utilizing managed care in the form of HMOs to provide health care coverage to Medicaid recipients by beginning it on a limited basis in the late 1980s. Like other states, Florida's ability to contract with managed care plans had been constrained because federal approval in the form of a Section 1115 Waiver of Social Security Act restrictions was necessary.[52]

In 1993, President Clinton streamlined the process of granting Section 1115 Waivers, opening the way for several states to apply and receive waivers. The Medicaid program prior to 1993 had experienced an annual growth rate of approximately 28% per year for the past five years. Medicaid at that time was consuming more than half of all new general revenue growth.[53] Moreover, the Florida Health Care and Insurance Reform Act of 1993 mandated that all Medicaid recipients be enrolled in a managed care program to the maximum extent practicable and permitted by federal law. The legislative goals at this time were to reorient the Medicaid system to emphasize the delivery of health care through entities and mechanisms designed to contain costs, to emphasize preventive and primary care, and to promote access and continuity of care. The concept of "managed care" was believed to embody these goals. Florida's federal waiver allowed enrollment of Medicaid beneficiaries in managed care plans, and Florida utilized managed care in the form of HMOs and the MediPass program.

Medicaid managed care in Florida has evolved into a case-management continuum of care. On one end of this continuum is the state's primary care case-management program, MediPass, and at the other end of the continuum, Medicaid Health Maintenance Organizations.

The "MediPass program" is the state's primary care case-management, fee-for-service managed care program for Medicaid recipients. The pilot program for MediPass began in 1991 and in 1993 the legislature mandated to move Medicaid into managed care, expanding the MediPass program. Aid For Dependent Children (AFDC) recipients were the first to be phased into the MediPass program, followed by Social Security Insurance (SSI) recipients with completion of enrollment scheduled for July 1996.[54]

An evaluation of the MediPass program published in December 1995 found consistently lower expenditures for services as compared to traditional fee-for-service recipients. The overall cost savings ranged from 8.5% to 19.1% for a 39-month period. Comparisons of spending between MediPass and capitated managed care programs [i.e., health maintenance organizations (HMOs) or pre-paid health plans (PHPs)] found large cost savings for MediPass children, but comparable savings for adults.[55]

Opposite MediPass on the case-management continuum of care are capitated managed care programs [i.e., health maintenance organizations (HMOs) or pre-paid health plans (PHPs)].[56] Florida began the shift toward capitated managed care programs in the late 1980s as a means of reducing Medicaid costs. Traditional HMOs perceived Medicaid recipients as poor health risks and therefore unprofitable. With the backing of the federal government, in the form of Section 1115 waivers, Florida sponsored the creation of "Medicaid HMOs." The state offered these new Medicaid HMOs attractive payment rates and relaxed standards compared to traditional HMOs, granting the majority of Medicaid HMOs three-year waivers from Florida HMO licensing laws.[57]

Medicaid HMOs are paid a monthly flat fee by the state for each patient. The Medicaid managed care recipient is assigned a primary physician, who acts as a gatekeeper to care. The primary physician must approve all referrals to specialists and for hospital care and treatment. The benefit for the recipient is continuity of care, a relationship with a primary physician, and improved access to care.[58] All eligible Medicaid managed care recipients have a choice of provider. Prior to May 1996 the recipient could choose a Medicaid HMO provider; if the recipient did not choose a HMO provider he or she would default to the MediPass program and would be assigned a primary care physician by the AHCA.[59]

As Florida moved rapidly into the capitated managed care system, the state experienced severe start-up problems, such as oversight difficulties, fraudulent marketing, substandard care, and enterprising health maintenance organization (HMO) entrepreneurs.[60] The start-up programs produced mixed results in the utilization of capitated managed care as a means of providing cost-effective health care to Florida Medicaid recipients. Yet, the state has saved $45.1 million in fiscal year 1992–1993 and reduced total program expenditures in fiscal year 1993–1994 by $54.5 million.[61]

Hopeful Realism Stage of Health Care Reform: Positive Results of Improvement Efforts

The third stage of the emotional cycle of change is "hopeful realism," when the temptation to quit is overcome and a sense of realistic hope emerges. Modifications to the process based on reality testing occur and the policy is changed to adapt to the reality of the situation.[62] The assumption for this stage of the cycle is that the level of pessimism or optimism about the policy is a function of the data available concerning the task requirements for the individual, the organization, or the state.[63] Florida experienced this stage during late 1994 and 1995 as reports and evaluations were conducted on the Medicaid programs to assess areas of difficulty and to make recommendations for improving the system.

Several reports regarding Medicaid fraud and abuse in Florida made recommendations to improve the current system. In April of 1994, the Florida Office of the Auditor General released the results of an audit of Medicaid's Program Integrity functions. The audit made specific recommendations to improve the AHCA's ability to determine Medicaid providers' fraud and abuse: (1) to refer all suspected cases of provider fraud to the Medicaid Fraud Control Unit; (2) to document sanctioning recommendations; and (3) to monitor providers who have a history of Medicaid abuse to prevent further abuse.[64]

This was followed by the *Fort Lauderdale Sun Sentinel* reports on Florida's Medicaid HMOs in December of 1994. This year-long investigation revealed HMOs' poor medical care, the use of questionable tactics to sign up new members, and extremely high salaries for HMO executives; and compiled reform suggestions from patient advocates, government regulators, and industry officials. Key points for reform were to: abolish the three-year waiver exempting Medicaid HMOs from commercial licensing standards; require Medicaid HMOs to be nationally accredited as are commercial HMOs; limit or ban HMOs from marketing at food stamp offices or door-to-door; address the issue of over-payment; conduct routine patient satisfaction surveys; utilize sanctions when appropriate; strengthen laws barring questionable individuals from operating Medicaid HMOs; and ensure that monitoring moves beyond "paper" monitoring. These recommendations for reform were echoed by state and federal audits and investigations.

A joint federal-state health care fraud and abuse task force examined the extent of both Medicare and Medicaid abuse in south Florida. The report released in March of 1995 focused on three processes: (1) provider enrollment requirements and procedures; (2) claims review policies and procedures; and (3) procedures and tools to deal with fraudulent or abusive providers. Identified were several factors that contributed to Medicaid's vulnerability to fraud and abuse in Florida, such as the ineffective use of data to detect fraud, light penalties for fraud and abuse, and extremely complex administration and coordination.[65] In its 1995 annual review, the state Agency for Health Care Administration found the average HMO failed 17% of 125 standards demanded by its state contract; and as a result of this review, a dozen of HMOs were fined a total of $522,000 and some were barred from expanding.[66]

The period from 1993 to 1996 revealed the harsh political realities of health care reform in Florida, defining the state's period of "uninformed pessimism" and "hopeful realism." The failure of the state to implement the Med/Access program to expand Medicaid coverage to those at 250% above the federal poverty level was a significant blow to the comprehensiveness of the program. The administrative hesitation in utilizing managed competition to purchase Medicaid managed care diminished the uniqueness of the Florida Medicaid program. Lastly, the findings that Medicaid fraud and abuse are significant in Florida have all served to define the stage of change when reality offers its challenge.

Informed Optimism Stage of Health Care Reform: The Medicaid Fraud and Abuse Act

The fourth stage of the emotional cycle of change is informed optimism manifested by a growing sense of accomplishment and a new burst of energy.[67] This can be seen in the passage, in May 1996, of the Medicaid Fraud and Abuse Act that addressed significant difficulties in the Medicaid system and generated optimism in making the system more responsive and accountable.

The federal Medicaid program enacted in 1965 was implemented in Florida on January 1, 1970. Included in the Medicaid legislation is a provision for the encouragement of investigation and criminal prosecution of Medicaid fraud. The federal government reimburses states 75% of the expenditures in establishing a state Medicaid fraud unit. The Florida Medicaid Fraud Control Unit (MFCU) was established in 1980 in the Auditor General's Office and in 1994 the unit was transferred to the Attorney General. The location of the unit complies with federal law requiring the fraud office be independent from the state agency that administers the Medicaid program. Florida statutes authorize the Attorney General to investigate (1) alleged abuse or neglect of patients in health care facilities receiving Medicaid payment; (2) possible criminal violations of laws pertaining to fraud in the Medicaid program; and (3) alleged misappropriation of patients' private funds in health care facilities receiving Medicaid payment. Also, prior to 1996, Medicaid fraud investigators in Florida were not classified as law enforcement officers. The 1996 legislation permits the investigators to become law enforcement officers. The intent of this legislation was to increase efficiency and effectiveness of the unit.[68]

In addition, the Florida legislature strengthened the ability of the Agency for Health Care Administration to identify abuse and fraud, issue sanctions, and terminate Medicaid contracts with fraudulent providers. The agency will conduct these activities in concert with the Medicaid Fraud Control Unit. The staff of the Office of Medicaid Program Integrity were charged with developing statistical methodologies to identify aberrant billing patterns, conducting investigations and audits based on this information, calculating provider overpayment and initiating recovery, and recommending provider sanctions and referral to the Medicaid Fraud Control Unit when abuse or fraud is suspected. To facilitate investigations providers are required to retain professional and financial records for five years.[69]

The Managed Care and Publicly Funded Primary Care Program Coordination Act of 1996 initiated several reform measures. First, the three-year waiver exempting Medicaid HMOs from commercial licensing standards has been abolished. Second, Medicaid HMOs are required to be nationally accredited in the same manner as commercial HMOs. Third, the AHCA will monitor HMO marketing at food stamp offices. Fourth, the AHCA will monitor and follow-up on overpayment for Medicaid services and utilize sanctions when appropriate, ensuring that monitoring moves beyond "paper" monitoring. Fifth, routine patient satisfaction surveys are to be conducted by the AHCA. Lastly, the laws barring questionable individuals from operating Medicaid HMOs have been strengthened.[70]

The legislation also mandated that Medicaid recipients be placed in a managed care program, either the MediPass program or enrolled in a capitated managed care program. For this legislation to be implemented an amendment to the current waiver from the federal government is required. The legislation requires eligible managed care recipients to make a choice, and if the recipients do not, the state will make the choice for them. The initial enrollment would be a 50/50 split assignment process between a Medicaid HMO or MediPass. After initial enrollment, the recipient would be assigned according to a ratio based on previous choice trends either into the MediPass program or a Medicaid HMO. Each eligible recipient would receive choice counseling information to assist them in making an informed choice. An eligible recipient may make a change within the first 60 days, if he or she is unhappy with the initial choice.[71]

This legislation reflects the many recommendations that have been made by governmental audits and investigations. The need for tighter control and increased authority for the governmental entities that are charged with this control are the key elements in this legislation. Florida's health care reform movement and the Medicaid program reflect with this legislation the stage of "informed optimism" in the emotional cycle of change, as the state moves competently to improve, modify, and implement the program. The state AHCA's 1996 annual review of 21 HMOs that have provided care for Medicaid patients, released on October 14, 1996, revealed that an average HMO failed 9.5 of 125 standards demanded by its state contract or an average score of 92%, as compared with 83% in 1995; and no fine was imposed on any HMO. This represents real "informed optimism" as Florida pays HMOs about $700 million a year to care for 385,000 Medicaid patients, about one-third of the state total Medicaid population.[72]

Rewarding Completion Stage of Health Care Reform:
Uncertainty of Health Care Reform

The final stage, "rewarding completion," occurs as successful change is made and the project is processed and closed. The final result of the change frequently is different from that which was originally expected, yet feelings of fulfillment and satisfaction predominate.[73] The current status of the Medicaid program in Florida is significantly different from the proposed sweeping reform program. The changes have been made, but Florida will probably never reach the stage of "rewarding completion" of health care reform. Based on the diversity of the state, the economics of health care, and the state's political climate, the health care reform process in Florida will continue to change and may start again the emotional cycle of change by trying a new approach to health care policy.

The political patterns that sustained health policy advances in Florida can offer insights about health policy reform. First, the use of "commissions" can educate, create a shared vocabulary, create a focus, and establish an intellectual foundation for the legislative process. Second, the deployment of policy "clubs" sustained by a substantial liberal constituency can keep the reforms on the policy agenda and force a persistent search for a middle ground. Third, Florida demonstrated the use of "consensus" in astute legislative-executive relations utilizing a strong governor and experienced policymakers committed to health care reform. Florida has demonstrated innovative health care policy reform, yet the state has largely dodged the toughest questions of how to finance universal coverage and how to keep it affordable.[74]

The managed competition model established in Florida has been advanced as a model of health care reform for the nation, but the model has yet to be used for the purchasing of Medicaid managed care. The significance of managed competition to the financing of Medicaid remains unexplored. These unresolved issues continue to plague the comprehensive health care reform attempted in Florida.

There are several obstacles to realizing the goal of expanded health care coverage. Fiscal constraints may come first in the form of increasingly limited savings from managed care. Second, the extent of funds from the disproportionate-share hospital payments depends on reducing the numbers of individuals who receive services for which hospitals are uncompensated. Florida plans to gradually divest disproportionate-share funds, avoiding dramatic decreases in funding to hospitals.[75]

Political and economic obstacles have stopped the implementation of the Florida Health Security Plan (Med/Access and Medicaid Buy-In). The changing political climate seen in Republican cost-cutting has removed one of the premier programs in the 1993 Health Care Reform legislation.

The political difficulties that Florida has experienced when enacting and trying to implement health care reform have been dramatic, and reform has often experienced setbacks. The managed competition plan enacted in 1992 contained an employer mandate, but the public opposition was so strong that the mandate was repealed in 1993 making employer contributions entirely voluntary.[76] With political difficulties limiting the comprehensive Florida Health Security Plan, the Medicaid program in Florida currently relies almost exclusively on the utilization of managed care in the form of capitated managed care programs (HMOs) and primary care case management by the state (MediPass). Florida's uniqueness in both its political climate and in its response to a health care crisis make it an appropriate case study for other states and the federal government in enacting health care reform.[77]

CONCLUSION

The case study of Florida using the model of the emotional cycle of change can provide other states with an understanding of the change process from the psychological perspective. The state's "uninformed optimism" seen in the sweeping reforms of 1992 and 1993 can prepare other states to anticipate this stage of reform. The implementation realities that moved the state into "informed pessimism" can be attributed to political changes and loopholes in the capitated managed care Medicaid system that permitted fraud and abuse. The ability of the system to respond adaptively moved the state into the "hopeful realism" stage of the emotional cycle of change. Responsive legislation in 1996, that directly addressed the identified problems, has led the state to the stage of "informed optimism."

The final result of the health care reform in Florida is different from that which was originally expected, yet a feeling of fulfillment and satisfaction predominates. According to Governor Chiles, Florida leads the nation in reforming Medicaid, having cut the rate of growth in half and reduced the cost through the use of managed care, saving over $1 billion a year.[78]

Florida health care reform demonstrates the potential and the limitations of a state to respond to a major societal issue such as health care. The Florida health care experience encompassing Medicaid was presented using a historical perspective and the emotional cycle of change. Florida can provide other states with valuable information on responding to the health care crisis, specifically Medicaid. The Medicaid program in Florida continues to evolve and adapt to the changing economic and political climate. However, the hopes of health care coverage for all Floridians have dimmed as the changing political and economic climate reduces the chance for the dream to come true.

NOTES

1. U.S. Department of Health and Human Services, Health Care Financing Administration, Medicaid Bureau, *Medicaid Statistics, Program and Financial Statistics Fiscal Year 1993*, HCFA Pub. No. 10129 (Washington, D.C.: Health Care Finance Administration, October 1994), 43, 64, 126. Quoted in Florida Medicaid Program Analysis, *Medicaid Statistics: Florida Medicaid Program* (January 1996): 22.

2. Lawrence D. Brown, "Commissions, Clubs, and Consensus: Reform in Florida," *Health Affairs* (Summer 1993): 7–26.

3. Teresa Coughlin, Leighton Ku, John Holahan, David Heslam, and Colin Winterbottom, "State Responses to Medicaid Spending Crisis: 1988 to 1992," *Journal of Health Politics, Policy and Law* 19, no. 4 (1994): 837–864.

4. Ibid.

5. Mark A. Peterson, "Political Influence in the 1990s: From Iron Triangles to Policy Networks," *Journal of Health Politics, Policy and Law* 18, no. 2 (1993): 399–438.

6. Ibid.

7. State of Florida Agency for Health Care Administration, *The Florida Health Security Plan: Health Homes 1994* (Tallahassee: State of Florida, 1993).

8. Peterson, "Political Influence," 403–404.

9. Teresa Coughlin, Leighton Ku, and John Holahan, *Medicaid Since 1980: Costs, Coverage, and the Shifting Alliance Between the Federal Government and the States* (Washington, D.C.: Urban Institute Press, 1994).

10. Brown, "Commissions, Clubs," 11.

11. Coughlin et al., "State Responses," 481.

12. Jan L. Shebel, "Necessity Gives Birth to Health Care Reform in Florida," *Benefits Quarterly* 9, no. 3 (1993): 32–40; *Florida Health Security Plan 1994*.

13. Brown, "Commissions, Clubs," 17.

14. Peterson, "Political Influence," 401.

15. Ibid., 419.

16. Brown, "Commissions, Clubs," 20.

17. Shebel, "Necessity," 33.

18. State of Florida Agency for Health Care Administration, *Project Narrative* (Tallahassee: State of Florida, 1993).

19. Peterson, "Political Influence," 430.

20. Brown, "Commissions, Clubs," 10.

21. Ibid., 14.

22. Shebel, "Necessity," 34.

23. Brown, "Commissions, Clubs," 3.

24. Ibid., 20.

25. Paula McAuley, Medical Health Care Program Analyst, Florida Agency for Health Care Administration, MediPass Unit, telephone conversation with Mary Ann Feldheim, June 5, 1996.

26. Shebel, "Necessity," 34.

27. Lawton Chiles, governor of Florida and Buddy MacKay, lieutenant governor of Florida, *The Governor's Budget Recommendations: FY 1994–95* (Tallahassee, 1993), xxxi.

28. Shebel, "Necessity," 35.

29. Brown, "Commissions, Clubs," 19.

30. Don Kelley and Daryl R. Conner, "The Emotional Cycle of Change," in J. E. Jones and J. W. Pfeiffer, eds., *The 1979 Annual Handbook for Group Facilitators* (San Diego, Calif.: University Associates, Inc., 1979).

31. Ibid., 118.

32. Shebel, "Necessity," 34.

33. Brown, "Commissions, Clubs," 23.

34. Ibid., 21–22.

35. Ibid.

36. Shebel, "Necessity," 36

37. Ibid., 37.

38. *Florida Statutes*, sec. 409.9121, 09.9122

39. Brown, "Commissions, Clubs," 23.

40. Kelley and Conner, "The Emotional Cycle," 119.

41. Lawton Chiles, governor of Florida and Buddy McKay, lieutenant governor of Florida, *The Governor's Budget Recommendations Fiscal Year 1993–94* (Tallahassee, 1992), 12.

42. Coughlin et al. "State Responses," 854.

43. *Florida Statutes*, sec. 409.9121, 409.9122.

44. John Holahan, Teresa Coughlin, Leighton Ku, Debra J. Lipson, and Shruti Rajan, "Insuring the Poor Through Section 1115 Medicaid Waivers," *Health Affairs* (Spring 1995): 199–216.

45. Ibid.

46. Peter Mitchell, "Chiles Appears Alone Pushing Insurance Plan," *Wall Street Journal* (August 23 1995), 1(F), 4(F).

47. John Holahan, Marilyn Moon, Pete W. Welch, and Stephen Zuckerman, *Balancing Access, Costs, and Politics: The American Context for Health Care Reform* (Washington, D.C.: The Urban Institute Press, 1991).

48. Holahan et al., "Insuring the Poor," 208.

49. Ken Terry, "Covering Small Businesses," *Florida Business Trends* 38, no. 6 (1995): 82–84.

50. *Florida Health Security Plan 1993*, G5.

51. John K. Inglehart, "Health Policy Report: The American Health Care System," *New England Journal of Medicine* 328, no. 12 (1993): 896–900.

52. John K. Inglehart, "Health Policy Report: Medicaid and Managed Care," *New England Journal of Medicine* 332, no. 25 (1995): 1727–1731.

53. *Florida Statutes 1995*, sec. 409.9121: 320.

54. Paul McAuley, telephone conversation.

55. Charles Barrilleaux, Susan Phillips, and Christopher Stream, *Florida MediPass Evaluation Report* (Tallahassee: Policy Sciences Center, Florida State University, 1995).

56. Ibid., 1.

57. Fred Schulte and Jenni Bergal, "Profits from Pain," *Fort Lauderdale Sun-Sentinel* (December 11, 1994), 1(A), 16(A), 17(A); and *Florida Statutes 1995*, sec. 641 Part III.

58. Schulte and Bergal, "Profits from Pain," 1(A), 16(A), 17(A).

59. McAuley, telephone conversation.

60. Inglehart, "Health Policy Report," 1729.

61. *Florida Health Security Plan*, 13.

62. Kelley and Conner, "The Emotional Cycle," 121.

63. Ibid., 118.

64. Senate Staff Analysis and Economic Impact Statement of *Florida Senate Bill 118*, February 2, 1996.

65. United States General Accounting Office report, "Medicare and Medicaid: Opportunities to Save Program Dollars by Reducing Fraud and Abuse," March 25, 1995, quoted in *Senate Staff Analysis and Economic Impact Statement Senate Bill 118* (February 2, 1996), 3.

66. *Sun-Sentinel*, October 15, 1996.

67. Kelley and Conner, "The Emotional Cycle," 121.

68. *Florida House Bill 573*, Analysis, 1996.

69. *Senate Bill 118*, Analysis, 2.

70. House Amendment to *Senate Bill 886*, May 3, 1996.

71. McAuley, telephone conversation.

72. *Fort Lauderdale Sun-Sentinel*, October 15, 1996.

73. Kelley and Connor, "The Emotional Cycle," 121.

74. Brown, "Commissions, Clubs," 25–26.

75. Holahan et al., "Insuring the Poor," 210.

76. Colleen M. Grogan, "Hope in Federalism? What Can the States Do and What Are They Likely to Do?" *Journal of Health Politics, Policy and Law* 20, no. 2 (1995): 477–484.

77. Russell Hanson, "Health-Care Reform, Managed Competition, and Subnational Politics," *Publius: The Journal of Federalism* 24 (1994): 49–68.

78. "On Block Grants: Excerpts from Remarks by Governor Chiles before National Press Club May 11, 1995," *The Florida Nurse* 43, no. 6 (1995): 2, 11.

7

Medicaid Reform in Kansas: A Cautious Approach

JOCELYN M. JOHNSTON, RAYMOND G. DAVIS,
AND MICHAEL H. FOX

Medicaid reform has been a cautious undertaking in Kansas, reflecting the unique geographic, political, and demographic influences in the state. Unlike other states which have developed stringent, centralized policy guidelines for serving diverse constituencies, Kansas has responded to community needs in a style which is partly reflective of its populist tradition. This style can be characterized as a decentralized means of developing and generating policy. As targeted needs within areas of the state have been identified for segments of the Medicaid population, the Kansas Department of Social and Rehabilitation Services (SRS), which administers the Medicaid program, has worked closely with community groups to see that these needs are met, but has also maintained tight control over policy implementation. Increasingly over the last three years, this process has taken the form of developing forms of managed care which can best maintain recipients' access to quality health care while pursuing strategies designed to contain Medicaid cost growth.

The state's moderate approach to Medicaid reform results from a combination of factors which have influenced the development, design, implementation, and administration of the reform process since the early 1980s. This chapter examines the reform process in Kansas, focusing on the following five themes. First, although Kansas is fiscally conservative, many citizens and political leaders would characterize Kansas as a socially responsive state. However, evidence suggests that in fact, Kansas is often less responsive to the health care needs of its poor than neighboring states in the plains region. Second, the state has a tradition of responding to local needs. Yet Medicaid administration is centralized, with limited opportunities for local input into program operation and implementation. Third, the Medicaid bureaucracy has struggled to manage and implement Medicaid reforms, with limited success. The ability of administrators to respond to the changes required by reform has been restricted by the structure of the bureaucracy and by chronically inadequate resources. Fourth, in its pursuit of reform, Kansas has followed the lead provided by other states, and by the private sector within the state. Fifth, efforts to privatize social services have dominated the current period of reform.

The framework in which these features will be examined includes discussions of the background to reform, the Medicaid bureaucracy, and physician supply and rural issues. In addition, the structure of the reform is described. The caution with which the state has approached reform is evidenced throughout the discussion.

INTRODUCTION

Kansas is a relatively prosperous but aging state. Although the poverty rate is lower than average (only 11.5% in 1990, relative to the nation's average of 13%), Kansas ranks eleventh among states with regard to the percentage of its population aged 65 or older (13.9% verses 12.6% nationally), and has the fifth highest percentage aged 85 or older.[1] In addition, Kansas has more nursing home beds and community hospital beds per capita than most other states. This is partly a function of the widely dispersed population in rural portions of the state, where there are often great distances between health care facilities and providers, and where communities strive to provide health services "close to home." The state is geographically large (the fifteenth largest in the nation), encompassing 105 counties, yet it contains only two major metropolitan areas. Consequently, efforts to reform Medicaid have had to balance those few areas in the state with sufficient provider supply with the many underserved areas. (Table 7.1 provides a statistical description of Kansas, its Medicaid program, and selected Kansas border states.)

In the primarily rural western half of the state, populations are declining, population densities average below ten persons per square mile (see Figure 7.1), and most county populations fall below 8,000.[2] On the other hand, rapid population growth characterizes the Kansas suburbs of the Kansas City metropolitan area, located in the northeastern portion of the state.[3] Located in the southwest corner of the Kansas City metropolitan area, these suburbs are experiencing healthy economic growth and comprise one of the fastest growing regions—in terms of both economic growth and population growth—in the nation. Wichita, the second major metropolitan area, is located in south central Kansas. The absence of other major population centers has generally discouraged broad adoption of managed care programs until recently.

In addition to its unique demographics, Kansas has political traditions which have contributed to its cautious approach in implementing Medicaid reform. Those traditions include a strong rural political base infused with the populist streak which has influenced Kansas politics since it was granted statehood in

Table 7.1
Selected Demographic, Health Service, and Medicaid Statistics, Kansas and Selected Border States[1]

	U.S.	Kansas		Nebraska		Iowa		Missouri		Oklahoma	
Fiscal Features											
Median Household Income, 1992	30,786	30,447	(24)	30,177	(27)	28,880	(32)	27,490	(38)	25,363	(46)
State-Local General Revenue, as % of Personal Income, 1991*	16.1	15.7	(30)	16.7	(19)	17	(18)	12.8	(50)	16.6	(21)
State-Local Taxes, as % of Personal Income, 1991	11.3	10.9	(28)	11.3	(21)	11.6	(18)	9.2	(49)	11.1	(25)
State-Local General Expenditures, as % of Personal Income, 1991	19.4	18.1	(39)	19	(33)	20.3	(22)	15.3	(50)	19.3	(30)
Demographic Features											
Poverty Rate, as % of Total Population, 1989	13.1	11.5	(31)	11.1	(33)	11.5	(30)	13.3	(18)	16.7	(10)
Poverty Rate, as % of Total Population Under Age 18, 1989	18.3	14.3	(34)	13.8	(38)	14.3	(33)	17.7	(22)	21.7	(11)
Aged 65+ as % of Total Population, 1991	12.6	13.9	(11)								
Aged 85+ as % of Total Population, 1992		1.74	(5)								
Physicians per 100,000 Population, 1992	204	165		167		139		188		141	
Eligibility and Program Coverage											
Med Beneficiaries per 1000 Poor	510	397		401		408		451		476	
Medicaid Eligibility (for AFDC), Income Limit as % of Federal Poverty Level, 1995,	44.2	43.6		37		43.3		29.7		47.8	
Medicaid Eligibility Levels for Pregnant Women and Children (Expansions), as % of Federal Poverty Level, 1995	169	150		133		185		185		150	

The Elderly and Long Term Care

Number of Nursing Facility (NF) Beds per 1000 Population Aged 65+, 1992	53	87.5 (1)	85.9 (2)	81.7 (4)	84.4 (3)	79.5 (6)
Average Number of Beds per NF, 1992**	102.4	70.2	80.9	74.2	98.6	81.9
NF Residents as % of Population Aged 65+, 1992	4.4	7.2 (49)	6.9 (47)	6.8 (46)	5.12 (32)	6.07 (42)
Average Medicaid Per Diem NF Costs, 1993***	71	43.5 (46)	57.4 (34)	4.02 (49)	45.8 (44)	36.44 (50)
Percent of Total Medicaid Expenditures Spent on Long Term Care	35	40	46	43	29	45
Home and Community Based Services as % of Total Medicaid Long Term Care Expenditures, 1992	13.2	6.2	15.2	4.3	8.5	12.5

[1]State ranks, where available, are in parentheses.

*Own source revenues.

**Ratio of average daily census to total facility beds, expressed as a percentage.

***In dollars.

Sources: The American Association of Retired Persons, *The State Economic, Demographic and Fiscal Handbook* (Washington, DC, 1993); Richard C. Lane, Robert Kane, Rosalie Kane, and Wendy Nielson, *State LTC Profiles Report* (Minneapolis: National LTC Mentoring Program, Institute for Health Services Research, School of Public Health, University of Minnesota, November 1995); Colin Winterbottom, David Liska, and Karen Obermaier, *State-Level Databook on Health Care Access and Financing, Second Edition* (Washington, DC: The Urban Institute, 1995); The Kaiser Commission on the Future of Medicaid, *Medicaid Expenditures and Beneficiaries: National and State Profiles and Trends, 1984–1993* (Washington, DC, July 1995); Teresa Coughlin, Leighton Ku, and John Holohan, *Medicaid Since 1980: Costs, Coverage, and the Shifting Alliance Between the Federal Governments and the States* (Washington, DC, 1994).

113

Figure 7.1
Population Density of Kansas Counties, 1990

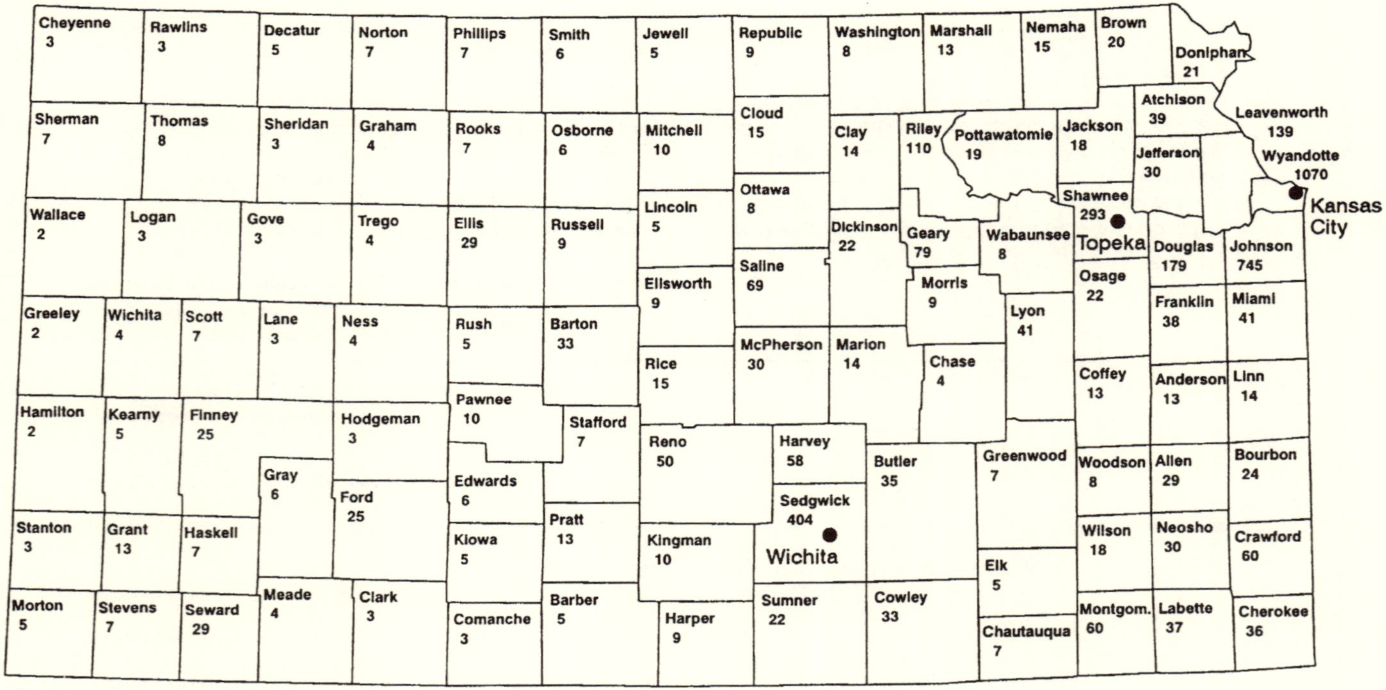

Figures are number of persons per square mile.
Source: Institute for Public Policy and Business Research, The University of Kansas; date from U.S. Bureau of the Census.

1861. Kansas is a fiscally conservative state, with tax burdens and spending levels which are lower than average, and lower than most other states in the region (see Table 7.1). Yet many Kansans consider the state to be socially responsive. The evidence, however, provides only partial support for this assessment, and Medicaid policy provides an example. Kansas has consistently offered more comprehensive coverage than required by federal law. Nonetheless, fiscal conservatism keeps the state's Medicaid generosity at or below average. For example, Table 7.1 reveals that Kansas Medicaid covers a smaller proportion of its poor population, relative to programs in neighboring states, and to the rest of the nation.

Since 1980, Kansas has made a number of careful incremental efforts to control Medicaid cost increases, including the establishment of more restrictive eligibility standards for certain segments of the population, such as AFDC recipients. Early reform efforts were hampered by an environment in which providers had little experience with managing patients and risk under a non-traditional reimbursement system. These problems were exacerbated by inadequate health data systems, which limited the state's ability to properly determine areas or populations with particular health care needs, and to subsequently evaluate the effectiveness of programs designed to serve them. More importantly, while legislators were willing to entertain alternative health care delivery methods with more ambitious cost control mechanisms, they were not prepared to radically alter the existing system, or to provide adequate resources for reform implementation.

More recently, Kansas has moved quickly to design and implement health delivery reforms for most segments of its Medicaid population throughout the state. Following the lead of other states, the state has built upon models developed elsewhere, flavored with adaptations to Kansas' unique needs, including its rural nature and aging population. Kansas' "wait and see" approach to Medicaid reform may allow the state to avoid some of the pitfalls associated with reforms enacted earlier in other parts of the nation.

THE BACKGROUND TO REFORM

Since 1967, Kansas health care for the poor has been driven largely by response to federal initiatives. Since that time, the state has adopted a largely reactive stance, responding to Medicaid federal policy initiatives, but pursuing relatively little in the way of state-originated reform. Over time, however, Kansas faced financing problems similar to those in other states, including increasing rates of Medicaid cost growth, which have caused the state to consider more proactive reform policies.

By the early 1980s, yearly Medicaid cost increases had reached a critical stage, prompting legislative action designed to contain costs. In 1984, the Kansas legislature reacted to early cost growth by requiring SRS to apply for a HCFA

Figure 7.2
Average Annual Growth in Medicaid Expenditures, 1988–1993

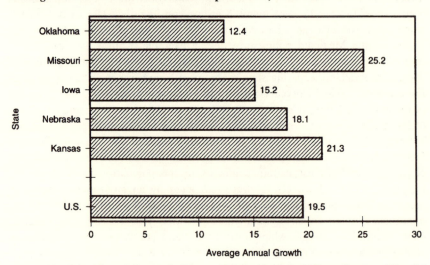

Source: The Kaiser Commission on the Future of Medicaid, *Medicaid Expenditures and Benefici-aries: National and State Profiles and Trends, 1984–1993,* Washington, D.C., July 1995.

Waiver which would permit operation of a modest Medicaid managed care pro-gram in a few selected counties. In addition, incremental reductions in the scope of services and eligibility standards for its Medi-Kan program (for General As-sistance (GA) recipients) were enacted. Although the legislature voted to abolish medical benefits for GA recipients, court challenges succeeded in protecting the program. Nonetheless, medical services are now provided to only a fraction of those GA recipients previously covered. These limited attempts to manage rising state health care costs were considered inadequate by the legislature, particularly in view of the fact that total federal and state Medicaid expenditures nearly doubled between 1985 and 1989.[4] Meanwhile, state leaders were increasingly aware of other states' experiments with mandatory comprehensive managed care programs for Medicaid populations, and with the high expectations associated with those programs.

In the early 1990s, program cost increases began to exceed growth in other state budget categories, with average annual expenditure growth exceeding 15% between 1988 and 1993. The cost growth occurred despite comparatively slow growth in beneficiary levels. During the same time period, average annual ben-eficiary growth averaged 7%, which was below the national average of 8%.[5] Figure 7.2 indicates that annual Medicaid cost growth in Kansas exceeded av-erage national growth, and the rates of growth in most neighboring states. More importantly, in 1990 and 1991, the state legislature was presented with requests

for supplemental SRS appropriations to meet program obligations. In each instance, the request exceeded $40 million, which represented over 20% of total
state general fund spending on medical assistance.[6]

In addition, the state failed to reap the large, controversial financial benefits
pursued by other states through disproportionate share hospital (DSH) payments
to hospitals serving large numbers of Medicaid recipients. In many other states,
DSH payments provided leverage to collect substantial levels of federal matching funds, especially between 1989 and 1992.[7] Kansas' initial failure to use the
questionable DSH payment system was at least partially intentional. One state
official suggested that "it just wouldn't be right" to engage in DSH activity,
thereby participating in what some now view as a violation of the spirit of
federal intent. However, Kansas *was* one of the first states to glean new federal
dollars through DSH payments to state mental health hospitals, beginning in
1991. As a result, joint federal-state spending on mental health inpatient care
increased in the state by over 250% between 1990 and 1992, with significant
net gains to the state. DSH payments were severely curtailed by Congress in
1991, a condition which created serious funding challenges for Kansas and other
states which had made extensive use of DSH payments. Nevertheless, a temporary provision in the new DSH law enabled Kansas to generate a temporary
DSH windfall.[8]

By 1994, frustrated by continued Medicaid cost growth and its perception of
inadequate action by SRS, and cut off from the lucrative federal match for DSH
payments which had existed for a few short years, the legislature mandated the
creation of a statewide managed care system, and imposed a firm implementation
schedule, starting July 1997.

BUREAUCRATIC FACTORS

In Kansas, social service programs are characterized by a centralized administrative structure, with Medicaid and most other public welfare functions operated by the Department of Social and Rehabilitation Services (SRS). County
responsibility for welfare functions ended in the mid-1970s. Most legislative
mandates concerning Medicaid reform have been directed to SRS, which has
administered the Medicaid program since its inception. These mandates have
provided significant design and implementation discretion to SRS. Although
state legislators wanted to generate the cost savings and other benefits associated
with managed care, and relied on SRS to design Medicaid reform from scratch,
they furnished few policy guidelines, and did not provide the resources required
to adequately equip the agency for this enormous task. SRS has been plagued
over the years by insufficient staffing levels, which have compromised the
agency's ability to adequately research Medicaid policy, including innovations
and programs in other states.

The agency has traditionally followed a "balkanized" structure, in which each of the five major SRS service functions (adult and medical; children and family; mental health and retardation; rehabilitation; and alcohol and drug abuse) operated with relative independence, and in relative isolation from one another. In light of this fragmented structure, which was tolerated and perhaps even encouraged by past SRS directors, coordination across service jurisdiction lines has posed continual challenges, especially for management of reform initiatives.

The structure of SRS has contributed to the absence of an effective advocacy for health care needs in the state. Until very recently, the state has lacked a strong, unified force dedicated to health needs among its poor. SRS has not worked closely with the Kansas Department of Health and Environment (KDHE) in the past; consequently, the fragmentation of health care administration has been extended across agencies as well as within SRS. There is no school of public health in the state. SRS has focused on social welfare issues, and has a working relationship with the University of Kansas' School of Social Welfare to help SRS staff in developing policy. Thus, the incorporation of health care into the state's social service strategy has muted SRS's role as an effective independent voice for health care issues.

More recently, SRS has worked hard to pursue a consensus strategy—both within the agency and with other Medicaid-related organizations—which has been fundamental to the Medicaid reform efforts. SRS has been careful to continue and strengthen the tradition of soliciting input from formal and informal citizen and professional advisory groups, and has worked to enhance its relationship with regional HCFA representatives. Consensus within the agency, and improved links to HCFA have been instrumental in enabling SRS to meet the Kansas legislature's Medicaid reform mandates. Furthermore, the current secretary of SRS is a former state legislator. The secretary's legislative experience, combined with her efforts to improve intra-agency coordination and external relations, have augmented the organization's capacity to design and adapt to new Medicaid systems.

PRIVATIZATION

One of the secretary's more visible social welfare initiatives concerns extensive privatization of existing SRS services. The term ''privatization'' appears frequently in press coverage of social welfare issues, and in the language used by SRS officials. At present, Kansas is engaged in developing contracts with private providers for foster care and adoption services currently provided by the state. SRS's Medicaid reforms also involve significant privatization activity. As a result of these efforts, significant portions of existing SRS staff were laid off. SRS shrunk not only because of anticipated contracts with private providers, but also because of some program transfers within state government. On July 1, 1997, program responsibility for Medicaid services for the elderly was transferred to the Kansas Department on Aging (KDOA). KDOA has designed and managed contracts with diverse private and nonprofit providers of direct health services for the elderly. KDOA and a number of the new contractual service providers have employed laid-off SRS employees. Consequently, many former SRS staff have continued to work with those clients and services for which they had responsibilities as SRS employees.

This strategy raises a number of issues, including the complications associated with monitoring state contracts with organizations employing significant numbers of former state employees. In addition, the limited number of available contract providers, particularly in rural areas, will pose additional challenges to those responsible for monitoring service contracts. The absence of adequate competition can seriously compromise the success of privatization efforts. In light of the current limited competitive environment in which Kansas health care providers function, and because of the inadequacy of provider supply in most areas of the state, this concern is particularly pertinent.[9]

PHYSICIAN SUPPLY ISSUES

Medicaid reform in Kansas has been hampered in part because the state has never been endowed with an oversupply of physicians, nor with an adequate distribution of those physicians among its population. Consequently, the competitive forces which foster more innovative forms of service delivery, and ultimately lower costs, are lacking. Fifty-four of the state's 105 counties have been identified as "critically underserved" with regard to primary care providers.[10] The distribution of both primary care and specialty physicians in the state is greatly skewed (see Table 7.2). Among the state's 105 counties, four urban counties account for 43% of the state's population. Fifty-seven percent of the state's licensed, nonresident primary care physicians practice in these four counties. This distribution, not surprisingly, is even more pronounced among specialists, with over 64% practicing in these largely urban enclaves of the state.

The result is that physicians are concentrated in very small geographic areas which serve a growing urban population. The distribution of physicians is complicated by Kansas' geographic expansiveness and its predominantly rural political base. This combination of factors has created a system which: discourages physician organization; forces communities and state policymakers to concentrate on recruitment and retention of physicians and other medical professionals in medically underserved areas of the state; encourages individual entrepreneurship among both primary and specialty physicians; and limits consumer choices, so that market-driven demand to generate new or different forms of healthcare delivery in many parts of the state is weak.

Without clear incentives or more immediate threats to their current status, physicians have been slow to position themselves to organize around a managed care agenda in Kansas. Accurately reflecting this constituency, the Kansas Medical Society has only recently organized a physician network (Heartland Health)

Table 7.2
Physician and Population Distribution in Kansas

	Johnson, Sedgwick, Wyandotte and Shawnee Counties*		Rest of State		Total
Population (%)	1.08 M	(43.7%)	1.4 M	(56.4%)	2.48 M
Licensed Primary Care Physicians (%)	891	(57.1%)	669	(42.9%)	1560
Ratio Population: Primary Care Physicians	1214:1		2086:1		1588:1
Specialists (%)	1517	(64.1%)	850	(35.9%)	2367
Ratio Population:Specialists	713:1		1642:1		1047:1
Total (%)	2408	(61.3%)	1519	(38.7%)	3927
Ratio Population:All Physicians	449:1		919:1		631:1

*These four counties contain the dominant metropolitan areas of the state: Wichita (Sedgwick), Topeka (Shawnee), and Kansas City (Wyandotte and Johnson).
Source: Kansas Licensing and Credentialing Boards, 1995 Renewals; U.S. Bureau of the Census, 1990.

to act as negotiating agent in managed care contracting within the state. The society has also expressed strong reservations about the prospect of monitoring physician performance at the state level, in the face of mounting evidence that such monitoring is crucial to effective state health reform. The Medicaid program, by slowly developing managed care programs based on clearly defined populations residing in portions of the state where physician supply is high, is attempting to redirect the policy discussion from that of physician autonomy to patient need; from access to services to quality and integration of care; from provider supply to consumer demand behavior. In effect, the individualistic nature of physician practice in Kansas has reinforced and encouraged the state's cautious, incremental approach toward Medicaid policy change.

REFORM IN A RURAL SETTING

Kansas Medicaid reforms have been shaped by its decentralized system of policy development, yet the reforms will operate through the state's centralized administrative structure. Experiences in other rural areas of the country suggest that centralized administrative models may hold limited potential for success. The evidence suggests that effective rural managed care programs should adopt strategies which permit maximum flexibility and promote local accountability, and which provide opportunities for local efforts to "develop solutions appropriate to local circumstances."[11] In Kansas, this has been partially reflected in nongovernmental, locally initiated endeavors to forge private provider systems in rural areas of the state. Private foundations, hospitals, and other providers have made incremental efforts to expand access to health care in sparsely populated areas, with some success. The Medicaid reforms, however, will require more fundamental changes in rural delivery systems. The state's new Peer Education and Resource Council (PERC), created to formalize program input from Medicaid providers and clients, may provide one method through which local needs can be accommodated. Nonetheless, the role of local needs and preferences in the reform implementation process is not clearly defined, although the effort to privatize services does provide one important potential method for local involvement.

The experience of rural New York State may offer some lessons for Kansas' reforms. New York's decentralized approach to disseminating managed care to rural areas of the state resulted in county innovations which surpassed the state's expectations, despite rural counties' lack of experience with managed care systems.[12] Such an option is not directly applicable to Kansas, primarily because counties in New York have always played a major role in social welfare service provision and financing, while Kansas has relied on a centralized administrative approach for over 20 years. Nonetheless, the flexibility afforded to local groups to adapt managed care to best meet local characteristics has been an important component of reform elsewhere, and Kansas could benefit from more systematic incorporation of these administrative methods into its own reform efforts. In fact, there is significant evidence that locally initiated health system integration efforts in Kansas have created models that the state could employ in advancing Medicaid managed care into rural areas.[13]

THE ROLE OF INFORMATION

Due primarily to influence from the private sector, and the leadership of a few members active in health issues at the national level, the Kansas legislature has come to realize the importance of data in order to sustain Medicaid health reform. Educating policymakers to recognize the uses of health information has been a slow and incremental process. Considerable study of experiences in other states has preceded this change. Although the use of health data in Kansas has traditionally centered around public health monitoring and resource allocation, much of the momentum tied to more recent reform has been driven by the private sector, a point which legislators have used to enhance the overall credibility of the issue. As in other states, Medicaid cost growth in Kansas has occurred in tandem with rising overall health care costs in the state. Health care cost inflation has led to a mutual interest on the part of many large Kansas employers to seek more information about how their benefits payments are being spent. The term ''value'' has frequently been used as a catch-all term for quality, cost, and overall satisfaction with health care delivery on the part of purchasers of health care in Kansas.[14] The Medicaid program has been a largely silent, though willing recipient of the products of this effort, and has benefited from the resulting private-public consensus on the usefulness of statewide service-based data to promote more efficient health care for Kansas residents.

This private sector recognition of the usefulness of data was expressed through public representation in 1990, when the legislature instructed the Kansas Insurance Department to develop a statistical plan for reporting, compiling, and analyzing accident and sickness insurance premium, loss, and expense data. As has been the experience in a number of states, however, Kansas' delegation of this role to a single state agency with limited guidelines and budget has had minimal initial impact.[15] Undaunted, the legislature significantly expanded this charge in 1993 with the establishment of a Health Care Data Governing Board to assist in the maintenance of a comprehensive health care database for the state. The Board's mission is to ''promote the availability of and access to health care data, to provide leadership in health information management and analysis, and to provide guidance in use of the data for policymakers, program managers and citizens to make informed health care decisions.'' In the year following creation of the Board, the legislature designated the state's Department of Health and Environment (KDHE) as the state agency responsible for analyzing data collected through its authority. The legislature intended that the Department would identify factors driving the cost of health insurance throughout the state.

However, attributing causal influences to explain cost increases was a major refinement of the original legislative intent. The state has begun to realize the potential management uses of data beyond monitoring and statistical reporting.

The private-public nature of this initiative extended to funding, with insurance companies, group self-funded pools, health maintenance organizations, and other large purchasers of health services required to pay annual fees based on premium volume, to cover the expenses of collecting and analyzing the information. Consultants working with both the Department of Insurance and the KDHE have advanced this effort still further in both 1994 and 1996, so that at present, detailed reporting specifications exist which will allow state agencies to collect data to monitor both premium levels and health performance indicators in ways which can benefit all consumers of health services in the state. Since 24% of all health services in Kansas are paid for through the state's Medicaid program, the imminent distribution of performance monitoring reports should prove extremely useful to program administrators, and should enhance their incorporation of improved data into their management and policy decisions.

Additional nongovernmental efforts to strengthen information processing include the establishment of the Kansas Health Institute. In 1994, the Institute was created and funded by the Kansas Health Foundation, a major grant-making and philanthropic organization based in Wichita. The Institute has a public health mission consistent with advancing health information and research that will be used to affect policies leading to improved health for all Kansans. It has begun to facilitate and coordinate the use of data in formats which can be used for policy development. The Kansas Health Institute provides an additional example of a system in which the state government will benefit from private initiatives. Because of the Institute, the Medicaid program stands to gain a better understanding of its covered populations and their needs. The state could therefore coordinate systematic Medicaid service delivery revisions with private and public data initiatives. It is unclear whether this will occur.

THE STRUCTURE OF MEDICAID REFORM IN KANSAS

The SRS privatization efforts are a prominent feature of Kansas' Medicaid reforms. Kansas' use of contractual arrangements for providing enhanced Medicaid services follows a well-established practice in the managed care programs nationwide. In Kansas, portions of this model have been incorporated into reforms for the long-term care component of Medicaid as well. Thus, Kansas reform efforts directed at families with children, and at the elderly and disabled, rely heavily on nongovernmental providers of case management and health related services.

Families and Children

Kansas has a lower-than-average child poverty rate. In 1992, 14% of Kansas children aged 18 and under lived in poverty, compared to a nationwide average of 18% (see Table 7.1).[16] Although Kansas' Medicaid program has typically exceeded federal requirements for benefits to families and children, Table 7.1 indicates that its coverage policies are less generous than those of most other states, including some of the neighboring plains states. The relative generosity of Kansas' Medicaid program is indicated by the following characteristics: (1) when OBRA 1987 permitted extension of benefits to pregnant women and infants with incomes up to 185% of the federal poverty level, Kansas opted to expand benefits, but selected a cut-off level set at 150% of the poverty level,[17] while nearly half of all other states used the more generous 185% of poverty Medicaid eligibility level; (2) one report ranks Kansas among the bottom ten states with regard to its "aggressiveness" in implementing expansions for pregnant women;[18] (3) in Kansas, Medicaid covers smaller proportions of the poor population than in most other states, and in most of its neighbor states.

The Kansas legislature has authorized an accelerated phase-in of other federally required expansions for children. Although federal guidelines (under OBRA 1990) currently require coverage of 14-year-olds under 100% of the federal poverty level, Kansas covers children in this category up to age 16, and coverage expansions in the state will remain two years ahead of the federal timeline. In addition, Kansas has historically included an optional, federally matched Medicaid program for the "medically needy" and has provided most optional services beyond the basic federally required group of Medicaid services. Furthermore, Kansas has provided Medicaid services to more of its AFDC population than most other states. Table 7.1 indicates that the Kansas AFDC eligibility level, through which most families qualify for Medicaid, equaled 44% of the federal poverty level in 1995. By comparison, the national average AFDC eligibility level in 1995 was slightly higher, and 26 states used less generous levels, relative to Kansas.[19] Nonetheless, the evidence suggests that compared to most other states, Kansas still lags behind with regard to extending coverage to greater numbers of poor pregnant women and children.

In the mid-1980s, Kansas began to experiment with nontraditional (i.e., other than fee-for-service) models of health care delivery for its Medicaid population. A primary care case-management (PCCM) pilot program, called PrimeCare Network (PCN), was implemented in 1984 in a few selected counties.[20] PCN appeared relatively early on the national managed care scene, but was very limited in geographic scope, and in its capacity to meet the demands of successful managed care.[21] PCN was a mandatory program, requiring enrollment of all eligible Medicaid recipients in its service area. From its inception, the program was plagued by inadequate provider supply in selected portions of the service area. Providers were reluctant to serve Medicaid recipients, and state efforts to recruit additional providers were frequently unsuccessful. The state was often unable to assign Medicaid recipients to providers, despite its requirement that recipients participate in PCN. Consequently, from the legislature's perspective, PCN failed to generate adequate cost savings. Although the underlying PCCM model is still used by the state, the seven-county PCN experiment has been judged as unsuccessful.

Kansas' initial adoption of the PCCM model reflected the state's cautious approach to alternative delivery models for Medicaid. However, evidence from other state efforts indicates that this venture was probably quite prudent. For example, Hurley, Freund, and Paul argue that evaluations of early Medicaid managed care programs confirm an important and significant role for programs such as PCN.[22] They concluded that in many states, cost savings in such programs was significant. Furthermore, they caution that more recent restrictive managed care models, such as capitated plans, are often confronted by skepticism and reluctance from Medicaid beneficiaries, and from health care providers. In fact, Hurley et al. suggest that PCCM plans may have had the potential to generate greater aggregate savings than capitated models, particularly in early nonmandatory Medicaid managed care programs.[23]

Kansas' inability to effect more significant cost savings through PCN is most likely due to a number of factors, including the following three: First, provider dynamics within the state, including relatively low competition among physicians; second, the state's inability and/or unwillingness to sufficiently promote the program among providers, and to more aggressively recruit providers (this reflected the traditional state disinclination to extend government into the domain of the private sector, including private practice physicians); third, inadequate provider incentives for participation (case management fees were set at $3 per Medicaid recipient). Thus, despite the potential success of PCCM models, the PCN version was saddled with a variety of liabilities which compromised its ability to effectively ''manage'' care for Medicaid recipients.

However, a new and revised PCCM program, called Health Connect, now forms the foundation for part of the statewide managed care system mandated by the legislature. One important difference between Health Connect and its predecessor, PCN, is the inclusion of nonphysicians as primary care providers. This component of Health Connect is crucial, in light of inadequate physician supply in many rural portions of the state. In addition, the state has incorporated new incentives to recruit adequate numbers of providers, with significant success. Thus, the Health Connect version of the PCCM model appears to offer greater potential for enhanced services and for cost savings. There is also evidence that national managed care trends, which have altered provider perceptions of managed care, have influenced those Kansas providers who were previously disinclined to participate in PCN. Within Kansas, private employer pressure on health insurers to reduce premium costs has induced increased provider participation in private managed care plans. Consequently, changes in the private sector have encouraged physician participation in the new alternative Medicaid delivery systems.

Health Connect has been extended to other parts of the state in a fairly short time frame. Since July 1995, Health Connect has been providing Medicaid managed care through a pilot program in two rural western counties. However, on

July 1, 1997, the program was implemented in the remaining 95 counties, by legislative mandate. Patient education, which is often problematic in managed care programs, was provided after November 1, 1996, by contract with Blue Cross/Blue Shield of Kansas, the state's new Medicaid fiscal agent. This transition could pose some temporary challenges, as the previous fiscal agent administered the state contract for fifteen years. With state oversight, Blue Cross/Blue Shield will be responsible for some components of program monitoring, administration of the Medicaid Management Information System (MMIS), collection of provider encounter data, and review of consumer complaints.[24]

For the most part, capitated managed care is a very new phenomenon in the Kansas Medicaid program. Unlike Minnesota and other states with well-established HMO providers, health care in Kansas has had only modest experience with HMOs.[25] Although the state has not been inclined to adopt capitation until recently, it is now moving very quickly. A capitated managed care plan was implemented in early 1996 in most urban areas of the state. Known as PrimeCare Kansas, this program contracts with licensed HMOs to provide case management, inpatient, and primary care for AFDC recipients and for pregnant women and children eligible through the Medicaid expansions (Poverty Level Eligible, or PLE). Although PrimeCare Kansas was implemented in late 1995 in Wyandotte County (which includes Kansas City, Kansas), most implementation activity took place between January and April 1996. During that period, PrimeCare Kansas went "on-line" in Johnson and Leavenworth counties, both of which include Kansas City suburbs and fringe areas, and Douglas and Shawnee (Topeka) counties, which are also located in the northeastern portion of the state.

In each PrimeCare county, the implementation of Health Connect is complete. In these counties, Medicaid recipients are required to enroll in a managed care plan, but they can choose either a PCCM or a capitated plan. However, Medicaid-eligible SSI recipients and GA populations eligible for medical assistance are restricted to the Health Connect plan. The new system incorporates incentives for AFDC and PLE families to select PrimeCare Kansas (the capitated plan) over Health Connect. The Health Connect option requires modest service co-payments, and provides a less comprehensive service package, compared to PrimeCare Kansas.

The one urban center not currently included in PrimeCare Kansas is Wichita. Instead, a separate waiver is currently under consideration for a unique capitated plan in this area. Known as Community Care of Kansas, this capitated model would serve the AFDC and PLE populations. Community Care of Kansas is a privately initiated proposal, submitted to the state by Wichita-area hospitals, the area medical society, and existing social service agencies. Community Care of Kansas, if implemented, would provide more comprehensive benefits than those currently provided by PrimeCare Kansas, including mental health services, and the plan would extend coverage to greater proportions of poor children. Another distinctive feature of Community Care of Kansas is that it would consist of a

Medicaid-only program. By comparison, PrimeCare Kansas contracts with existing HMOs which also serve other health consumers. At present, negotiations continue between the proposed Community Care of Kansas providers, the state, and HCFA. The anticipated implementation date of January 1996 was not met. Current negotiations focus on the state-provider contract; potential Community Care of Kansas providers have asked the state to reconsider their originally proposed contract terms. If these negotiations fail, the state anticipates extension of PrimeCare Kansas coverage to Wichita-area Medicaid recipients.

The July 1997 legislative deadline has established a statewide system of mandatory managed care for all nonelderly Kansas AFDC, SSI, and GA recipients (see Figure 7.3). For the foreseeable future, the Kansas managed care program will consist primarily of the PCCM model, which deviates least from traditional fee-for-service delivery. Capitated managed care will operate primarily in the state's few urban areas. However, as private HMOs become more firmly established in nonurban portions of the state, Kansas is likely to undertake efforts to extend capitated Medicaid managed care into as many locations as feasible. One HMO currently providing services through PrimeCare Kansas has expressed an interest in extending services into rural areas.

The Kansas legislature's managed care implementation mandates are indicative of the state's recent lack of patience with Medicaid cost growth, but they also reflect Kansas' desire to maintain, and possibly enhance medical services for its poor. It is likely that the state could now embark on a relatively rapid effort to extend capitated models throughout the state. Until now, Kansas' careful consideration regarding capitated plans has provided the state with opportunities to take advantage of HMO refinements and improvements undertaken elsewhere. For example, SRS officials emphasize that their contract negotiations with HMOs were greatly facilitated by information about experiences in other states. In light of recent complaints about HMOs by both enrollees *and* HMO health care providers nationwide, Kansas' inclination to extend HMO-style managed care into rural areas deserves careful scrutiny.[26]

The Elderly

Kansas' population is relatively elderly. Nonetheless, until recently, the state has failed to successfully adapt its Medicaid program to better address the needs of the elderly, and to incorporate cost savings methods which are well established in other states. The task of reforming Medicaid for the elderly is complicated by the fact that Kansas has 87.5 nursing home beds per 1,000 population—more than any other state—compared to a national average of 54 (see Table 7.1). Note that the other plains states also have high numbers of nursing home beds per capita. In addition, there is a high likelihood that elderly population growth will place Kansas at the top of the list of states most in need of innovative and effective long-term care services.

Unfortunately, a recent report ranks Kansas 38th in the nation with regard to progress toward a less costly Home and Community-Based Services (HCBS)

Figure 7.3
Medicaid Managed Care in Kansas, June 1996

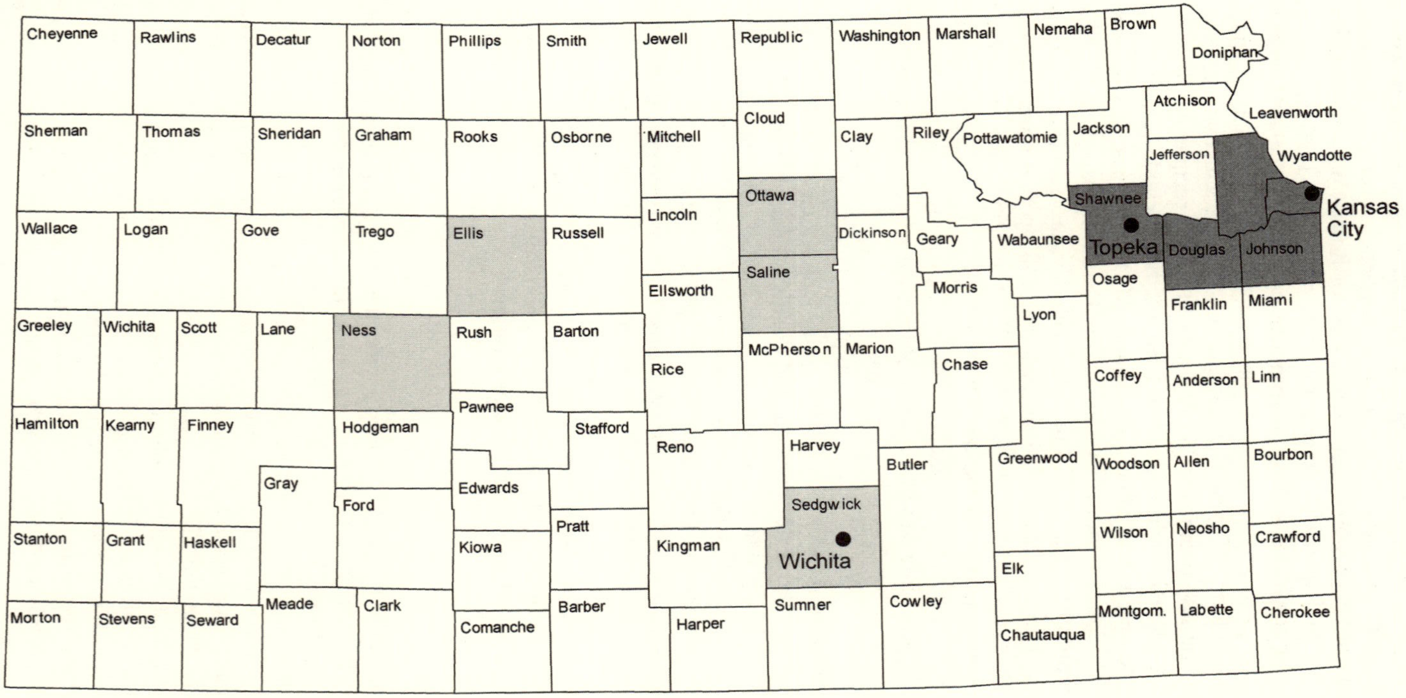

Source: Kansas Department of Social and Rehabilitation Services.

KEY

Primary Care Case Management
(Health Connect) Only

Capitated HMO (PrimeCare Kansas) and
Primary Care Case Management (Health Connect)
Available

system of long-term care for its elderly. Table 7.1 indicates a number of factors which led to this ranking, including the following: Kansas has more of its population aged 65+ living in nursing facilities (NFs) than all but two other states; the average functioning level of these residents is quite high, indicating that costly institutional care is probably unnecessary for a large portion of current NF residents;[27] despite the fact that Kansas' per diem NF costs are below average, the state doubled its expenditures on NFs between 1985 and 1989;[28] traditionally, more of Kansas' total Medicaid funds have been devoted to long-term care than average (40% of total Medicaid spending, compared to a nationwide state average of 35% in 1993);[29] and most importantly, Kansas has spent far less of its Medicaid long-term care funds on HCBS than average (6%, compared to a nationwide average of 13%).[30]

The state has addressed these issues with a new initiative directed toward its Medicaid elderly. The Living Independence for Everyone (LIFE) program, authorized through a HCFA Waiver, was implemented in January 1997. LIFE relies on a uniform, aggressive case-management system to identify those Medicaid recipients at risk of institutionalization, and it incorporates a comprehensive package of home and community-based services for this population, reserving NF care for those unable to remain in their homes.[31]

From the state's perspective, privatization is a vital component of LIFE. All direct care services for the Medicaid elderly, and all case management services for this population, were privatized effective January 1, 1997. The case management functions have been assigned to contracts with Area Agencies on Aging (AAAs), which are non-profit organizations currently providing a number of services to the elderly.[32] Direct care services such as home health care are now provided by a variety of private contractors. SRS caseworkers and direct care employees previously assigned to the Medicaid elderly have been laid off. Many of those laid off have been employed by new contractual providers, and some have transferred to KDOA. On July 1, 1997, administrative responsibility for Medicaid services for the elderly was transferred from SRS to KDOA. KDOA will reimburse the AAAs for case management services on an hourly basis, and LIFE's direct care service contractors will be reimbursed according to a fee schedule.

The transition from the current system to LIFE has the potential to drive many nursing homes out of business. In order to minimize such dislocation, the state is presently encouraging nursing homes to diversify their services, and to submit bids for contracts with the AAAs to provide nonresidential LIFE services for the elderly. Although Kansas has more licensed home health agencies than most other states, they are concentrated in the urban areas of the state. Inadequate supply of LIFE providers in the more sparsely populated areas of the state is a concern. However, SRS has been encouraged by numerous contacts from registered nurses in rural areas interested in establishing home health agencies to provide LIFE nonresidential direct services.

SRS officials recognize that cost containment is an important objective of the

new LIFE initiative, but they emphasize that LIFE will also respond to preferences expressed by the elderly Kansas population. The desire of elders to remain
in homes and in the community is a key preference. Therefore, LIFE attempts
to meet the dual objectives of providing solutions to satisfy elderly consumer
preferences, and reducing state Medicaid costs for elderly enrollees.

The Disabled

Kansas SSI recipients eligible for Medicaid services will be enrolled in a
program similar to LIFE, upon HCFA approval of a proposed waiver. Modeled
on a New Hampshire program, the new program, to be administered by SRS,
emphasizes home and community-based services (HCBS) for the physically disabled, and offers a number of services suggested by a task force assembled to
advise SRS in its formulation of the waiver application.[33] The range and selection of services to be provided for each recipient will be determined by an
Independent Living Counselor (case manager), but the determination will be
made with significant recipient input. All services, including case management,
will be furnished through contracts with private providers. SRS officials imple-
mentated this new program in early 1997.

Kansas has been less inclined to undertake major reforms for Medicaid mental
health patients. However, the state has altered its approach to mental health
treatment. Large institutions in which mental patients have often been treated
will be reduced in number. The locus of care has been shifted to local (county
and regional) community mental health agencies. Kansas' caution in the area of
Medicaid mental health is not surprising; in other states, this component of
health care has typically been addressed only when general acute and long-term
care issues have been resolved. The shift from large institutional treatment to
local mental health facilities may provide an opportunity for the state to use the
new delivery system to offer case-management options for its Medicaid mental
health patients. Thus far, however, the state's Medicaid reform efforts have
excluded services for mental health patients, which suggests that the state is not
yet prepared to include all health services in its reform, and is susceptible to
"carve out" pressure from special interests which stand to lose funding under
a managed care system. Meanwhile, the state is in the early stages of discussion
concerning reforms for other Medicaid-related needs, including those of foster
children, and alcohol and drug abuse patients.

CONCLUSION

Medicaid reform in Kansas has been characterized by both cautious observation and incorporation of reforms tried in other states. In its pursuit of contained Medicaid costs and adequate levels of services, Kansas has followed the
lead established not only by other states, but also by private sector health care
delivery and information management initiatives within the state. The legislature

has relied heavily on the state's Department of Social and Rehabilitative Services (SRS) to achieve reform objectives, but has been reluctant to provide adequate policy direction or resources for this purpose. The agency is now moving forward quickly, due in part to recently enacted legislative implementation deadlines, and is building its Medicaid reforms on a foundation of privatized service delivery for most of its Medicaid population. The state's tradition of decentralized social policy development, combined with its centralized administrative model, will pose challenges to the implementation process. However, the reforms will benefit from recent changes in the views of health care providers with regard to managed care, and from the growth of capitated, HMO styles of health care delivery in the private sector.

Most recently, Kansans have questioned the effectiveness of an incremental approach to Medicaid reform. The state has reached a critical point, and has become uncharacteristically aggressive in changing the Medicaid health service delivery system. Medicaid cost pressures have prompted the state to embrace the broad, forceful reforms undertaken in other states in an effort to assert greater fiscal control while maintaining service levels.

Much of the reform process has been shaped by the combined values of fiscal conservatism and social equity which drive state policy decisions. Kansas may very well provide a useful example of the benefits associated with restraint in the midst of fundamental change. In the context of Medicaid, Kansas has been watching and waiting until very recently, and Kansans may be better off as a result.

NOTES

We wish to thank Laura Poracsky for preparing the maps included in this chapter.

1. The American Association of Retired Persons, *The State Economic, Demographic & Fiscal Handbook* (Washington, D.C.,) 199; and Raymond G. Davis, "Public Health Policy: Perplexing Problems and Proximate Policies," in H. George Frederickson, ed., *Public Policy and the Two States of Kansas* (Lawrence: University of Kansas Press, 1994). See also Richard C. Ladd, Robert Kane, Rosalie Kane, and Wendy Nielson, *State LTC Profiles Report* (Minneapolis: National LTC Mentoring Program, Institute for Health Services Research, School of Public Health, University of Minnesota, November 1995).

2. Although Kansas is the 15th largest state, geographically, it is the 32nd largest in terms of population.

3. Thelma Helyar, ed., *Kansas Statistical Abstract, 1992–1993* (Lawrence: The University of Kansas, Institute for Public Policy and Business Research).

4. See Davis, "Public Health Policy," p. 69.

5. The Kaiser Commission on the Future of Medicaid, *Medicaid Expenditures and Beneficiaries: National and State Profiles and Trends, 1984–1993* (Washington, D.C., July 1995).

6. See Davis, "Public Health Policy," p. 72. Between 1986 and 1990, Medicaid spending as a share of Kansas personal state income grew by 45%, relative to a national average of 27%. See Victor J. Miller, "State Medicaid Expansion in the Early 1990s:

Program Growth in a Period of Fiscal Stress,'' in Diane Rowland, Judith Feder, and Alina Salganicoff, eds., *Medicaid Financing Crisis: Balancing Responsibilities, Priorities, and Dollars* (Washington, D.C.: American Association for the Advancement of Science, 1993).

7. For a comprehensive discussion of DSH payments, see Rowland, Feder, and Salganicoff, *Medicaid Financing Crisis*; and Leighton Ku and Teresa Coughlin, ''Medicaid Disproportionate Share and Other Special Financing Programs: A Fiscal Dilemma for States and the Federal Government,'' prepared for The Kaiser Commission on the Future of Medicaid, Washington, D.C., December 1994.

8. One of the more controversial components of the DSH story in Kansas is the fact that some of the revenue windfall was used to provide one-time funding to state higher education capital projects, which struck some professionals in the mental health field as inappropriate use of funds. In fairness, the decision to use the funds in this way may have been required by the one time nature of the DSH windfall.

9. For a discussion of privatization issues related to social services, see Donald F. Kettl, *Sharing Power: Public Governance and Private Markets* (Washington, D.C.: The Brookings Institution, 1993).

10. Kansas Department of Health and Environment, Bureau of Local and Rural Health Systems, *Primary Care Underserved Areas Report*, Topeka, Kansas, 1996.

11. See Jon Christianson and Ira Moscovice, ''Health Care Reform: Issues for Rural Areas,'' Sheps Center for Health Policy Research, University of North Carolina at Chapel Hill, 1996; and Andy Coburn et al., ''The Rural Perspective on National Health Reform Legislation: Addressing the Critical Rural Issues,'' prepared for the Congressional Rural Caucus and the House Rural Health Care Coalition, Rural Policy Research Institute, Columbia, Missouri, 1994.

12. See Mary K. Bliss et al., ''Adapting Managed Care to Rural Delivery Systems: A Decentralized Approach to Medicaid Reform,'' Rural Health Research Center working paper series, Working Paper #9, New York Rural Research Center, State University of New York, Buffalo, February 1996.

13. One such system, Med-Op, headquartered in Oakley, Kansas, offers such a model.

14. Reforming State's Group. Proceedings of Conference: ''Public and Private Collaboration on Health Information Policy.'' Sponsored by Milbank Memorial Fund, Topeka, Kansas, March 8, 1996.

15. Intergovernmental Health Policy Project, ''The Death of a Data Commission: A Cautionary Tale from Colorado,'' *State Health Notes* 16, no. 21 (September 4, 1995).

16. See Colin Winterbottom, David Liska, and Karen Obermaier, *State-Level Databook on Health Care Access and Financing*, 2nd ed. (Washington, D.C.: The Urban Institute, 1995).

17. Twenty-three other states had opted to use the more generous 185% level. See Congressional Research Service, *Medicaid Source Book: Background Data and Analysis (A 1993 Update)* (Washington, D.C.: U.S. Government Printing Office, 1993). Prior to the expansions, federal law required coverage only for AFDC recipients.

18. See Rachel Benson Gold, Susheela Singh, and Jennifer Frost, ''The Medicaid Eligibility Expansions for Pregnant Women: Evaluating the Strength of State Implementation Efforts,'' *Family Planning Perspectives* 25 (1993): 196–207; and Sara Rosenbaum, ''Medicaid Expansions and Access to Health Care,'' in Rowland, Feder, and Salganicoff, *Medicaid Financing Crisis*.

19. See Gold, Singh, and Frost, ''The Medicaid Eligibility Expansions for Pregnant

Women,'' 196–207; and Rosenbaum, ''Medicaid Expansions and Access to Health Care.''

20. Primary care case management models pay managing providers, or ''gatekeeper'' physicians, a case management fee, and reimburse through fee-for-service methods for services rendered to Medicaid recipients. For a detailed description, see Robert Hurley, Deborah Freund, and John Paul, *Managed Care in Medicaid: Lessons for Policy and Program Design* (Ann Arbor, Mich.: Health Administration Press, 1993).

21. Primary Care Network was operational in seven counties, each of which had a major population center. By 1993, approximately 52,000 enrollees, roughly 21% of the total Medicaid population, participated in PCN. See The Kaiser Commission, *Health Needs and Medicaid Financing: State Facts*; and also The Kaiser Commission on the Future of Medicaid, *Policy Brief: Medicaid and Managed Care* (Washington, D.C., April 1995).

22. See Hurley, Freund, and Paul, *Managed Care in Medicaid: Lessons for Policy and Program Design.*

23. For a description of a more recent successful PCCM initiative in Maryland, see Paul Valentine, ''Health Plan Saved Maryland $21 Million,'' *Washington Post* (November 18, 1994).

24. In addition to its role as the state's Medicaid fiscal agent, Blue Cross/Blue Shield of Kansas will provide direct Medicaid services through a number of its existing HMOs. This situation poses a potential conflict of interest, and could present difficulties for the state in terms of contract monitoring and management.

25. In 1990, Kansas general health HMO membership per 1,000 population was 80.7, compared to a nationwide average of 151.4. At that time, there were only eight established HMOs in Kansas, and all were in the eastern section of the state. See Pamela Loprest and Michael Gates, *State-Level Databook on Health Care Access and Financing* (Washington, D.C.: The Urban Institute, 1993).

26. See, for example, Milt Freudenheim, ''HMOs Cope with a Backlash on Cost Cutting,'' *New York Times* (May 19, 1996).

27. Ladd et al., *State LTC Profiles Report.*

28. Ibid.

29. Winterbottom et al., *State-Level Databook.*

30. Ladd et al., *State LTC Profiles Report*; and Teresa Coughlin, Leighton Ku, and John Holohan, *Medicaid Since 1980: Costs, Coverage, and the Shifting Alliance Between the Federal Governments and the States* (Washington, D.C.: The Urban Institute, 1994). Kansas ranks 42nd out of the 52 states in terms of the proportion of its long-term care Medicaid expenditures devoted to home and community-based health services.

31. LIFE services include wellness monitoring, adult day care, adult day treatment, medical attendant care, nonmedical attendant care, respite care, medical alert devices, and residential personal care.

32. The Area Agencies on Aging rely on a diverse set of state and federal funds at present, including funding under the federal Older Americans Act. Although the rhetoric associated with the use of ''privatization'' in the state suggests extensive transfer of program functions to the private sector, it appears that for the elderly, the bulk of this transfer will accrue to nonprofits, many of which have been providing similar or supplemental services. Thus, the use of the term ''privatization'' may be inaccurate—a better

description might focus on the state's divestiture of the direct service function. In any event, from a political perspective, one of the largest state bureaucracies will have been significantly diminished, at least in size.

33. The services include personal and assistive services for the physically disabled.

8

Managed Care or Managed Politics? Medicaid Reforms in Maryland

THOMAS R. OLIVER AND KAREN ANDERSON OLIVER

INTRODUCTION

As midnight approached on April 8, 1996, the last day of the legislative session, the Maryland General Assembly took its final actions for the year. By a unanimous vote in both houses, the conference committee report on Senate Bill 750 was enacted into law. With the signature of Governor Parris Glendening, Maryland joined the growing number of states planning major expansions of managed care in their Medicaid programs.

The new legislation authorized the Secretary of Health and Mental Hygiene to create a "research and demonstration" project under Section 1115 of the Social Security Act.[1] The Department of Health and Mental Hygiene (DHMH) promptly came forward with its Medicaid demonstration proposal to the federal Health Care Financing Administration (HCFA) on May 3, 1996, and HCFA gave its final approval on October 30, 1996. The new program, called HealthChoice, began in June 1997 and will ultimately enroll about 80% of the Medicaid population in capitated managed care organizations.[2]

In this chapter, we describe the recent evolution of the Maryland Medicaid program and the logic of the policy designs put forward by state officials. The 1996 initiative builds on a rapidly developing track record in managed care in the state as a whole and for Medicaid in particular. It culminates a series of initiatives in the last five years to transfer the organizational and financial features of managed care from the private sector to the public sector. We also examine the fiscal pressures and changes in federal and state political leadership that led to stronger and broader efforts to slow the growth of spending in the Medicaid program. The unanimous support for the 1996 legislation reflected a broad consensus that an expansion of managed care is appropriate for Medicaid, but the superficial unanimity can obscure the contentious politics of managed care within the Maryland health policy community. It is likely that without compelling external forces and considerable commitment from political leaders, legislators would have deferred action on the major reform package at least one year and possibly longer. We identify several areas in which policymakers attempted to accommodate special interests and the considerable sources of tension remaining as implementation proceeds. Finally, we explore the implications of these reforms for the performance of the Medicaid program in Maryland and in other states.

THE MARYLAND ECONOMY AND MEDICAID GROWTH

The primary factor driving the Maryland Medicaid program toward managed care was an extended budget crisis during the early 1990s. Maryland was one of the states hit hardest by the national recession at the beginning of the decade. As Cold War levels of federal defense spending declined and its construction and service industries suffered setbacks, the state lost 109,600 jobs from 1990 to 1992, equivalent to 5% of its workforce. The economic slide caused both slower growth of state revenues and increased growth in state spending.[3]

This period was a dramatic reversal from the state's economy during the 1980s. During fiscal years 1981–1990, general revenues rose by an average of 8.7% annually. This growth rate dropped to 3.5% during fiscal years 1991–1993, even after transfers from the state revenue stabilization fund (from previous budget surpluses) and increases in income and sales taxes.[4]

In a span of less than three years, Governor William Schaefer (D) and legislators struggled through seven rounds of cost containment to balance the state budget during regular and special sessions of the General Assembly. The Medicaid program helped to bring about that struggle and, not surprisingly, it became a prime target of the effort to bring state spending into alignment with lower than projected revenues.[5]

The proximate problem was the rapidly increasing size of the Medicaid program in recent years. The Maryland Department of Fiscal Services reported that a major factor in the general fiscal crisis from 1991–1993 was unanticipated growth in entitlements, specifically the number of state residents eligible for public assistance and Medicaid.[6] Statewide program enrollment was fairly steady during the late 1980s at about 340,000. But in 1991, the economic recession led to a substantial increase in enrollment and there was no decline as the economy improved. (Some of this increase was due to expanded eligibility for women and children under federal legislation in the 1980s.) By fiscal year 1994, the average monthly enrollment in the Maryland Medicaid program was 443,908, or about 9% of the state's population. The pattern of enrollment indicated wide economic and geographic disparities throughout the state, as the average enrollment rate ranged from 2.9% of the population in Howard County to 25.6% in Baltimore City.[7]

The combination of rising enrollment and general health care inflation led to a doubling of the Medicaid budget between 1989 and 1994.[8] The fiscal year 1994 budget was $2.02 billion, the largest single expenditure of state government (about half was paid by the federal government). In Maryland and many other states, Medicaid reform has become a leading example of what Jack Walker referred to as "problemistic innovation," part of the governmental agenda driven by frequently recurring problems. The tremendous growth in the Medicaid program has made its goals and performance almost permanent issues on the state agenda.[9] Increasingly, Medicaid, like entitlement programs at the federal level, is dealt with as a fiscal issue rather than a health issue.[10] Indeed, it may be that perceived budgetary crises are the only predictable opportunities for health care reform; and that cost containment is the dominant and only certain goal of reform.

MEDICAID MANAGED CARE INITIATIVES

Managed care was well underway in the state of Maryland and in its Medicaid program before the most recent reforms. As of 1994, 1.8 million people in Maryland, or 36% of state residents, were enrolled in HMOs. This proportion of HMO enrollment was third highest in the nation, only slightly behind California and Oregon. The state Medicaid program had contracted with HMOs for 20 years, primarily in Baltimore City. Between 1988 and 1995, an HMO option became available statewide and enrollment increased nearly fourfold. By late 1995, over 126,000 beneficiaries had voluntarily elected to obtain their Medicaid coverage through HMOs.[11] Capitation payments to HMOs in fiscal year 1993 totalled approximately $192 million, or 9.1% of all Medicaid spending, though close to 20% of program beneficiaries enrolled in HMOs. Overall Medicaid payments to HMOs more than tripled in the four years from 1990 to 1994.[12]

The trends in HMO participation suggest that continuing growth of managed care was inevitable in the Maryland Medicaid program. The combination of higher voluntary HMO enrollment and program initiatives in the early 1990s increased the technical and political feasibility of the current plan to institute mandatory managed care for Medicaid patients. The sections below will briefly describe the first initiative and then analyze why and how Maryland devised more complex approaches to manage its Medicaid services and budget. The key steps toward a comprehensive managed care program are summarized in Figure 8.1.

THE MARYLAND ACCESS TO CARE PROGRAM (1991)

The first responses of state officials ordered to reduce Medicaid spending were to cut back eligibility to the minimum required by federal law, eliminate coverage of some services, and reduce payments to some providers.[13] Further re-

Figure 8.1
Key Activities in the Maryland Medicaid Reform Process

Winter and Spring 1994
· Pilot study of high risk patient management under grant from the Robert Wood Johnson Foundation

· Development of Department of Health and Mental Hygiene budget proposal for the High Cost User Initiative under Secretary Nelson Sabatini

· Approval of High Cost User Initiative by Maryland General Assembly in Governor William Schaefer's final budget bill

Summer 1994
· Creation of the Center for Health Program Development and Management at the University of Maryland Baltimore County

· Submission of Section 1115 Waiver proposal for High Cost User Initiative to the Health Care Financing Administration (HFCA)

Fall 1994
· Development of proposed regulations for implementation of Integrated Care Management Systems

· Election of Governor Parris Glendening

· Republican majorities elected to U.S. Senate and House of Representatives

Winter 1995
· Development of Integrated Care Management Systems suspended by new Secretary of Health and Mental Hygiene Martin Wasserman

· Decision to pursue Section 1115 Waiver for new systemwide Medicaid managed care program

· Introduction of Senate Bill 694 by Senator Paula Hollinger with support from the Department of Health and Mental Hygiene

Spring 1995
· Adoption of Senate Bill 694 by the Maryland General Assembly, directing the Secretary of Health and Mental Hygiene to formulate plans for comprehensive reforms in the state Medicaid program.

Summer and Fall 1995
· Public hearings throughout the state to receive preliminary input and identify key issues
· Appointment of Waiver Advisory Committee and schedule of issue-oriented meetings
· Community forums with Medicaid beneficiaries
· Development of recommendations by the UMBC Center for Health Program Development and Management in consultation with the Department of Health and Mental Hygiene
· Approval of the High Cost User Initiative waiver proposal by the Health Care Financing Administration

Figure 8.1 (continued)

Winter and Spring 1996
- Submission of legislative proposal for Medicaid reform from the Department of Health and Mental Hygiene to the Maryland General Assembly
- Executive and legislative modifications to the DHMH proposal
- Passage of House Bill 1051 and Senate Bill 750 and appointment of conference committee to resolve differences
- Adoption of Senate Bill 750 by Maryland General Assembly and approval by Governor Glendening
- Submission of new waiver proposal to the Health Care Financing Administration

Summer and Fall 1996
- Development of Medicaid regulations for implementation of sytstemwide managed care reforms
- Approval of waiver proposal by the Health Care Financing Administration

Winter and Spring 1997
- Scheduled implementation of the Maryland Medicaid Managed Care Program (in January 1997, the start of program implementation was delayed until June 1997)

trenchment in these areas became difficult or impossible for legal, political, or ethical reasons. To achieve still deeper cuts in the projected growth of Medicaid costs, policymakers needed more creative changes in the program.

The first breakthrough came in 1991 in the form of the Maryland Access to Care program (MAC). The MAC program did not change any Medicaid eligibility requirements or covered services. Instead, it simply assigned each Medicaid beneficiary to a primary medical provider—an individual physician or clinical group to serve as the "medical home" and as a "gatekeeper" to specialty services. Emergency rooms and other specialty service providers needed to obtain a referral or authorization from a patient's primary medical provider to receive payment from the Medicaid program.

Under MAC, primary medical providers were reimbursed on a fee-for-service basis. Fee levels for most services were increased to encourage provider participation. The goals of the program were to improve access to primary and preventive services, encourage more appropriate use of services, improve continuity of care, increase provider participation, and reduce Medicaid expenditures.

All Medicaid beneficiaries were enrolled in MAC except for voluntary HMO enrollees, individuals receiving institutional or hospice care, and those in special programs for diabetes, sickle cell, and corrective case management. In December 1992, twelve months after its inception, the program enrolled 300,000 individuals, or 70% of the Medicaid-eligible population.[14] A preliminary evaluation of the MAC program found there was greater access to the federally mandated

Early, Periodic Screening, Diagnosis, and Treatment (EPSDT) and other preventive services for Medicaid-eligible children. There was no large impact on the frequency of inappropriate emergency room visits, although there was some evidence that they declined the longer patients were enrolled in the MAC program. Finally, the evaluation estimated that the MAC program saved approximately $35 million on patient services during its initial year of operation, compared with predicted Medicaid expenditures without the new program.[15]

With the inception of the MAC program, Medicaid beneficiaries no longer had a "Gold Card," as one official put it, to seek any provider and service of their choice. Yet a primary care network, even if it worked properly, was an imperfect solution to many problems of health services delivery to the Medicaid population. Many patients still suffered from poor continuity of care and supervision, since the primary care provider often did not follow them into the hospital. The primary care providers had no strong financial incentive to hold down the costs of services; nor was there any incentive for hospitals and specialty providers to hold down the volume of services, since Medicaid still made payments on a fee-for-service basis.

Furthermore, even conscientious primary and specialty providers were unable to prescribe support services for Medicaid patients who repeatedly cycled through the health care system because inadequate housing, nutrition, counseling, supervision, or multiple health conditions affected their compliance with medical orders and reduced the efficacy of treatment plans. These deficiencies impinged on their health status and generated additional program costs as well.[16]

It was to the needs of these individuals and other high-cost Medicaid patients with intensive needs that policymakers turned next. Officials in Maryland sought to introduce nonmedical services that would prevent costly medical complications and introduce management procedures and incentives to provide more efficient care once high-risk patients entered the medical care system.

THE HIGH COST USER INITIATIVE (1994)

The High Cost User Initiative was predicated on the knowledge that a very small proportion of patients generate the vast majority of health care costs, and the prospect that the state could design interventions to improve treatment outcomes and reduce costs for patients with chronic or catastrophic illnesses.

In 1992, Secretary of Health and Mental Hygiene Nelson Sabatini requested an analysis of Medicaid expenditures from his Medical Care Finance and Compliance Administration. The subsequent report indicated that, in a given year, 5% of Medicaid beneficiaries accounted for roughly 50% of program spending, and 10% of beneficiaries accounted for 70% of the annual costs. A few cases each year were extraordinarily costly: in fiscal year 1993, 784 Maryland Medicaid patients each incurred costs of more than $100,000 for the year.[17] Most of them suffered from chronic or multiple ailments related to conditions such as low birth weight, AIDS, drug and alcohol dependence, mental illness, respiratory illness, and severe disabilities.

The basic data were hardly novel, since a skewed distribution of program spending is inherent in any system of health insurance, public or private. The response of Maryland officials to the data was highly innovative, however, as the highest cost cases caught Sabatini's attention and established a focal point for problem definition and policy design.

Conception and Design of High Cost Patient Management Systems

Sabatini called upon Mary Stuart, the director of the Health Policy and Statistics Administration in the Department of Health and Mental Hygiene (DHMH), to design a system to better manage services for high cost Medicaid patients. Sabatini wanted the new system to perform four functions: (1) identify current and potential high cost patients; (2) give providers greater flexibility in prescribing the most appropriate combination of medical and nonmedical services; (3) give providers financial incentives to deliver and coordinate care for seriously ill patients, with savings to be shared between providers and Medicaid; and (4) monitor patient outcomes to guarantee the quality of care.[18]

The pressure from Sabatini represented a "politics-driven opportunity" for advocates to come forward with preferred solutions to the problems described above.[19] What is striking is that Stuart and her staff could not find any readily available policy alternatives that met Sabatini's criteria; even just a few years ago, the health policy community had not worked out the underlying technical issues of how to assess patient risks and needs, organize an integrated set of health and social services, or establish procedures to assure appropriate quality and cost outcomes. So Sabatini's request had no immediate results, but instead set off a lengthy search for a viable set of program components. It would take nearly two years to translate the basic idea into a concrete policy proposal.[20]

The High Cost User Initiative began to emerge out of a combination of activities involving state health agencies, foundations, hospitals, and researchers. The preliminary work in 1993–1994 helped resolve some issues of feasibility and provided a much greater understanding of the types of patients and problems involved in catastrophic episodes of illness. The process of program design was far more inductive than deductive, more pragmatic than idealistic. The participants started with concrete problems to be rectified and worked backwards to the proper delivery system. They used ideas based on discussions with providers about their clinical experience and organizational problems, studies of actual high cost cases, and exploratory data analysis to define workable groups of patients and services.

The ultimate design of the High Cost User Initiative called for two basic interventions: "enhanced case management" and "integrated care management systems.'' Each would provide a broader set of covered services and create new financial incentives. These interventions were designed to save Medicaid money by reducing hospital readmission rates through more complete discharge planning and use of community-based services, and by maintaining patients in the lowest cost setting of care appropriate to their needs.[21]

The plan was to screen almost all Medicaid patients upon hospital admission. Those whose medical history, diagnosis, complexity of illness, or demographic makeup indicated they were likely to end up in the top 6% of cases based on treatment costs were then referred to one of the two interventions.[22]

First, some patients would enter into an enhanced version of case management similar to that used by some private health plans. Teams of nurses and social workers would review all Medicaid patients within 24 hours of hospital admission and work up discharge plans for those cases. Pending the approval of the federal government, the state planned to pay for a wide range of supplemental ''waiver services'' that could enhance the quality and efficiency of the treatment plan. These services included acupuncture, chiropractic services, behavior management, occupational and physical therapy, outpatient addiction therapy, dental care, nutritional supplements, assisted living services, respite care, hospice, assistive equipment, family training, transportation, environmental modifications, and others.[23]

Second, the initiative called for placement of certain patients in an integrated care management system (ICMS). This was essentially a specialty HMO that would receive partial or full capitation payments for the comprehensive care of patients who fit into ''clinically focused groups'' with a history of high cost episodes, based on studies of Medicaid claims. Plans suggested that different ICMSs would be organized to serve patients with uncontrolled hypertension, complications from diabetes, chronic obstructive pulmonary disease, congestive heart failure, high risk pregnancy, premature birth, pediatric asthma, mental illness combined with medical problems, traumatic head injury, spinal cord injury, late stage cancer, and AIDS.[24] As with case management, the ICMSs would use interdisciplinary teams to develop treatment plans, coordinate the provision of health and social services, and monitor patient progress.

The ICMS concept reflected Sabatini's insistence on creating new systems with broader scope of services, financial risk-sharing with providers, and continuous responsibility for patient management. It was assumed that short-term case management alone would be insufficient for many patients with chronic conditions; yet few general HMOs had the expertise and none had financial incentives to establish long-term relationships with high risk patients under the existing Medicaid program. The ICMS provisions also gave academic health centers and other institutions with established expertise and commitment to these specialized populations an opportunity to participate in the rapid movement away from fee-for-service medicine toward prospective payment and managed care.

Another notable feature was the decision to create the Center for Health Program Development and Management (CHPDM) and locate it on the campus of the University of Maryland Baltimore County (UMBC). The new center was to develop the state's application to HCFA for the waivers needed to implement the interventions. It would then operate the High Cost User Initiative and serve as an ongoing source of technical assistance to the state health department and Medicaid program. It would: (1) supervise patient screening, assessment, and referral to case management and ICMSs; (2) run the case management program; (3) construct and refine data bases to track patient utilization, costs, and outcomes; (4) develop payment methods and set rates for different types of high cost patients; and (5) evaluate provider performance.

The partnership with UMBC offered several advantages for DHMH. It provided a way for the Medicaid program to hire additional staff during a state hiring freeze for permanent civil service positions. The contract for program operations could be developed through an interagency agreement rather than the usual nine-month procurement process involved with private sector contractors. The university would have greater flexibility than DHMH in personnel decisions and setting staff salaries and, in addition, the academic setting might help attract a higher quality staff.[25] Yet because of reduced overhead charges the program costs would still be lower under this arrangement than if the state used private consultants. Daniel Fox, who was president of the Milbank Memorial Fund and lent support to the High Cost User Initiative, suggested that this arrangement deviated from the usual administrative decision to "make or buy" services; DHMH officials would in essence be "renting" resources from another state agency.[26]

Leadership and Strategy in Policy Innovation

At its inception, the High Cost User Initiative was not controversial and did not have a high profile in the political process. As work progressed on the technical and organizational details, Sabatini met with Governor Schaefer in the fall of 1993 and received permission to include the initiative in the administration's budget proposal for fiscal year 1995. Sabatini had used this strategy for other program changes and it was more likely to succeed than independent legislation for several reasons. The budget is a must-pass piece of legislation and the process is streamlined—a single bill is presented by the governor to the General Assembly and considered by only one committee in each house, so there is no jurisdictional conflict or shared authority, as often occurs in other legislation. Also, the executive branch has an unusually strong constitutional position on budgetary matters in Maryland: the General Assembly can only reduce the amount proposed for appropriations by the governor; it cannot add or transfer funds from one program to another. Thus, the new Medicaid initiative for high cost patients could not be held hostage to other legislative priorities.

The spending plans in the initiative also contributed to its success. The

DHMH proposal did not call for any additional appropriations, but instead for a reallocation of program funds. It was advertised as a way for Medicaid to put taxpayer dollars to better use. Even though its creators and advocates hoped the initiative would improve the quality of care and patient outcomes, they were required to save the state at least as much money as it cost to run the initiative. The waiver proposal to HCFA actually projected that the High Cost User Initiative would save $114 million over its first five years.[27]

A large proportion of the reallocated funds—several million dollars each year—was to go to program staff and operations based at UMBC. In 1994, the Senate was the lead house on the budget bill and Barbara Hoffmann (D), who represents parts of Baltimore County and takes a special interest in the UMBC budget, was vice chair on the Senate Budget and Taxation Committee. Hoffman has long been active on education and health issues and is one of the key legislators credited with smoothing the way for the DHMH budget proposal and monitoring the subsequent performance of CHPDM.[28]

After a routine legislative hearing, the High Cost User Initiative passed the Maryland General Assembly as part of Governor Schaefer's final budget in the spring of 1994. Legislators were evidently impressed by Sabatini's personal commitment and by the interest of national foundations in the Maryland experiment.[29]

Operating on a tight timeline, CHPDM staff and DHMH officials completed a waiver application to HCFA after only a few weeks. The proposal sought federal agreement to pay for the supplemental services needed to replace or prevent higher cost care and to allow mandatory reassignment of potential high cost patients from MAC providers to ICMSs. The Maryland proposal went to HCFA on July 7, 1994.

Implementation Successes and Failures

In the summer and fall of 1994, the screening and case management components of the program got underway in earnest. Despite some operational complications, case management proved even more successful than imagined as a cost control device.[30] Originally, CHPDM staff believed that the greatest savings in the High Cost User Initiative would come from ICMS services. Before a single ICMS was organized, however, it was case management that revealed how inefficient the existing system was for high risk patients.

Even though only a fraction of eligible Medicaid patients were being screened and referred to case management, the early implementation produced enough estimated savings to more than offset the cost of all CHPDM operations. For fiscal year 1996, Medicaid saved an estimated $8.6 million, or $2.30 for every dollar spent on the CHPDM operations.[31]

The waiver proposal submitted to HCFA called for a full year of ICMS planning and implementation of services beginning in July 1995. The ICMS was the hallmark innovation in the High Cost User Initiative and, indeed, had no organizational counterpart in the private sector or in other states. These specialized systems of managed care promised a lot: better care at lower cost for an extremely needy segment of the population. The program designers believed that ICMSs would provide immediate benefits to the Medicaid population, and in time their operation might have provided useful information for improving virtually all managed care programs.

The potential significance of this innovation did not guarantee its survival, however. By the end of 1994, plans for ICMS development were dead. The High Cost User Initiative lost political momentum in its first few months and the seeds were sown for a much broader and less specialized system of managed care for the Medicaid population. A number of factors contributed to the early demise of ICMS development and the eventual death of the entire initiative.

The first sign of strain was external resistance from health care organizations that were expected (and needed) to establish and operate ICMSs. The Maryland Association of Health Maintenance Organizations expressed concern that ICMS sponsors would not be reviewed by the state insurance department and would not have to meet the same financial and quality assurance requirements as regularly licensed health plans.[32] The High Cost User Initiative would effectively allow physician and hospital groups to form their own managed care organizations without full legislative consideration of the issue. Even with the built-in advantages of their existing provider networks and experience with capitation payments, HMOs saw the ICMS plans as an entry point for "unfair" competition.

Health care providers had quite different concerns and constituted a more formidable source of opposition to ICMS development. Most providers, including those whose staff had worked closely with DHMH on the preliminary design, expected there would be a trial period to test the feasibility of the ICMS concept and different payment arrangements. The original budget proposal put forward by Sabatini said that the project would begin with pilot testing in only three institutions in Baltimore—Johns Hopkins Hospital, University of Maryland Hospital, and Mercy Hospital—and only after a year would it expand to other institutions throughout the state.[33] By the fall of 1994, however, it appeared that Medicaid would begin statewide implementation of ICMSs in mid-1995 without a smaller-scale trial.

The atmosphere became contentious after CHPDM and DHMH officials announced the draft regulations for ICMS operations and payments in September 1994. The ICMS guidelines stated that Medicaid would negotiate capitation rates for the different patient groups. This worried hospital officials who believed the initial payments should be based on an individual provider's historical payments under the existing fee-for-service system. They wanted capitation rates to be phased in, and a guarantee that those rates would be adjusted to cover "social costs" such as graduate medical education and charity care. There was a further concern that even if adjustments were included in the basic capitation rate, there would still be a financial incentive for Medicaid to eventually compress capitation payments toward the lowest negotiated rate or direct patients away from institutions with teaching programs or high volumes of uncompensated care.[34]

This fear was compounded because DHMH and CHPDM would be in charge of screening patients and referring them to an appropriate ICMS. In fact, the draft regulations and a subsequent letter of clarification stated that ICMSs with lower capitation rates would be rewarded with a higher volume of patients.[35] The two academic medical centers in Baltimore, which received almost one-third of all Medicaid general hospital revenues under the existing system, were concerned that a selective contracting process would emerge and many patients would be referred to lower cost providers without regard to geographic location or historical service to the Medicaid population.

The staff from CHPDM and DHMH held a public meeting on October 25, 1994, to discuss concerns with the draft regulations. The state response, which accompanied a cover letter on December 16, 1994, listed "several important proposed changes" for the regulations. It expressed a willingness to consider risk-sharing between Medicaid and providers and suggested methods such as a stop-loss mechanism where the state would pick up individual patient costs above a certain amount, or "risk corridors" where Medicaid and the ICMS would share a specified proportion of the difference between the capitation rate and the actual costs incurred for patient services.[36]

The misunderstandings between providers and Medicaid staff appear to reflect differences in both substance and style. The High Cost User Initiative was intended to create more sensible and compassionate health services for seriously ill individuals and their families; at the same time, it was designed to make the state a more prudent purchaser of services and encourage market forces in the larger health care system. This policy preference put Medicaid officials at odds with providers who hoped to maintain the relatively insular and anti-competitive culture that has distinguished Maryland health policy for decades. This culture was already eroding because of competition among insurers and providers for employer health coverage and disputes over how the state hospital rate-setting system covers the costs of teaching and uncompensated care.[37] The new Medicaid plan threatened one of the few remaining areas of relatively stable coverage and financing. These substantive differences were exacerbated by poor communication as program development moved from DHMH to CHPDM. Many of the CHPDM staff were newcomers to the state's health policy community and did not sense the importance of consulting with key leaders and organizations before recommending options for implementation.

While discontent grew on the outside, there were divisions within DHMH as well. Some Medicaid officials questioned whether an experimental program concentrated on a small number of beneficiaries was worth all the technical and political difficulties it created for them. There was a sense that the High Cost User Initiative was "pie in the sky," devoted more to research and development than to solving immediate problems in Medicaid operations. The argument for establishing the growing staff, data systems, and other departmental operations at UMBC was not universally accepted. Finally, some officials felt that limiting the initiative to a small, high risk population put excessive pressure on DHMH to accurately estimate the necessary services and capitation payments. They came to prefer a broader initiative because they believed it would be simpler for DHMH to administer. Enrolling most Medicaid patients in larger health plans would spread the actuarial risk more broadly than in the ICMSs under the High Cost User Initiative and presumably create more economic slack for providers, health plans, and the Medicaid program.[38]

The ambivalence and dissent surrounding ICMS development might not have made much difference had HCFA conducted a more timely review of the Maryland waiver proposal. The federal waiver arrived in December 1995—over seventeen months after the original request—and HCFA officials were surprised to learn that there were no longer any plans for ICMS development. There is a feeling among CHPDM staff that the Maryland plan, because it dealt with only a portion of the Medicaid population, was treated as a ''small'' waiver and was put at the end of the queue while HCFA devoted itself to proposals from other states with broader policy and political implications.

The fate of the High Cost User Initiative and the subsequent course of the Maryland Medicaid program are most easily traced to political events in November 1994. The national election swept Republicans into majority control of both houses of Congress for the first time in two generations. The results of that turnover in leadership would be felt a few months later. Of more immediate consequence was the narrow victory of Parris Glendening (D) in the race to succeed retiring Governor Schaefer. He selected Martin Wasserman, a physician and career public health officer, as the new Secretary of Health and Mental Hygiene.[39] Nelson Sabatini arranged to leave DHMH and have his successor appointed in December 1994, even before the new governor took office. The High Cost User Initiative lost its champion with his departure. Within weeks, word passed from DHMH to CHPDM to the health care community that ICMS development would be suspended and the state would undertake a new managed care initiative.

MARYLAND MEDICAID MANAGED CARE PROGRAM (1995– 1996)

The change in administration provided an opportunity to reconsider the entire Medicaid program. Even though the MAC program was a modest success, DHMH officials believed it would not produce major cost savings. With Sabatini gone, the state trade associations for HMOs and hospitals appealed to Wasserman to reconsider the scope and timing of the High Cost User Initiative.[40] There was already support within DHMH, as noted above, to stop tiptoeing into managed care through conventional HMO contracts and specialized programs and seek greater savings through a comprehensive managed care program.[41] The Glendening transition team report included a recommendation to move additional components of the Medicaid program from fee-for-service into managed care.[42]

As he prepared to take office, Wasserman attended a conference that discussed Medicaid managed care initiatives taking shape in other states. So he was somewhat aware of Section 1115 Waivers when state Senator Paula Hollinger (D) urged him to consider a new round of Medicaid reform based on mandatory enrollment in managed care organizations (MCOs).[43] The new governor had other agenda priorities and was not ready to take the lead on health care, but was willing to let Hollinger and DHMH move forward.

Policy Ideals and Political Realities

Wasserman's main interest in a new initiative was to consolidate several highly specialized waiver programs for high cost patients and conditions such as diabetes, sickle cell anemia, and lead-paint poisoning into a single managed care program that could serve all Medicaid beneficiaries. Hollinger sought a new system for somewhat different reasons. She was a nurse by profession and a prominent legislative advocate of better health services for the poor. Over the past few years, Hollinger had met periodically with officials from other states who were active in health care reform. In the immediate wake of the Clinton administration's failed attempt at national reform, she believed that, through Medicaid reform, states could still achieve modest but important gains.

Many states have initiated Section 1115 demonstrations under the premise that managed care is the "magic bullet" and will yield cost savings that can be used to expand Medicaid eligibility to populations that were previously uninsured or underinsured—in other words, to simultaneously improve the efficiency and the equity of their health care systems.[44] Hollinger originally hoped to pursue the same "more with less" strategy in the 1995 legislative session, during a brief period after the 1994 election when Medicaid managed care was still thought of as a progressive tool of health care reform.[45]

Those aspirations were short-lived, of course. Any plans to expand insurance coverage disappeared in the face of congressional proposals to severely restrict the growth of federal contributions to the Medicaid program in the spring of 1995. Once Congress turned from the largely rhetorical actions on the "Contract with America" to a spending plan necessary to reduce the federal deficit and finance tax cuts, state policymakers were forced to think of Medicaid in very different terms. Hollinger began to focus on ways that Maryland might react constructively to federal cutbacks in order to avoid what she believed were ill-considered reductions in Medicaid eligibility or services.

So Hollinger, a proud liberal and staunch advocate of tax-financed national health insurance, became the leading voice in the legislature for building a new

Medicaid system built around managed care. Her alliance on the issue with Wasserman, the public health doctor, may have struck some observers as the health care equivalent of Richard Nixon opening diplomatic relations with Communist China.

Neither DHMH nor CHPDM gave any formal indications there might be a delay or reconsideration of implementation plans for the High Cost User Initiative released in September 1994. At some point in January 1995, however, Wasserman "suspended" ICMS development and announced plans for a new Section 1115 Medicaid Waiver. According to officials at DHMH and CHPDM, the two decisions were basically linked together with pursuit of a new waiver as the driver; it was only logical to put ICMS development on hold and integrate services for high cost patients into a systemwide managed care program. The opposition of health care organizations appears to be a supporting, not determining factor in Wasserman's decision on ICMS implementation. None of the parties outside of DHMH has seen official documentation of this change in policy or the precise rationale for it.

With strong support from DHMH, the Maryland General Assembly passed Senate Bill 694 and Governor Glendening signed it on May 25, 1995. It directed the Secretary of Health and Mental Hygiene to formulate plans for comprehensive reforms in the state Medicaid program and submit those plans to the legislature for action during the 1996 session. The statute endorsed a stronger effort to slow the growth of spending in the Medicaid program by moving the great majority of beneficiaries from a fee-for-service system into prepaid managed care plans. Upon legislative approval, DHMH would develop a new Section 1115 demonstration proposal to the federal government.[46]

The Process of Public Input and Policy Formulation

During the 1995 deliberations over Senate Bill 694, Wasserman promised a meeting of advocacy groups that once the bill passed they would be consulted on the design of the upcoming waiver proposal. They would then have further input after the proposal was sent back to the legislature for approval. In retrospect, Maryland officials took considerable precautions to create the best possible conditions for success of the reform proposal. The formulation of the new plan was a delicate technical and political exercise that took a full year. Medicaid documents contend that Maryland used "the most extensive and inclusive public process for developing the waiver of any state in the country."[47] According to Barbara Shipnuck, Deputy Secretary at DHMH, officials at HCFA praised the Maryland proposal for its clarity and conciseness and consider the public process to be a model for other states to follow.

In the spring of 1995, DHMH set up a contract for technical assistance with CHPDM. The center was given the responsibility of running meetings and developing preliminary recommendations to DHMH for design of the new managed care system. In addition, CHPDM was to help state officials draft program regulations and the waiver application to be sent to HCFA upon approval of the General Assembly.[48]

In an effort to gain a broad base of input and also secure political support for the Medicaid reform proposal prior to the legislative process, Wasserman directed that public hearings be held to solicit information and gain a preliminary sense of what key issues would need to be addressed in the process of policy development. Eleven public hearings were conducted in every region of the state in June and July 1995. Over 1,000 people attended the hearings and CHPDM and DHMH staff heard testimony from 228 individuals.[49]

To follow up on that general base of input, Wasserman appointed a 131-member advisory committee and created a highly organized process for identification and deliberation of issues and policy options. The 1115 Waiver Advisory Committee (Advisory Committee) was composed of elected officials and representatives of MCOs, medical care providers, Medicaid beneficiaries, state and local governmental agencies, and a variety of advocacy groups. Wasserman sent personal letters of invitation to members and asked for their collaboration to improve the overall quality of care for the Medicaid population and help curtail rising costs in the program.

A group of 45 state agency experts was to assist in the development of policy options to be presented to the Advisory Committee, conduct research, and track legislation regarding changes in the Medicaid program at the federal level.

Medicaid beneficiaries were invited to small community forums to meet directly with CHPDM staff members and discuss their priorities for the new system. Six forums with Medicaid beneficiaries were held in September 1995 in the most populous counties in the state.[50] The privacy of these forums made them a valuable supplement to public meetings where "consumer" input is solicited by policymakers. This approach required CHPDM staff to augment their role as technical analysts and consultants; this new role meant they were also responsible for identifying and representing beneficiary interests throughout the process.

Even with the emphasis on inclusion and representation, most stake-holders were reacting to an agenda established by the state health department and the legislature in Senate Bill 694. Louis Hays, Director of Operations for CHPDM, set the political tone at the first meeting of the Advisory Committee by stating that Secretary Wasserman and the center agreed that the proposed system would focus on providing more services, providing them more efficiently, and operating at a lower total cost to the state. They assumed that most Medicaid beneficiaries would be enrolled in managed care and few, if any, services would be carved out. Anyone advocating the exclusion of any services from the managed care program carried the burden of proof that a carve-out was the best alternative for the state.[51]

The participation and solidarity of key legislators on the Advisory Committee also proved instrumental in keeping the members focused on system performance and encouraging mutual cooperation.[52] The elected officials communicated the message that they supported the move to managed care and if groups wanted to influence the waiver, they had to offer suggestions that were not merely self-serving. Success would largely depend on convincing other committee members to adopt their position, and building strategic coalitions.

As the summer progressed, the Advisory Committee paid increasing attention to federal funding cuts and the potential impact on the waiver process. Members received repeated reminders that proposals for federal budget cuts and block grant caps meant that expanding Medicaid eligibility was not an option. John Folkemer, Deputy Director of the Medical Care Policy Administration in DHMH, reported that Congress had adopted a budget resolution cutting $181.6 billion from the federal Medicaid budget over seven years. Folkemer said the proposed cuts could result in an estimated $2.8 billion of lost revenue to Maryland over a period of seven years.[53] The possibility of such sizable federal funding cuts was the final ingredient needed to ensure that a vast majority of committee members continued to accept the basic concept of mandatory managed care for Medicaid beneficiaries. The discussion focused on the need to expand managed care to simply maintain current levels of eligibility and benefits.

Possibly the most controversial problem the Advisory Committee faced was setting the terms of provider participation in the new managed care system. The question was whether Medicaid should require MCOs to contract with certain providers or allow them to organize MCOs on their own. For most providers, the mission was simple: If the state was to enroll Medicaid beneficiaries into managed care, those who had served this population in the past should be able to do so in the future.

In contrast to states like Tennessee, the vast majority of Maryland providers who participated in the waiver development process sought inclusion in the system.[54] In particular, African-American physicians expressed difficulty negotiating with MCOs for inclusion in their networks, and local health departments and Federally Qualified Health Centers believed that MCOs would resist contracting with them.[55] Participation in Medicaid was also crucial for the two academic medical centers in the state, at Johns Hopkins University and the University of Maryland in Baltimore. In fiscal year 1994, the Johns Hopkins and University of Maryland hospitals accounted for 17% of the Medicaid general hospital discharges, about one-quarter of the general hospital days, and about 30% of Medicaid expenses on general hospital services.[56] Ultimately, the Advisory Committee and policymakers would have to choose between two disparate views regarding historic providers. The first view was that the state should focus on identifying necessary services and ensuring access to those services;

the second view was that it was truly important what providers render the services.

On September 21, 1995, the Advisory Committee held its last formal meeting to help develop recommendations for the 1115 Waiver application. That input served as the basis for CHPDM to draft a preliminary reform plan for Secretary Wasserman. Dozens of members of the Advisory Committee reconvened in downtown Baltimore three weeks later for a review of the draft proposals.

The CHPDM recommendations introduced several trial balloons into the policy process and allowed DHMH officials to observe the reaction of interest groups before adopting the recommendations as their own. The CHPDM recommendations established the basic framework of the waiver proposal. The guiding principles were to establish a "medical home" for patients, promote a prevention-oriented system of care, get better value for state funds, and make MCOs accountable for quality. CHPDM staff projected that the overall plan would save the Maryland Medicaid program a total of $1.3 billion over six years. The CHPDM plan set the stage for several innovations in the Maryland reforms and many of the major recommendations carried through to the final reform plan in 1996.

State and Federal Approval of Systemwide Managed Care

The legislative proposal by DHMH was announced on January 11, 1996. Shortly thereafter, it was introduced as House Bill 1051 and Senate Bill 750 in the Maryland General Assembly. During legislative hearings in late February and early March, many members of the Advisory Committee offered testimony supporting a systemwide expansion of Medicaid managed care. Many interested organizations and groups, including some groups represented on the advisory committee, offered amendments calling for major or minor modifications to the DHMH proposal.[57]

The large number of proposed amendments indicated that while there was little opposition to the basic policy, there was still considerable disagreement about critical details of organization and financing. Officials in DHMH worked with interest groups and incorporated many of the proposed amendments into revised bills in January, prior to legislative hearings. Nonetheless, individual groups and coalitions pushed many amendments not supported by DHMH forward into legislative deliberations. Many of the controversial provisions continued to be debated as the bills from each house went to conference committee. After a drawn-out conference, agreement was reached on a modified version of Senate Bill 750 and sent back to the floor of each house at the very end of the legislative session. Medicaid officials commented that this had been an extraordinarily difficult process and that, in ordinary circumstances, legislation with so many contested amendments would be rejected or returned to the summer session of the legislature for further study and development of consensus.[58]

Figure 8.2
Key Features of the Maryland Medicaid Managed Care Program

· Beneficiaries guaranteed eligibility for six months
· Guaranteed participation for historic providers
· Risk-adjusted capitation rates using Ambulatory Care Groups (ACGs)
· Special capitation payments for (1) Centers for Disease Control–defined AIDS patients, and (2) pregnancy and delivery services
· Stop-Loss Case Management
· Rare and Expensive Case Management
· Mental health services carve-out administered by the Mental Hygiene Administration in conjunction with local Core Service Agencies
· Additional quality standards for seven special populations
· Self-referral provisions for family planning, school health services, and HIV/AIDS diagnostic and evaluation services
· State-administered enrollment and prohibition of direct marketing by MCOs
· MCO mandate for patient outreach
· Local ombudsman program for relations between Medicaid beneficiaries and MCOs

The final version of Senate Bill 750 was passed by unanimous vote in both houses of the General Assembly near midnight on April 8, the final day of the session, and was signed into law by Governor Parris Glendening on May 14, 1996.[59] Within weeks of enactment, CHPDM and DHMH polished the final details of a new Section 1115 Waiver proposal and sent it to HCFA. The proposal received a favorable review and HCFA sent preliminary approval with attached terms and conditions on September 19, 1996.

Secretary of Health and Human Services Donna Shalala gave her final approval to the Maryland waiver proposal on October 30, 1996, and state officials announced plans to begin implementing the new managed care program in February 1997.

Key Features of the HealthChoice Program

The new Maryland Medicaid Managed Care Program, renamed HealthChoice, includes several notable features summarized in Figure 8.2. If the system operates as planned, it will integrate and strengthen services for most if not all beneficiaries. It will also cost less to operate than the existing set of programs. The waiver application to HCFA estimates that the new program will save $541 million over five years from 1997 to 2001.[60]

The only major improvement in access is a guarantee of six months' coverage once beneficiaries become eligible for Medicaid. The legislature rejected any expansion of benefits in order to meet projected savings and directed that MCOs cover only the current benefits under the fee-for-service MAC program.[61]

Beneficiaries may self-refer for family planning services and certain services performed at school-based health centers. Also, patients diagnosed with HIV/AIDS may self-refer for an annual diagnostic and evaluation service. MCOs are required to reimburse out-of-plan providers for these services.

To assure that most Medicaid beneficiaries can remain with their current provider if they wish to, DHMH will designate health care professionals and institutions with a demonstrated history of providing services to Medicaid beneficiaries before July 1995 as "historic providers." Those who meet the Medicaid quality standards are entitled to be assigned by the state to at least one MCO provider panel if the provider has unsuccessfully attempted to join the panels of all MCOs in their service area. In addition, providers will be allowed to establish their own MCOs if they meet state guidelines for quality and financial security. Through this policy, Maryland has elected to join other states in offering providers a chance to maintain autonomy rather than be integrated into conventional MCOs that have not historically shown a commitment to providing services for the underserved.[62]

In contrast to current Medicaid HMO operations, MCOs will not be permitted to engage in direct, face-to-face marketing to beneficiaries. To reduce the likelihood of risk-selection practices among MCOs, DHMH will distribute comparable information on available health plans and administer enrollment.

The MCOs will be required to contact enrollees who are difficult to reach or who miss appointments, and attempt to bring them in for care. MCOs may enlist assistance from local health departments if their documented attempts for patient outreach are unsuccessful. DHMH will also contract with local health departments or other community agencies to run an ombudsman program to assist beneficiaries and handle disputes with health plans.

The new system sets limits on administrative expenses in MCOs. Managed care plans must use at least 85% of the money they receive from Medicaid for patient care, and no more than 15% for administration and profits.

The new plan will include a novel "mental health services carve-out" and the creation of a Specialty Mental Health System designed and administered by the state Mental Hygiene Administration in conjunction with local Core Service Agencies. The Medicaid reform process presented an opportunity for the agency to implement a managed care system for *all* publicly funded mental health services. The plan blends together funds from Medicaid, Medicare, Mental Hygiene Administration grants, forensic care appropriations, self-pay, and private sector reimbursement. It will use a private behavioral health company only for administrative services. The Mental Hygiene Administration considers the new system a "profound paradigm shift for the public mental health system as it will now perform as a purchaser rather than simply a provider of services."[63]

One of the novel features of the Maryland program is the attention devoted to special patient populations. Advisory groups composed of clinical experts, advocates, beneficiaries, and health plan representatives will develop new access and quality standards that MCOs must meet for seven groups with special needs: (1) children with special health care needs; (2) individuals with a physical disability; (3) individuals with a developmental disability; (4) pregnant and postpartum women; (5) individuals who are homeless; (6) individuals with HIV/AIDS; and (7) individuals with a need for substance abuse treatment. The MCOs are required to submit treatment protocols and demonstrate the adequacy of their provider network for serving these special populations, including circumstances under which patients would be referred to outside specialists.[64]

Maryland Medicaid will use innovative methods to set MCO capitation rates. It will phase in use of the Ambulatory Care Group (ACG) case mix system developed at Johns Hopkins University to set adjusted rates for beneficiaries with at least six months of claims data in the fee-for-service program. For new enrollees or enrollees currently in Medicaid HMOs for whom there are insufficient data to use the ACG risk-assessment system, rates will be adjusted for age, gender, and region. There will be special capitation rates for AIDS patients, and a lump-sum payment for pregnancy-related costs including delivery. Since the mental health services will be delivered in a separate system of care, MCOs will not receive payments for these services in the capitation rates. This change is substantial for the HMOs that currently serve the Medicaid population, as mental health expenditures represent 10–12% of the total Medicaid budget.[65]

There are two case management programs in the new reform plan: (1) Rare and Expensive Case Management (REM); and (2) Stop-Loss Case Management (SLM). Secretary Wasserman has designated UMBC to operate these programs for DHMH. The REM program provides focused management and access to specialized networks of care for patients with conditions such as pediatric AIDS, congenital anomalies such as cleft palate and spina bifida, metabolic diseases such as cystic fibrosis, selected degenerative diseases, and hemophilia. Rare and expensive diagnoses were determined by claims analysis and input from clinicians familiar with the treatment needs. The program makes fee-for-service payments for services authorized by case managers. It is essentially a small population carve-out, since REM patients are not enrolled in regular MCOs.

Finally, an MCO shall qualify for protection under the Stop-Loss Program if the inpatient hospital costs of an enrollee exceed $61,000 in one contract year. Beneficiaries whose care exceeds the stop-loss threshold enter into case management and subsequent care must be deemed medically necessary and appropriate. Medicaid will pay 90% of inpatient hospital charges according to established Medicaid fee-for-service rates above the stop-loss limit throughout the remainder of the year. Stop-Loss patients continue to be enrolled in their MCO, which must cover the remaining 10% of inpatient hospital charges and 100% of all other medical care services in the Maryland Medicaid benefits package.

Next Steps

The timetable for implementing the new Maryland Medicaid program is still undergoing change. The state originally hoped to complete all phases of implementation during the first six months of 1997. In January 1997, however, Secretary Wasserman announced that HealthChoice would not begin operations until June 2, 1997. The delay allowed state officials to secure the participation of managed care organizations in the new program, assure the capacity of new provider-sponsored plans, and supervise enrollment procedures. A memorandum to the governor's cabinet argued that the delay was needed to correct "demonstrated deficiencies" in MCO applications so that DHMH would be able to authorize a sufficient number of participating organizations to guarantee high quality and assure continuity of care for beneficiaries.[66]

The new program represents only the first step toward a comprehensive system of managed care for all health services in Maryland. Senate Bill 750 directed DHMH to establish a "long-term managed care advisory committee" to help develop a managed care proposal to cover the Medicaid population excluded from the first phase of reform (mainly patients who are eligible for both Medicare and Medicaid and those receiving institutionalized care). In June 1996, the long-term care committee heard public testimony, conducted public meetings around the state, and prepared a report that was presented to Secretary Wasserman in November 1996.

Wasserman presented a DHMH proposal on managed long-term care to the governor on January 30, 1997. The Phase II plan proposed five initiatives: (1) encourage enrollment of persons who are dually eligible for Medicaid and Medicare in managed care plans; (2) supervise privately initiated pilot projects that integrate acute and long-term care; (3) develop or expand DHMH-sponsored demonstration projects; (4) promote long-term care insurance options for public and private employees in Maryland; and (5) commission a public education campaign to emphasize the importance of individual long-term care planning.[67] Legislators will not take action on the Phase II plan until 1998 at the earliest, when the first phase of the HealthChoice program is complete.

LESSONS FROM MEDICAID REFORM IN MARYLAND

We now turn to examine what lessons might arise from the recent changes to the Medicaid program in Maryland. First, we identify some important sources of innovation in the policy-making process—factors that influenced how participants perceived the series of situations and available options in the policy process. Then we consider what issues remain unresolved as managed care advances in Medicaid and other parts of the health care system.

The latest round of reform was in part a legacy of earlier health care developments in the public and private sectors. The fact that over one-third of all

Maryland residents were already enrolled in managed care plans of some kind by 1994 made it much easier to require managed care for Medicaid beneficiaries. There were clearly spillover effects on Medicaid policy from a perception that the public sector was behind in the organization and delivery of efficient health care systems.

In addition, Maryland was part of a wave of states reforming their Medicaid programs. Between 1991 and mid-1995, the number of Medicaid beneficiaries enrolled in managed care rose from 2.7 to 11.6 million. A total of 27 states have now implemented or applied for managed care research and demonstration waivers under Section 1115 of the Social Security Act.[68] The recent rush to institute Medicaid waiver programs constituted a response to the failure of federal efforts to solve pressing problems in the health care system. States reacted by exerting control over the part of the health care system they have substantial power over as a major purchaser.

Within the Maryland Medicaid program itself, over 100,000 individuals, or close to a quarter of all beneficiaries, were already voluntarily enrolled in HMOs. The MAC program had assigned Medicaid patients to primary care providers as gatekeepers to improve continuity and reduce inappropriate self-referral to specialty or emergency services. The systemwide managed care program is viewed by some state officials as an extension of those efforts to establish a "medical home" for Medicaid patients.[69] Finally, the plans under the High Cost User Initiative for integrated care management systems and capitation payments prepared most providers and health plans for a greater emphasis on managed care for Medicaid beneficiaries.

It is important to recall that early on, the Maryland managed care reforms had progressive goals and were not merely reactionary moves by state policymakers. The introduction of support services under the High Cost User Initiative reflected the vanguard of thinking about how health services can be made more efficient and more humane at the same time. Similarly, it is easy to forget the optimism of state officials in early 1995 that Medicaid managed care could achieve the "impossible solution" of greater insurance coverage and cost containment.[70] Although the goal of expanding coverage fell victim to budgetary projections soon after the 1995 legislation was introduced, those motivations helped broaden interest and sharpen thinking about policy design across partisan lines and interest groups.

The successful conversion of societal forces and institutional opportunities into policy innovation depends on skilled leadership. Leaders clarify policy goals, recognize opportunities, search for feasible alternatives, and generate political resources in the policy-making process. The substantive course of Medicaid reforms in Maryland was inextricably tied to the vision and energy supplied by Nelson Sabatini and Mary Stuart to the High Cost User Initiative, and Martin Wasserman and Paula Hollinger to the new systemwide managed care program. Their ideas and strategies led Maryland to first attempt a unique and untried experiment in managed care for the seriously ill, then incorporate many of the ideas from that unfinished experiment into a more universal approach resembling Medicaid reforms in other states. The leaders' styles and strategies—Sabatini as the consummate insider and Wasserman as the public communicator—reflected their different professional experience and programmatic priorities; but they also demonstrated a common ability to follow a process required by the timing and scope of the proposed reforms.

The process of policy formulation and public deliberation was crucial in shaping the ultimate design and improving the political feasibility of the new systemwide reforms. Many states with significant health care reforms have used commissions to expand the scope of conflict and enhance the voice of normally disadvantaged groups.[71] These institutional devices also can bring contending parties face-to-face in reasoned discussion and discourage isolated lobbying of policymakers. In Maryland, the broad representation on the advisory committee and technical advisory group meant that from the start, traditional providers of Medicaid services and patient advocates had a strong position relative to managed care organizations. The policy process was not restricted to the bureaucracy, a handful of health-minded legislators, and leaders of "peak associations" representing physicians, hospitals, and insurers. There was extraordinary weight of discussion on preserving existing patient-provider relationships to assure the accessibility and appropriateness of services, compared to discussion of mechanisms to improve efficiency and cost containment. In addition, there was considerable discussion devoted to protecting "special populations."

The relatively inclusive and visible process offered a clear contrast to the "stealth reform" in Tennessee, and to the formulation of the High Cost User Initiative as well.[72] It was also a politically savvy response to the criticisms levied against the Clinton administration in its abortive attempt at national reform. The careful, measured process allowed advocates for all groups and types of services to mobilize before the policy was developed, not afterwards. A satisfactory outcome to the advisory process was not preordained—interest groups still sought out special provisions from legislators and an extraordinary number of changes were incorporated into the final statute and regulations. In retrospect, however, the process produced less resistance to the final waiver proposal and it should facilitate implementation of the new system.

An important reason why the broad-based commission did not produce an unwieldy and deadlocked debate was the sense of urgency regarding federal proposals to restrict future Medicaid spending and possibly end entitlements. The 1995 congressional budget resolutions increased pressure on officials in Maryland and other states to design a system that would save money without reducing eligibility, services, or payments to providers. The federal deliberations represented a new type of "policy club" cited as instrumental in other state health care reforms, where credible threats of worse alternatives help instill political commitment and facilitate cooperation among potential opponents of reform.[73]

The success of the process to date does not guarantee that the performance of Maryland's new Medicaid managed care program will live up to policymakers' expectations, for "it is less difficult to bring together a talented group for designing a new program than it is to hold one together for the arduous task of program implementation and refinement."[74] In Maryland and other states, the ongoing interaction between policy goals, administrative resources, and political support will determine how well the new system serves individual beneficiaries and the greater polity.

The impact of managed care on Medicaid will depend on the resolution of three key issues. First, what is a realistic balance between the goals of efficiency and appropriateness? The practices of MCOs may achieve short-term economies and profits for corporate managers and shareholders but fail to achieve long-term efficiency for individuals and society. Enrollment in managed care creates the promise of a better system for many Medicaid beneficiaries;[75] yet health care studies continue to find evidence that managed care produces worse outcomes for vulnerable groups—the chronically ill, elderly, and poor—than fee-for-service medicine.[76] The problems of seriously ill individuals led to the High Cost User Initiative and will continue to be a challenge for the new Medicaid program.

The political drive for budgetary savings must be reconciled, therefore, with the ideal of equal access to health care and a social responsibility to meet urgent human needs. In the typology articulated by Daniel Fox, Medicaid managed care reforms represent an effort to impose an "economizing" paradigm on an anti-poverty program rooted in a "social conflict" paradigm.[77] Introducing stronger monetary incentives for the providers of care for this population invites either a destructive collision or a constructive synthesis of the two competing paradigms.

The Maryland Medicaid reforms demonstrate that there are sufficient doubts about the motives and capacities of MCOs to warrant dozens of requirements for their clinical and administrative practices. Providers and advocacy groups have successfully pressured politicians to adopt what one might regard as heroic measures to manage the managers. With stipulations such as the explicit treatment and referral protocols for the seven "special population" groups, MCOs must feel like modern-day Gullivers being strapped down by the Lilliputians. If the idea is to create a more streamlined and efficient system of services, why all the micromanagement?

The attention paid to ensuring that special populations receive appropriate care is laudable. On the other hand, the special provisions raise the question of whether major savings are possible. Within a year, savings estimates for the new waiver dropped from $1.3 billion over six years to $541 million over five years to $56 million per year. If the latest estimate holds up, the annual savings to the state and federal government will be less than 3% in a Medicaid budget that now exceeds $2 billion. Because of the collision between economics and politics in program design, the achievements of the new system will have to be justified in terms of quality as well as economy.

The second issue is whether states have the technical resources needed to bridge the potential gap between economic incentives and social needs in a managed care system for the poor. The Maryland approach contradicts the conventional idea that privatization of governmental functions will allow states to streamline their operations and reduce personnel. In fact, states will likely have to transform their Medicaid agencies from what James Q. Wilson calls procedural organizations to craft organizations.[78] They must shift from tasks involving relatively routine oversight and claims processing to much more sophisticated responsibilities in quality assurance, risk adjustment, patient advocacy, and economic evaluation. This will require a more skilled, and possibly larger, management staff.[79]

In Maryland, contracting out the technical assistance to the UMBC Center for Health Program Development and Management gave Medicaid officials sufficient expertise and control over technical design issues and a rapid turnaround time for some very complex projects. It also allowed DHMH to direct interest group concerns to CHPDM, create an early warning system of political intelligence, and establish some political independence from the initial recommendations for reform. CHPDM performed very much the same functions as the staff of the Physician Payment Review Commission performed for Congress in the Medicare physician payment reforms in the late 1980s.[80]

The third and final issue is what role politics will play in a new era of health policy innovation. As the United States heads toward a more organized and competitive health care system, politics is simultaneously an accelerator and brake on restructuring in that system. Nowhere is this more evident than in the rush of the states to institute mandatory enrollment of Medicaid patients in managed care plans. The main factor accelerating governmental endorsement of managed care and market competition is the perception that those policies will slow budget growth and reduce the pressure for tax increases. While the concerns of advocacy groups and some public officials for special populations are certainly a modest brake on the movement to managed care, the real constraints are those applied by providers attempting to preserve their professional and economic status in the health care system.

Despite the successful legislative record, the recent Maryland Medicaid reforms demonstrate the difficulty of initiating major system change through government. Although the political economy of health care in Maryland is changing, health policy is still made in a "negotiated regime" that must accommodate traditional health care organizations rather than a regime imposed by government.[81] The power of the health care establishment manifested itself in the death spiral of the High Cost User Initiative. A few key institutions reacted to uncertainties in the policy design by first demanding accommodation, then undermining the initiative when the process and substantive responses did not fit their customary expectations. In the systemwide managed care reform now underway, a somewhat broader set of Medicaid providers have had a major influence in the rules regarding historic providers, sponsorship of MCOs, prohibition of selective contracting, and limits on administrative expenses and profits. The delay in implementing the HealthChoice program is a sign that the Medicaid program is having difficulty persuading major managed care organizations to even play in the system under its new rules.

Some of the MCO regulations can be interpreted as a way to ensure that certain professional and group values are maintained in the new system. The guarantees for historic providers and the ceiling on administrative expenses appear to be proxies for a much deeper concern in the Maryland health policy community, however. These rules help preserve local control over the health care system in an era when large regional and national managed care plans are a greater threat to provider autonomy than state government.

There is an ironic twist in the passage of the Maryland Medicaid program to managed care. When some providers decided to play hardball to slow or defeat the High Cost User Initiative in 1994, they got what they wanted in the short run. But they were thinking only one step at a time and in one dimension; and when the Clinton plan and its stronger governmental regulation gave way to Republican plans to radically deregulate and defund government, the federal budget proposals made the status quo an untenable position in the state Medicaid debates in 1995 and 1996. Managed care has expanded and continued to squeeze providers in the private insurance market and now in the Medicaid and Medicare programs as well. For the past year, the Maryland Hospital Association has been proposing a near-equivalent of the High Cost User Initiative, but all of the old skirmishes over risk adjustment and capitation rates are now taking place on a much larger battlefield with more enemies and greater stakes. The early victories of providers in the policy process cannot restore the political economy of health entering the 1990s and they are unlikely to alter the passage to relatively open market competition and a subsequent consolidation of health care institutions.

The ongoing challenge for policymakers is to channel legitimate professional and local concerns into a more patient-centered and more accountable health care system that is an improvement for all jurisdictions and medical conditions. The process of introducing managed care into the Maryland Medicaid program is a reminder that the problem of improving health system performance is not entirely, and perhaps not mainly, a problem of technique. The problem is creating institutional and political resources to achieve policy goals. The lesson we draw is that the potential of managed care and competition is at least as ambiguous in the Medicaid program as in other parts of the health care system. Whether managed care constitutes the "unbungling" or "rebungling" of health care, after a quarter century of refinement the design of an ideal system remains a work in progress.[82]

NOTES

We gratefully acknowledge the support of the Milbank Memorial Fund and the many individuals in the Maryland health policy community who shared their personal knowledge and documentary information on the state Medicaid reforms. This chapter is adapted from a report, *Reflections on the "Revolution" in Maryland: The Collision of Economics and Politics in Medicaid Managed Care*, submitted by the first author to the Milbank Memorial Fund in October 1996.

1. Because many of the programs now being approved by the federal government apply to all or most Medicaid beneficiaries and are adopted statewide, there are no direct control groups to assess how the new system works compared to the old system. These reforms are entirely new policies, not experiments to test ideas for improving old policies.

2. Maryland Department of Health and Mental Hygiene (DHMH), and the Center for Health Program Development and Management, University of Maryland Baltimore County (CHPDM), "Maryland Medicaid Section 1115 Health Care Reform Demonstration Proposal," application for waiver to the U.S. Health Care Financing Administration, May 3, 1996, 2.

3. Maryland Department of Fiscal Services, *Major Fiscal Issues: A Four Year Summary, 1991–1994 Sessions, Maryland General Assembly* (Annapolis, Md.: Department of Fiscal Services, 1994), 3.

4. Ibid.

5. Ibid, 8–9.

6. Ibid., 7.

7. Maryland Department of Health and Mental Hygiene, *Maryland Medical Care Programs: Year in Review, Fiscal Year 1994*, 2–4.

8. Maryland Department of Health and Mental Hygiene (DHMH) and the Center for Health Program Development and Management (CHPDM), Section 1115 Medicaid Waiver Application, May 3, 1996, 9.

9. Jack L. Walker, "Setting the Agenda in the U.S. Senate: A Theory of Problem Selection," *British Journal of Political Science* 7 (October 1977): 423–445. This is a sharp contrast to instances of "slack innovation" where leaders have greater leeway to set the policy agenda and respond to problems or opportunities that are highly original or that occur only infrequently. There is presumably greater reward in the effort to bring a National Football League team back to Baltimore, for example, than dealing with another proposal to restructure Medicaid organization and financing—particularly when the outcome is zero-sum or worse for patients and providers.

10. For example, see Thomas R. Oliver, "Health Care Market Reform in Congress: The Uncertain Path from Proposal to Policy," *Political Science Quarterly* 106 (Fall 1991): 453–477; John F. Hoadley, "The Fruits of Reform: A New Payment Scheme," in Jonathan D. Moreno, ed., *Paying the Doctor: Health Policy and Physician Reimbursement* (New York: Auburn House, 1991).

11. DHMH and CHPDM, Section 1115 Medicaid Waiver Application, May 3, 1996, 10–11.

12. Maryland Department of Health and Mental Hygiene, *Maryland Medical Care Programs: Year in Review*, Fiscal Year 1994.

13. Maryland Department of Fiscal Services, *Major Fiscal Issues*, 10.

14. Julie A. Schoenman, William N. Evans, Claudia L. Schur, and Leigh Ann White, "Evaluation of the Maryland Access to Care Program: Managed Care for Medicaid Recipients. Interim Report on the First Year of the Program," project produced by Project HOPE under Cooperative Agreement No. 18-C-90142/3–01 with the Office of Research and Demonstrations, U.S. Health Care Financing Administration, October 14, 1994, 1–2.

15. Ibid., vii.

16. Interview with Mary Stuart, Director, Health Policy and Statistics Administration, Maryland Department of Health and Mental Hygiene, March 19, 1996.

17. Maryland Department of Health and Mental Hygiene, "Demonstration of Integrated Care Management Systems for High-Cost/High-Risk Medicaid Beneficiaries," Application for waiver to the U.S. Health Care Financing Administration, submitted July 7, 1994, 7.

18. Interview with Mary Stuart, August 8, 1995.

19. A "window of opportunity" is an important element in John Kingdon's model of governmental agenda-setting and policy innovation. John W. Kingdon, *Agendas, Alternatives, and Public Policies* (Boston: Little, Brown, 1984). For a model of the strategies policy entrepreneurs use to exploit politics-driven opportunities, see Thomas R. Oliver, "Conceptualizing the Challenges of Public Entrepreneurship," in Chris E. Stout, ed., *The Integration of Psychological Principles in Policy Development* (Westport, Conn.: Praeger, 1996), 5–31.

20. Kingdon and other scholars of the policy process make the point that an opportunity created by political leadership may not produce policy change if there are not reasonably well-developed alternatives to match the acknowledged problem and political climate. See also Walker, "Setting the Agenda in the U.S. Senate"; Robert Eyestone, *From Social Issues to Public Policy* (New York: John Wiley and Sons, 1978); and Jack L. Walker, "The Diffusion of Knowledge, Policy Communities, and Agenda Setting: The Relationship of Knowledge and Power," in John E. Tropman, Milan J. Dluhy, and Roger M. Lind, eds., *New Strategic Perspectives on Social Policy* (New York: Pergamon Press, 1981), 75–96.

21. Maryland Department of Health and Mental Hygiene, Policy and Health Statistics Administration, "Maryland Medicaid High-Cost/High-Risk Patient Management Initiative," grant proposal submitted to the Robert Wood Johnson Foundation, July 1993.

22. DHMH, "High-Cost/High-Risk Waiver Application," July 7, 1994, 2. The original DHMH budget proposal called for case management of the top 10% of high-cost cases, but the high-cost group was reduced under the subsequent waiver plan approved by the HCFA.

23. A general list of supplemental services planned under the waiver appears in: DHMH, "FY 1995 Budget Initiative: High Cost Patient Initiative" (Mimeo, 1994), 3; and DHMH, "High-Cost/High-Risk Waiver Application," July 7, 1994, 26. The full set of planned waiver services is described in CHPDM, "Answers to Maryland Medicaid High Cost User Initiative Questions/Comments" (undated mimeo provided to the Health Care Financing Administration), 31–36.

24. DHMH, "High-Cost/High-Risk Waiver Application," July 7, 1994, 20–21.

25. Interview with Nelson Sabatini, former Secretary of Health and Mental Hygiene, February 22, 1996.

26. Personal communication from Daniel M. Fox, president, Milbank Memorial Fund, January 3, 1995.

27. DHMH, "High-Cost/High-Risk Waiver Application," July 7, 1994, 4.

28. While there was little concern expressed about the purpose of the High Cost User Initiative, there were naturally questions about why the department was establishing the research and development operations at UMBC. The University of Maryland medical school and other health sciences programs in downtown Baltimore, and the private Johns Hopkins University, could both claim greater experience and expertise in health care

research. The creation of CHPDM was a major boost to the health policy activities at UMBC, therefore, but an ongoing source of tension between the academic institutions and their political benefactors.

29. The interest of national foundations in the High Cost User Initiative was cited as a helpful, though not crucial, factor in legislative deliberations over the Medicaid budget. The Robert Wood Johnson Foundation had already given its blessing by funding the pilot study for the initiative, and Milbank Memorial Fund president Fox came to Maryland to join Sabatini and give favorable testimony to legislators at the budget hearing in the spring of 1994. Interview with Mary Stuart, August 8, 1995.

30. Some of these early operational problems are detailed in Maryland Department of Health and Mental Hygiene, Interim Report to the Robert Wood Johnson Foundation on Grant 22905, "Maryland Medicaid High-Risk Patient Management Initiative" (1995), 12–13.

31. University of Maryland Baltimore County, Center for Health Program Development and Management, *Maryland Medicaid High Cost User Initiative Case Management and Cost Savings Annual Report: Fiscal Year 1996*, October 1996 (draft), Executive Summary. These savings were based on the case managers' estimates of the cost of their care plans compared to an estimate of what would have been delivered without management. Although this method is often used in the private sector, these estimates have not been validated by claims analysis of the amount actually spent by Medicaid. Some of the case management savings might be attributed to incentives introduced by the procedures that directly confronted case managers with the financial implications of their therapeutic preferences. At the same time they drew up their patient care plans, they were responsible for calculating the savings to Medicaid and, therefore, justifying their worth to the program.

32. These concerns are summarized in a letter from Geni Dunnells, executive director of the Maryland Association of Health Maintenance Organizations, to incoming Secretary of Health and Mental Hygiene Martin Wasserman, dated January 12, 1995.

33. Maryland Department of Health and Mental Hygiene, "FY 1995 Budget Initiative: High Cost Patient Initiative" (Mimeo, 1994), 3.

34. Interview with Gerard Reardon, consultant at Arthur Andersen, February 26, 1996. Reardon was director of patient care services at the Johns Hopkins Hospital during the planning and development of the High Cost User Initiative. This rationale was incorporated into a report on "A Conceptual Approach to Medicaid Managed Care" by the Maryland Hospital Association, draft dated August 16, 1995.

35. Maryland Department of Health and Mental Hygiene, "Notice of Proposed Action on Integrated Care Management System" (Draft), September 13, 1994, 26. Open letter with "Proposed Changes to Draft ICMS Regulations" from John Folkemer, Deputy Director, Medical Care Policy Administration, and Louis Hays, Director of Operations, UMBC Center for Health Program Development and Management, December 16, 1994.

36. Open letter with "Proposed Changes to Draft ICMS Regulations" from John Folkemer and Louis Hays, December 16, 1994.

37. Academic medical centers and other teaching institutions want to replace the procedure that set their rates higher to cover those "social costs"; they wanted those costs spread across rates of all hospitals so that the rates would more accurately reflect the true efficiency of patient care and make them more attractive to managed care plans.

38. Interview with Lawrence Triplett, Director, Medical Care Finance and Compliance Administration, Maryland Department of Health and Mental Hygiene, February 23, 1996;

phone interview with Joseph Millstone, Director, Medical Care Policy Administration, Maryland Department of Health and Mental Hygiene, March 18, 1996.

39. Wasserman also holds a law degree.

40. Letter from Geni Dunnells, executive director of the Maryland Association of Health Maintenance Organizations, to Secretary of Health and Mental Hygiene Martin Wasserman, dated January 2, 1995; letter from Cal Pierson, president, Maryland Hospital Association, to Secretary of Health and Mental Hygiene Martin Wasserman, dated January 3, 1995.

41. Medicaid officials argued that HMOs were overpaid under the existing system (a small discount of average per capita expenses under the fee-for-service), an assertion that supported a move to a more sophisticated system of capitation payments that more accurately predicted resource use.

42. *Maryland Forward: Moving into the 21st Century*, Human Services and Neighborhood Revitalization Executive Summary, 3–4.

43. Most waivers associated with demonstration projects under Section 1115 of the Social Security Act enable states to bypass federal regulations that ordinarily give Medicaid patients, like those on Medicare, free choice of health care providers. Normal federal rules also prohibit health plans from enrolling more than 75% of their patients from the Medicaid program in an effort to ensure that Medicaid beneficiaries will receive "mainstream" care.

44. Alpha Center, "More for Less? Increasing Insurance Coverage through Medicaid Waiver Programs," *State Initiatives in Health Care Reform*, Number 10 (January/February 1995): 1–3. In fact, the literature and experience to date suggest that cost savings from the expansion of managed care in Medicaid programs are likely to be very limited. Prior managed care programs for the Medicaid population have achieved savings of 5–15% relative to costs in the fee-for-service system; but these estimates overstate the savings potential since most managed care programs have primarily enrolled the younger and healthier individuals in the Medicaid population, especially women and children. Kaiser Commission on the Future of Medicaid, 1995, *Medicaid and Managed Care: Lessons from the Literature* (Menlo Park, Calif.: Henry J. Kaiser Family Foundation, March 1995).

45. Interview with Maryland state Senator Paula Hollinger, February 26, 1996.

46. Medical Assistance Program, Eligibility, Managed Care Plans, Ch. 500, 5lr, 1394 (1995). Codified as amended at Health-General § 15–101.

47. DHMH and CHPDM, "Section 1115 Medicaid Waiver Application," May 3, 1996, 5.

48. Although Wasserman could have turned to other consultants, it was natural to use CHPDM because its staff and operations were already covered by the Medicaid budget; CHPDM could simply shift much of its staff and analytical work from the High Cost User Initiative to development of the new systemwide managed care program.

49. DHMH and CHPDM, "Section 1115 Medicaid Waiver Application," May 3, 1996, 6.

50. In these forums, beneficiaries expressed concerns with ensuring that their children had access to high-quality care, maintaining their current provider relationships, assuring reasonable waiting time for appointments, providing for patients with serious diagnoses such as mental illness or HIV infection, and securing access to care for beneficiaries who are homeless. Other concerns included transportation to and from appointments, the need for a simple enrollment and disenrollment process, an effective grievance system to lodge

complaints about services, and a fair appeals process. UMBC Center for Health Program Development and Management, "History of the 1115 Waiver Process" (Mimeo, 1995), 29.

51. Minutes for the 1115 Waiver Committee, July 20, 1995, 2.

52. The key legislators on the advisory committee were Maryland state Senators Paula Hollinger, Barbara Hoffmann, and Larry Young. Hollinger was the chief legislative sponsor while Hoffmann and Young were leaders on important legislative committees.

53. Minutes for the 1115 Waiver Committee, August 3, 1995, 25. Testimony of John Folkemer. The congressional budget bill and provisions for major changes to the Medicaid program were subsequently vetoed by President Clinton.

54. A key provision in Tennessee required providers to participate in TennCare if they wished to participate in the lucrative state employee health program. Thus, providers who ordinarily would not accept Medicaid patients were induced to do so. David M. Mirvis et al., "TennCare—Health System Reform for Tennessee," *Journal of the American Medical Association* 274, no. 15 (1995): 1235–1242.

55. Minutes for the 1115 Waiver Committee Meeting, July 27, 1995, 23.

56. Maryland Department of Health and Mental Hygiene, *Maryland Medical Care Programs: Year in Review, Fiscal Year 1994.*

57. See testimony on House Bill 1051, House of Delegates, Environmental Matters Committee, February 27, 1996. See also open testimony, Senate Bill 750, Senate Finance Subcommittee, March 1, 1996.

58. Phone interview with Joseph Millstone, March 18, 1996.

59. Medical Assistance Program—Managed Care Organizations, Ch. 500, 6lr, 2794 (1996). Codified as amended at Health-General § 15–101.

60. DHMH and CHPDM, "Section 1115 Medicaid Waiver Application," May 3, 1996, 129.

61. Ibid., 57.

62. Michael S. Sparer, "Medicaid Managed Care and the Health Reform Debate: Lessons from New York and California," *Journal of Health Politics, Policy and Law* 21 (Fall 1996): 433–60; Helen Halpin Schauffler and Jessica Wolin, "Community Health Clinics under Managed Competition: Navigating Uncharted Waters," *Journal of Health Politics, Policy and Law* 21 (Fall 1996): 461–488.

63. It was decided that MCOs can contract with the Mental Hygiene Administration to provide specialty mental health services for their regular enrollees. In order to do that, MCOs would have to offer mental health services to patients other than their own enrollees, including non-Medicaid patients eligible for public mental health services. The Mental Hygiene Administration would contract with MCOs on a fee-for-service basis for the first year with the possibility of capitation payments thereafter.

64. *Maryland Register*, volume 23, issue 25, December 6, 1996, 1745.

65. Karen Anderson Oliver, "Maryland Medicaid Expenditures for Mental Health Services: Fiscal Years 1993–1995," Center for Health Program Development and Management, University of Maryland Baltimore County (Mimeo).

66. Memo to Cabinet Officers from Marty Wasserman, Secretary, Department of Health and Mental Hygiene, January 9, 1997 (Mimeo).

67. Martin P. Wasserman, "Plan for Long Term Managed Care in Maryland," January 30, 1997 (Mimeo).

68. David Liska, Karen Obermaier Marlo, Anuj Shah, and Alina Salganicoff, *Medicaid Expenditures and Beneficiaries: National and State Profiles and Trends, 1984–1994*, 2nd ed. (Washington, D.C.: Kaiser Commission on the Future of Medicaid), 124, 129.

69. Interview with A. Michael Collins, Director of Research and Development, Center for Health Program Development and Management, University of Maryland, Baltimore County, February 23, 1996; DHMH and CHPDM, "Section 1115 Medicaid Waiver Application," May 3, 1996, 13–14.

70. John Golenski and Stephen Thompson, "The Impossible Solution: Expanding Access to Health Care While Reducing Costs," *Stanford Law & Policy Review* 3 (Fall 1991): 73–80.

71. Lawrence D. Brown, "Commissions, Clubs, and Consensus: Reform in Florida," *Health Affairs* 12 (Summer 1993): 7–26; Thomas R. Oliver and Pamela Paul-Shaheen, "Translating Ideas into Actions: Entrepreneurial Leadership in State Health Care Reforms," *Journal of Health Politics, Policy and Law* 22 (June 1997): 721–788.

72. G. Gordon Bonnyman, Jr., "Stealth Reform: Market-Based Medicaid in Tennessee," *Health Affairs* 15 (Summer 1996): 306–14. A process characterized as "ready, fire, and then aim" has its merits in many situations, however, and is typical in many state and local programs recognized by the Ford Foundation as significant innovations. See Martin A. Levin and Mary Bryna Sanger, *Making Government Work: How Entrepreneurial Executives Turn Bright Ideas into Real Results* (San Francisco: Jossey-Bass, 1994).

73. Brown, "Commissions, Clubs, and Consensus: Reform in Florida."

74. Harvey Sapolsky, James Aisenberg, and James A. Morone, "The Call to Rome and Other Obstacles to State-Level Innovation," *Public Administration Review* 47 (March/April 1987): 135–142.

75. Jane E. Sisk, Sheila A. Gorman, Anne Lenhard Reisinger, Sherry A. Glied, William H. DuMouchel, and Margaret M. Haynes, "Evaluation of Medicaid Managed Care: Satisfaction, Access, and Use," *Journal of the American Medical Association* 276 (July 3, 1996): 50–55.

76. Mark Schlesinger and David Mechanic, "Challenges For Managed Competition from Chronic Illness," *Health Affairs* 12 (1993 Supplement): 123–137; John E. Ware, Jr., Martha S. Bayliss, William H. Rogers, Mark Kosinski, and Alvin R. Tarlov, "Differences in 4-Year Health Outcomes for Elderly and Poor, Chronically Ill Patients Treated in HMO and Fee-for-Service Systems: Results From the Medical Outcomes Study," *Journal of the American Medical Association* 276 (October 2, 1996): 1039–1047.

77. For a fuller analysis of contending perspectives in the analysis and politics of health policy, see Daniel M. Fox, "Health Policy and the Politics of Research in the United States," *Journal of Health Politics, Policy and Law* 15 (Fall 1990): 481–499.

78. James Q. Wilson, *Bureaucracy: What Government Agencies Do and Why They Do It* (New York: Basic Books, 1989), 154–175.

79. A similar argument about new administrative expenses associated with Medicaid managed care programs appears in Michael S. Sparer, *Medicaid and the Limits of State Health Reform* (Philadelphia: Temple University Press, 1996), 154.

80. Thomas R. Oliver, "Analysis, Advice, and Congressional Leadership: The Physician Payment Review Commission and the Politics of Medicare," *Journal of Health Politics, Policy and Law* 18 (Spring 1993): 113–174.

81. Robert S. Hackey, "Regulatory Regimes and State Cost Containment Programs," *Journal of Health Politics, Policy and Law* 18 (Summer 1993): 491–502.

82. Paul M. Ellwood, Jr., and George D. Lundberg, "Managed Care: A Work in Progress," *Journal of the American Medical Association* 276 (October 2, 1996): 1083–1086.

9

Economic Constraints and Political Entrepreneurship: Medicaid and Managed Care in Michigan

MICHAEL HARRIS AND RHONDA S. KINNEY

MEDICAID IN MICHIGAN: AN OVERVIEW

In Michigan, the Medicaid program is administered by the Medical Services Administration (MSA), a unit of the newly created state Department of Community Health. Until April 1996, when the state's executive departments were reorganized, the MSA was part of the Department of Social Services. The reorganization centralized all of Michigan's various health care assistance and prevention programs into a single umbrella department.

At any given time about 11–13% of the Michigan population is eligible to receive Medicaid benefits. Currently, as Table 9.1 indicates, that translates into an average of over 1.1 million persons per month, the eighth highest state total in the United States.[1] Michigan obviously covers groups that are federally required: persons receiving Aid to Families with Dependent Children (AFDC); people who receive Supplemental Security Income (SSI); families with medical expenses that depress their income and assets below a certain level. However, the state has extended eligibility to other groups including many low-income pregnant women and young children living in low-income homes as well as to children in protective care.

As in other states, the Michigan Medicaid program is a central part of the state's budget resource allocation process. The program began with a gross expenditure of $157 million in FY 1967[2] and was slated to spend a total of nearly $5.9 billion dollars in FY 1996,[3] an increase of nearly 3750%. Clearly, this nominal dollar increase does not control for inflation, but does demonstrate the huge increase in the size of the Medicaid program in Michigan over time.

Another indication of the growth of Medicaid over time is that the program has also increased its relative share of the state's budget. In 1980, it totaled

Table 9.1
Number of Michigan Medicaid Eligibles, 1988–1997

Year	Average Monthly Total
1988	916,243
1989	926,081
1990	976,503
1991	1,066,988
1992	1,105,981
1993	1,161,770
1994	1,194,822
1995	1,178,895
1996*	1,140,000
1997*	1,143,000

*Michigan Medical Services Administration Estimates

Source: "Michigan Department of Community Health FY 97 Executive Budget Recommendations, Senate Appropriations Subcommittee Meeting on Medical Service Administration." Prepared by Michigan Medical Services Administration (MSA) for presentation March 1996.

8.3% of the general fund, while in FY 1997 it comprised 18%. This is the highest percentage ever, and Medicaid continues to grow as does its share of the budget.

These costs translate into roughly $2,800 per Medicaid recipient. These expenditures per recipient are relatively moderate compared to other states. They are $330 below the national average and nearly $630 below the region average.[4] The Engler Administration has identified three general factors that have contributed to Medicaid expenditure increases over time: broadening of eligibility, increases in the costs of services, and increased utilization of services.

Figure 9.1
Medicaid Recipient Groups

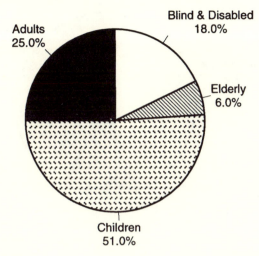

Source: Michigan MSA.

As Figure 9.2 indicates, nearly 75% of total Medicaid funds were spent on elderly, blind, and disabled clients. What is interesting here is that these recipients comprise only 24% of the persons receiving benefits in Michigan (see Figure 9.1). In other words, one-fourth of the program's recipients are responsible for nearly three-fourths of the program's costs.

Michigan currently receives matching funds from the federal government at the rate (FY 1996) of 56.77% but the matching rate is slated to drop to 55.20% in FY 1997 and to 53.58% in 1998 under current law.[5] The state's current governor, John Engler, was prominently involved in efforts to change Medicaid funding at the federal level. His efforts centered on several items: passage of the Medicaid Restructuring Act vetoed by President Clinton in 1995; the agreement on Medicaid restructuring adopted by the Governors Association in February 1996; and the Medicaid Restructuring bill introduced in Congress, May 1996. None of these items, however, were subsequently passed into law.

Michigan had a contingency plan in place in the event of the bill's failure. The budget director called it the "lockbox strategy." They set up a Medigrant surplus fund of $400 million, which was their estimate of the difference between what Michigan would have received under the bill and what they would get under current law. Because the formula in the proposed bill relied on older data, Michigan would have benefitted greatly under the proposed new bill. The budget director was authorized to invoke the contingency plan in the event the bill did not pass. He invoked the lockbox on October 1, 1997.

Figure 9.2
Medicaid per Capita Expenditures

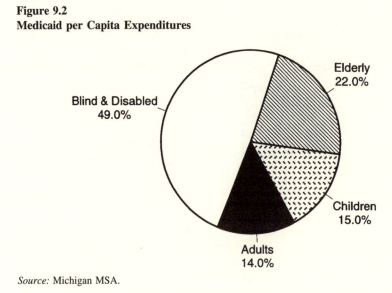

Source: Michigan MSA.

While national reform efforts continue, most innovative change in Medicaid has occurred at the state level. Michigan has been actively involved in implementing Medicaid changes, especially the use of alternative delivery systems such as managed care programs. We turn now to a brief discussion of the state's political and economic backround before we detail Michigan's state-level Medicaid reforms. This discussion provides a framework for analyzing the state's efforts.

MICHIGAN POLITICS AND ECONOMIC PICTURE

The political backround of Michigan is largely a tale of Republican leadership with intermittent periods of Democratic competitiveness. Republicans dominated Michigan politics through most of the early twentieth century. Michigan went largely unaffected by the national shift in party identification that created a Democratic majority in 1932. Democrats only became competitive in the state around 1948 when they were able to capture the governorship.[6]

Democrats held the governorship from 1948 until 1962 when a relatively liberal, progressive Republican Party emerged in the state. George Romney was elected governor in 1962, holding the post until 1968 when he left to serve in the Nixon administration. Another progressive Republican, William Milliken, served out Romney's term and remained governor until he retired in 1982. Romney, in particular, had openly rejected the conservative, ideological wing of his party.

In 1982, Michigan began to see hints of the more ideological and conflictual partisan politics that are present in the state today. It was at this time that both Republicans and Democrats became more openly partisan and the debate between them more acrimonious. Democrat James Blanchard won the 1982 gubernatorial race, but a conservative wing in the Republican Party gained strength in the state throughout the economically difficult 1980s. During this period, Michigan voters often split tickets resulting in intermittent divided state government.[7]

Upon taking office in 1983, an important event occurred when Blanchard raised state income tax rates. In the ensuing uproar, Republicans were able to force a recall election, gaining two important seats in the state senate. The two seats gave Republicans control of the senate and John Engler, a relatively unknown conservative Republican, was chosen majority leader.

In 1990, amid continuing tough economic times and facing a growing state budget deficit, Engler unexpectedly defeated Blanchard in the race for governor. The election was one of the closest in Michigan history. Republicans were also able to maintain their control of the state senate. Their wins were solidified in 1994 when Engler was overwhelmingly reelected and Republicans gained control of both chambers of the state legislature. Republicans comfortably held the senate by a 22–16 margin and the house by a closer 56–54 count.

We concentrate on the governorship here because in Michigan the office is central to understanding the power structure of the state. The institutional powers of the office are sufficient to rate Michigan's governor as relatively strong when compared to other governors.[8] The state's 1963 Constitution gives the governor traditional executive powers such as proposing the state's annual budget and appointing officials to bureaucratic positions. However, the governor also possesses broad powers to reorganize agencies of the executive branch. Along with the power to veto entire bills, he can reject individual line items of the budget passed by the legislature.

As in most areas, politics and economics are closely tied together in Michigan. Several gubernatorial elections in particular have turned on economic conditions in the state. Michigan's economy is highly cyclical and seasonal.[9] In fact, to a significant degree, the linkage between politics and economics in the state can be attributed to the state's boom-and-bust economy.[10]

The boom-and-bust cycle in Michigan is especially pronounced due to the state's dependence on the automobile industry. The economy is simply not all that diversified. Until the 1960s, this dependence served Michigan well, allowing the state to enjoy a long cycle of economic prosperity based on a growing automobile industry. By 1960, the state's per capita income was among the highest in the world. These conditions allowed for a wide variety of state-provided social services and welfare benefits such as substantial workers' compensation benefits, unemployment insurance, and cash welfare benefits. Michigan's residents grew accustomed to the ability of the state to provide generous services. Leaders continued this high expenditure/high expectations pattern throughout the 1960s, even as the state's revenue base faced great instability in the latter part of the decade.[11] The oil shocks of the 1970s and their resulting high rates of inflation, interest rates, and unemployment hit Michigan and the automobile industry especially hard. It has been observed that "when the nation gets a cold, Michigan gets pneumonia."[12] Back-to-back recessions in 1979 and 1981 were especially severe—the worst in the state's history. Unemployment topped out at 19% with nearly 13% of the state's residents receiving welfare benefits. The state's once high per capita income dropped to 7% below the national average.[13]

These recessions had a lasting impact on the state's economic condition. People migrated away from Michigan for the first time in search of lost, well-paying industrial jobs. Also, the state's economy began to shift away from relatively high-paying manufacturing jobs toward lower-paying, service-oriented jobs.[14] When John Engler was elected in 1990, the state faced a budget deficit of $1.8 billion and a citizenry accustomed to the high level of government services that had been provided for decades. Michigan was left to grapple with questions of what the state government should and could still do.[15]

MEDICAID REFORMS

Medicaid reform efforts in Michigan have been closely associated with the cyclical downturns in the economy discussed earlier. The origin of current managed care reforms in Michigan can be traced to the recession of 1979–1981. The economic downturn increased demands on the state's Medicaid program while decreasing the state's revenues and ability to deal with the problem. It became clear to Governor Milliken, his administration, and the state legislature that budget cuts would be necessary in order to deal with the situation.

Preliminary plans to cut the Medicaid program budget centered on cutting fees and eliminating benefits. But the state also initiated discussions with health care providers about possible alternative routes to reducing costs. For the first time, in July 1982, a small managed care program—a physician-sponsor plan—was implemented in lieu of reducing fees paid to providers. This plan focused on physicians acting as authorizing agents for all medical care program clients received.

The state's Medical Society, Hospital Association, and the Medical Services Administration worked together on formulating the plan. They formed a lasting partnership that has greatly facilitated Michigan's later, successful effort institute statewide managed care to all eligible program recipients. While the relationship between these groups has not been without ups and downs, the pragmatic needs of each have dictated a great degree of cooperation.[16]

Michigan's initial program was limited to its most populous county, Wayne County, which contains Detroit, the state's largest city. The county was, and is, the largest in terms of demands placed on the Medicaid system. In 1996, Wayne accounted for more than 40% of the state's total program recipients. The initial small-scale managed care effort was voluntary to recipients and remained the sole reform effort undertaken until the late 1980s, when the scope of the program was expanded slightly to include portions of five other counties. In the early 1990s, for the first time, the efforts included rural areas where enrollment was made mandatory for selected participants in these counties. Further, some recipients were required to work in order to continue coverage.

As with many Medicaid program reforms, these late 1980s changes were made possible by federal 1915(b) Waivers. No additional program revisions were undertaken until 1990, when the reform-minded Engler was elected governor. Democrats had stumbled badly during the campaign. With a recession in progress and state budget deficits climbing, Blanchard, the incumbent Democrat, chose to replace his older female lieutenant governor with a younger woman, angering many. Blanchard had also alienated many others in his own base constituency, including the powerful mayor of Detroit, Coleman Young. He had raised taxes in 1983 leading to a recall election that had given Republicans control of the state senate.[17]

Engler ran on a clear platform for his administration: (1) property tax reduction, (2) increased educational spending, (3) smaller, more efficient government. Upon his election, facing an impending budget deficit,[18] Engler quickly made moves to implement changes on all of these fronts. He introduced and passed a large property tax reduction, shifted funds into educational programs, and began downsizing state government. In particular, he began a process of entitlement reform by eliminating General Assistance (GA), a program that provided small, subsistence-level grants to unemployed persons in the state.[19] In the fight to end GA, Engler took effective advantage of his substantial executive powers, including his power to reorganize and create new executive units.

As part of this comprehensive welfare reform and budget-cutting strategy, Engler reignited Michigan's drive toward a managed care Medicaid system. In 1991, Gerald Miller, the state's Director of Social Services, and Vernon Smith, the director of the Medical Services Administration (MSA), assessed the state's budget situation and success of earlier managed care efforts. The two set an ambitious long-term goal of full mandatory enrollment of 100% of program recipients into managed care systems. Governor Engler concurred and encouraged the directors' efforts. The rationale behind the full-scale implementation clearly centered on the ability provided by managed care systems to better predict and control program costs. They also believed that managed care systems would place the state in a better position to foster greater access to coverage for a larger number of groups and allow more efficient ways of monitoring the amount and quality of care provided through the program.[20]

Since setting this goal in 1991, Michigan has made a great deal of progress toward its achievement. The overall approach has been one of conservative but steady, staged implementation over time. County infrastructures were put in place to enroll recipients and monitor the program. Offices and personnel were put in place first, and efforts moved on from there. As soon as county infrastructures were in place, voluntary encouraged enrollments were begun there among targeted recipient groups. Finally, managed care enrollment was made mandatory statewide for these targeted populations only.

Since August 1995, Michigan has had mandatory enrollment in managed care for all "targeted" eligibles in all of the state's 83 counties. Targeted eligibles include all program recipients except those in nursing homes, those with dual Medicaid-Medicare eligibility, those with partial Medicaid "spend-down" eligibility, and others who may have been specifically exempted (i.e., those who require continuity of care such as children in the CSHCS program).

Targeted Michigan Medicaid recipients are provided three managed care choices: (1) physician sponsor plans (PSPs), where recipients choose from participating physicians who are reimbursed directly by the state for services provided; (2) HMOs, where the state contracts with private HMOs and Medicaid recipients enroll like all other HMO participants; and (3) clinic plans, where providers offer primary and specialized care and the state assumes partial risk for hospital stays. The clinic plans in particular are unique to Michigan.[21] The state refers to the physician sponsor plans as a "gatekeeper" form of managed care. Physicians are paid a $3 capitation rate per enrolled client and then are paid negotiated, reduced fees for services. All authorized care provided by others is paid fee-for-service at the Medicaid rate. The HMO plan is a strictly capitation plan where HMOs are paid a contracted rate per enrolled client. Clinic plans are capitated for primary and specialized care and fee-for-service in the case of hospital and emergency care.

Once a client's (individual or family) Medicaid program eligibility is established, they are notified that they must enroll in a managed care plan. They are allowed to choose for themselves which plan option they wish, but if they do not notify the state of their choice within the enrollment period (30 days) they will be assigned one of the plan options. All members of a case family are required by the state to choose the same managed care plan option. Provisions for moving from plan to plan vary across the managed care options.

Physician Sponsor Plan. Under these plans the physician acts as the recipient's health care coordinator, providing or authorizing nearly all care. However, there are a number of covered services that do not require PSP authorization including emergency services, family planning obtained at authorized clinics, Community Mental Health and substance abuse services, as well as dental, podiatric, chiropractic, and hearing services. Under this plan, each case member is allowed to select his or her own PSP participating physician and may change doctors at any time. Recipients choosing this option may also change to another managed care plan at any time. Physicians who participate in the program are required by the state to provide recipients with access to in-person medical advice 24 hours a day, 7 days a week.

Health Maintenance Organization (HMO). HMOs provide or authorize all health care services within their provider network. Medicaid recipients who join HMOs are to receive the same care and treatment as other HMO members. If Medicaid recipients choose this option, all family case members must belong to the same state-approved HMO. Recipients must select an HMO that has contracted with the state to provide Medicaid patient care. Each case member may choose a different doctor within the HMO and members are free to change their primary care doctor within the HMO in accordance with HMO procedures. Recipients in this plan are also required by the state to have access to medical advice 24 hours a day, 7 days a week.

Ability to change plans is more limited under this option than under the physician sponsor plan. Case families may disenroll from the HMO in the first 30 days of enrollment. They also may change options during twice-a-year enrollment periods—May and November. Recipients must remain in the HMO under all other circumstances until the next enrollment period.

Clinic Plan. The clinic plans are a hybrid, combining aspects of both managed care and fee-for-service medical coverage. To recipients the clinic plan seems similar to an HMO; all health care is authorized or provided by the state-authorized Clinic Plan within its network of providers, and members belong to a single clinic plan and may switch among plan doctors as desired. Here, however, the level of risk assumed by participating physicians is reduced from that of HMOs. Under the Clinic Plan, physicians provide primary and most specialized care for the contracted rate. However, the state assumes partial risk for the cost of inpatient hospital care. The state of Michigan pays hospital fees directly for these services and shares in cost savings achieved by the plans. Recipients choosing this option can change to other plans at any time.

Under all three of the plans one provider (physician or medical group) provides or authorizes medical care and services covered are the same. Access to medical advice is available to recipients 24 hours a day, 7 days a week. There are no co-payments for recipients enrolled in managed care except for dental procedures. Also, a great deal of choice remains. One plan must be chosen but each case member may choose his or her own doctor within the plan.

Currently, nearly three-fourths of all Medicaid eligible persons in Michigan are required to enroll (or they will automatically be enrolled) in managed care. These targeted groups include recipients in the following categories: AFDC and related programs, Medicaid for persons under 21, Mich-Care Eligibles, Healthy Kids, SSI, and related programs. Some Medicaid eligibles have the option to voluntarily enroll in managed care if they wish: hospice patients, children in foster care, department/court wards, migrant population, persons with joint Medicare/Medicaid coverage. And certain client groups are *not* eligible at this time: long-term care patients, state Family/Medical Assistance Program participants, as well as recipients not entitled to full state Medical Assistance coverage (e.g., Spend Down Cases and Illegal Aliens).[22]

Progress to Date

Figure 9.3 illustrates that as of early 1996, nearly 96% of currently targeted recipients are enrolled in one of the state's three managed care systems, a percentage still in place in 1997. As the graph indicates, the state has made steady but regular progress over time in enrolling targeted populations. As late as January 1993, only 32% of recipients were enrolled. By the time enrollment in a managed care option was made mandatory for all targeted populations in all counties (August 1995), the state had already enrolled over 80% of recipients (please refer to Figure 9.2).

As you can see in Figure 9.4, the largest number of targeted recipients— 504,847—are enrolled with doctors in the physician sponsor plans. An additional 282,405 are enrolled in HMOs, with only 41,241 participating in clinic plans. While enrollment in all three plans has increased over time, the growth rate in the PSPs far outdistances the other plans. In April 1993, 43% of total clients were enrolled in PSPs, 52% in HMOs, and 5% in Clinic Plans. Two years later in 1995, a significant change had occurred in the overall picture; now 59% of clients were in PSPs, 36% in HMOs, and 5% in Clinic Plans. This trend continued into the early months of 1996, when 61% were enrolled in PSPs, 34% in HMOs, and again 5% in Clinic Plans. In 1997, 48% were enrolled in PSPs, 41% in HMO's, and 11% in Clinic Plans. Growth in managed care participation has come primarily in the gatekeeper plan where participation has tripled in three years. The rate of growth has been far slower in the capitation plans. These numbers in part reflect mandatory enrollment in nonurban counties not served by HMOs. In 1996 only 16 of Michigan's 83 counties were served by HMOs enrolling Medicaid eligibles (please refer to Figure 9.3).

The Michigan approach of steady, well-planned, staged implementation of Medicaid reform can be seen in how mandatory enrollment in managed care occurred at the local level. The MSA carefully built the administrative infrastructure needed to enroll recipients in each county before mandating recipient participation there.[23] The number of counties, as well as the percentage of recipients within each county participating, grew steadily throughout the period from 1993 to present. Now all 83 of Michigan's counties have an infrastructure in place to facilitate enrollment in the systems. The question now becomes to what degree have costs been contained as a result of these increased enrollments in managed care? We know that Medicaid program expenditures have stabilized in Michigan as well as in the nation as a whole. In FY 1994, Michigan's Medicaid spending on actual service-related accounts increased 10.4% from the previous year. However, in FY 1995, these accounts increased only 3.5%.

Unfortunately, Michigan does not maintain databases sophisticated enough to statistically measure whether the stabilization and decrease in the growth of the Medicaid program are actually due to more eligibles enrolled in managed care

Figure 9.3
Percentage Enrolled in Managed Care Programs

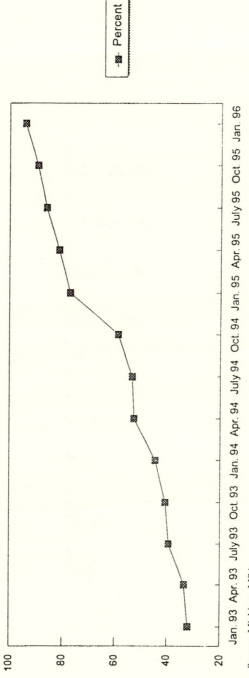

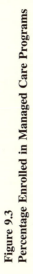

Jan. 93 Apr. 93 July 93 Oct. 93 Jan. 94 Apr. 94 July 94 Oct. 94 Jan. 95 Apr. 95 July 95 Oct. 95 Jan. 96

Source: Michigan MSA.

Figure 9.4
Targeted Group Enrollment by Plan

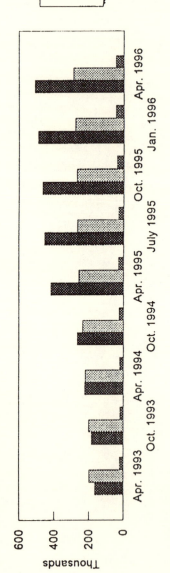

Source: Michigan MSA.

plans or to other contributing factors. What the available data does show is a decrease in inpatient hospital and emergency room usage and a modest increase in outpatient hospital spending. These declines may be reflective of managed care's ability to control costs through preventative approaches and using primary gatekeepers that can limit unnecessary hospital utilization. The lack of sophisticated data also limits the state's ability to effectively evaluate the relative annual costs and benefits of the various funding plans that may or may not be passed at the national level. So where do Michigan and the Engler administration plan to go from here?

Plans for the Future

The record of the Engler administration in accomplishing its goals has been mixed. First, plans to enroll "in managed care, those persons not currently targeted (e.g., persons in nursing homes, those with Medicare as well as Medicaid, or spend down eligibility)" have not been met.[24] No additional targeted groups have been incorporated into the system. Hearings were held about managed care for long-term care clients but no final action has occurred. Second, intentions to move clients into capitated plans from the gatekeeper plan (PSP) and phasing out clinic plans in favor of HMO's have only been partially met. In 1996, Engler's budget recommendations stated that . . . "while Michigan already is a leader in Medicaid managed care programming, it is clear that the state must move toward a comprehensive, capitated (fixed) managed care system if Medicaid costs are to be held to an acceptable level."[25] But 1997 enrollments in PSP's have declined, and enrollments in HMO's and clinic plans have increased. Clinic plans are still in existence, however, and have not been phased out. Third, introduction of competitive bidding for HMO services has only just begun. As of July 1, 1997, the state has awarded competitively bid contracts for HMO services in a few counties (Wayne, Oakland, Macomb, Washtenaw, and Genesee) and will continue expansion in the months ahead. Fourth, plans to allow AFDC recipients to "buy in" to Medicaid and continue coverage by paying premiums, have been accomplished through a $6 million general fund allocation for fiscal year 1998. This fund provides financial assistance to AFDC recipients in order to pay for Medicaid premiums when their transitional welfare health coverage ends.

In April 1996, the policy areas of mental health, public health, and Medicaid were combined into a new Department of Community Health. The new department director, James K. Haveman, Jr., established five workgroups to move toward implementation of these goals. These workgroups were to focus on achieving capitated health plans for (1) the regular Medicaid population; (2) children with special health care needs; (3) behavioral health; (4) the developmentally disabled; and (5) patients in long-term care. These plans are still in progress.

Some of these goals presented greater roadblocks than have been experienced in the past. Bringing mandatory managed care to long-term care clients seemed particularly problematic. In 1990, one of the few conflicts between the state and health care providers erupted. In two separate lawsuits, one by two nursing home associations and the other by the Michigan Hospital Association, it was argued that the state's Medicaid reimbursement rates did not meet federal law. Michigan was ordered to raise reimbursement rates. Without the previous cooperation from providers the state may experience greater difficulties implementing managed care reforms.

Further despite the fact that long-term care clients are a relatively small part of the Medicaid population, they are responsible for a significant share of the program's expenditures. Developing a quality capitated plan has yet to be accomplished.

On Michigan's side is the fact that the aging population is not growing as fast in the state as in the nation as a whole. Michigan is not a traditional retirement state. In addition, the migration of Baby Boomers out of the state during the 1980s decreased the size of this population group in the state. Michigan can delay dealing with these issues far longer than can the nation as a whole.

Another difficulty is likely to arise in moving clients from the PSPs into fully capitated managed care plans. Issues of choice and quality of care have increasingly been raised in connection with HMOs. Also, as we noted above, clients, when given a choice, clearly prefer the more flexible PSPs. So while the Michigan approach has resulted in rather smooth implementation over time, rougher waters may lie ahead.

DISCUSSION AND CONCLUSIONS

Clearly, Medicaid managed care reforms are not unique to Michigan. There are, however, several unique points that need to be highlighted about the implementation of managed care reforms to the program in Michigan.

First, Michigan began implementation of small-scale managed care efforts a decade before more comprehensive reforms were attempted in the early 1990s. The early reforms had an impact on later evaluations of the efficacy of implementing managed care on a larger scale. Michigan already had a tested program to learn from when larger-scale reforms were needed. It was easier to plan with previous information and experience to build on. In particular, the initial efforts gave the state an idea of what infrastructure needed to be in place in order to implement managed care on a large scale. Providers also had experience and a familiarity with managed care in the Medicaid program.

Further, an effective partnership between private health care providers, professional health care organizations, and the state was formed amidst the 1981 reform process. The state continued to effectively rely on this partnership in planning and implementing the larger managed care efforts that followed. This is not to say that the relationship between these groups has not been without its difficulties, but the overall interaction over time has greatly facilitated Michigan's reform efforts.

Another point that needs to be made about the Michigan experience regards the number of choices provided clients. Clients are given three managed care plan options, and each plan contains flexibility with regard to physician choice. Implementation was eased by the availability of options for individual clients.

The staged approach of full-scale managed care also facilitated the relatively smooth implementation of managed care reforms in Michigan. The MSA focused on developing infrastructure first and quick implementation thereafter. The implementation process was gradual compared to other state plans that moved more quickly. Tennessee, for example, made the decision to mandate managed care and implemented the requirement with less than two months to put administrative structures in place to carry out the new program.

Finally, one cannot ignore the role of a motivated policy entrepreneur like John Engler. The reform efforts were clearly related to the changing economic situation and budget pressures in the state. However, Engler skillfully used the opportunity provided by the economic distress and the institutional resources provided him as governor to fundamentally restructure the Medicaid system. Further, he had the cooperation of a Medicaid staff that had developed a high level of competence in the administration of large-scale managed care systems for this population. Along with these factors, Engler had a comprehensive plan relating Medicaid reforms to other entitlement reforms. While we have focused on a single program here, Engler integrates his discussion of welfare programs, SSI, Medicaid, Medicare, state assistance programs into a larger agenda.

The story of Medicaid managed care reform in Michigan is not yet complete. Our analysis highlights the close relationship between economic and political variables. Clearly, managed care reforms were initiated in response to economic realities. However, successful implementation of these efforts would have been much less likely without motivated and skilled political leadership.

NOTES

The authors would like to acknowledge the assistance of Dr. Vernon Smith, Mike Frederick, Farah Arabo, and Don VeCasey. Their willingness to share information, data, and their thoughts about managed care progress in Michigan significantly improved our work. We also wish to thank state Senator Alma Wheeler Smith and Representative Kirk Profit for their input. Previous works that contributed to this chapter were presented at the annual meetings of the Michigan Political Science Association, November 1995, and the annual meetings of the Michigan Academy of Science, Arts and Letters, March 1996.

1. Kathleen O'Leary Morgan, Scott Morgan, and Neal Quinto, *State Rankings 1994: A Statistical View of the 50 United States* (Lawrence, Kans.: Morgan Quinto Corporation, 1994), 479.

2. Public Sector Consultants, Inc., *Michigan in Brief: 1992–93 Issues Handbook* (Grand Ledge, Mich.: Millbrook Printing Company, 1993), 276.

3. Michigan Department of Management and Budget, *Executive Budget, Fiscal Year 1996, State of Michigan, John Engler, Governor* (Lansing, Mich.: Department of Management and Budget, 1996), G-10.

4. Michigan Department of Community Health, "Michigan Department of Community Health FY 97 Executive Budget Recommendations, Senate Appropriations Subcommittee Meeting on Medical Services Administration, March 6, 1996" (Lansing, Mich.: Medical Services Administration, 1996), photocopied, 11.

5. Ibid., 5.

6. William P. Browne, Kenneth VerBerg, Albert F. Palm, and Gregg W. Smith, "Inescapable Partisanship in a Ticket-Splitting State," in William P. Browne and Kenneth VerBerg, eds., *Michigan Politics and Government: Facing Change in a Complex State* (Lincoln: University of Nebraska Press, 1995), 196.

7. William P. Browne, Kenneth VerBerg, Bernard Klein, and Joseph Cepuran, "The Politics of Gubernatorial Leadership," in Brown and VerBerg, eds., *Michigan Politics*, 77.

8. Ibid., 76; Browne, VerBerg, Palm, and Smith, "Ineseapable Partisanship," 366.

9. Lyke Thompson, "The Death of General Assistance in Michigan," in Donald F. Norris and Lyke Thompson, eds., *The Politics of Welfare Reform* (Thousand Oaks, Calif.: Sage Publications, 1995), 79.

10. William P. Browne and Kenneth VerBerg, with contributions from David Murphy, Noelle Schiffer, William Sederburg, and David Verway, "Economic Problems: Issues and Policy," in Browne and VerBerg, eds., *Michigan Politics*, 256.

11. Public Sector Consultants, 33–35.

12. Ibid., 4.

13. Ibid., 5.

14. Ibid., 399.

15. Ibid., 5; Browne and VerBerg, with Murphy, Schiffer, Sederburg, and Verway, "Economic Problems," 254.

16. Vernon Smith, Director, Medical Services Administration, interviewed by authors, Brighton, Michigan, January 23, 1996 and Lansing, Michigan, February 27, 1996; Tom Wolff, Chief of Physician Organization and Legal Affairs, Michigan State Medical Society, interviewed by Michael Harris, May 29, 1996.

17. Thompson, "The Death," 85.

18. Public Sector Consultants, 5.

19. Carol S. Weissert, "Michigan: No More Business as Usual with John Engler," in Thad Beyle, *Governors and Hard Times* (Washington D.C.: CQ Press, 1992); see also Thompson, "The Death," 79.

20. Vernon Smith, interviewed by authors, Brigthon, Michigan, January 23, 1996 and Lansing, Michigan, February 27, 1996. See also "Michigan Medicaid Managed Care Program Summary of Benefits (Lansing, Mich.: Department of Social Services, 1995), photocopied.

21. Information on these plans is drawn primarily from "Michigan Medicaid Managed Care Program Summary of Benefits (Lansing, Mich.: Department of Social Services, 1995), photocopied. Additional information obtained from "PSP, Physician Sponsor Plan: Medicaid answers your questions on PSP" (Lansing, Mich.: Department of Social Services, 1995), photocopied; "HMO: Health Maintenance Organization: Medicaid answers your questions on HMOs" (Lansing, Mich.: Department of Social Services, 1995), photocopied; and "CP, Clinic Plan: Medicaid answers your questions on CPs" (Lansing,

Mich.: Department of Social Services, 1995), photocopied; "Medical Assistance Program Physician Sponsor Plan Contract" (Lansing, Mich.: Department of Social Services, 1995), photocopied.

22. "Michigan Medicaid Managed Care Program Summary of Benefits (Lansing, Mich.: Department of Social Services, 1995), photocopied.

23. Vernon Smith, interviewed by authors, Brigthon, Michigan, January 23, 1996 and Lansing, Michigan, February 23, 1996.

24. Michigan Department of Community Health, 25.

25. Michigan Department of Management and Budget, G10.

10

New York: Medicaid Managed Care in the Empire State

KENT GARDNER AND DAVID BOND

THE POLITICS OF NEW YORK MEDICAID

Like the streets of New York City, the politics of New York health care are turbulent, noisy, and difficult to navigate. Sheer size, the extent of need among its poorer citizens, the political power of its health care industry, and the crude disparity of legislative votes among New York City (NYC), NYC suburbs (including Long Island), and upstate cities and counties combine to belie any simple explanation of Medicaid policy. A thorough explanation of New York's Medicaid morass would require lengthy speculation on relative political power, administrative expediency, and misplaced idealism, followed by lengthy comments on the "law of unintended consequences."

With just over 18 million residents, New York is the third largest state in the nation (just smaller than Texas). The state's Medicaid establishment serves 2.5 million individuals who either qualify through their eligibility for the former Aid to Families with Dependent Children (AFDC) program, Supplemental Security Income (SSI), New York's income maintenance program for singles and childless families, Home Relief (HR), or who are deemed medically needy but do not qualify for cash assistance programs.[1] New York City accounts for the largest concentration of need. With 40% of the state's population, NYC accounts for 68% of Medicaid eligibles and 66% of total spending (see Table 10.1).

New York State has long exercised strict control over its health care industry. New York and Maryland are the last two states to directly regulate hospital rates, although New York's system ended January 1, 1997. As is often the case with regulated industries, health care providers wield tremendous political power in New York and can bring it to bear when the industry's position is threatened. Industry associations and health care unions are experienced advocates, quite

Table 10.1
Medicaid Eligibles in New York State (1994)

Region	AFDC Eligibles	HR Eligibles	SSI Eligibles	MA Only Eligibles	Total Eligibles
Upstate	361,552	59,534	119,304	292,600	832,990
NYC	840,124	164,441	365,048	373,415	1,743,028
State Total	1,201,676	223,975	484,352	666,015	2,576,018

capable of reminding state legislators that the industry employs 741,500 potential voters statewide.[2]

Efforts to reform Medicaid in New York have often foundered as the governor, the state assembly, and the state senate act to protect their traditional constituencies. Geographically, traditionally Democratic NYC holds the largest voting block in the state legislature. Of 150 assembly seats, NYC elects 60, Long Island and the two closest suburban counties (Westchester and Rockland) elect an additional 32, leaving 58 for the rest of the state. Of 61 senate seats, NYC controls 25, Long Island and the two closest suburban counties elect another 12, and 24 remain for the rest of the state (see Figure 10.1).

The two houses of the legislature are each controlled by one of the major parties. The Democrats have firm control over the assembly and the Republicans control the state senate. Courtesy of arcane election laws and blatant gerrymandering, incumbents are difficult or impossible to dislodge. Between 1986 and 1990, 98% of all incumbents were reelected.[3] In the nationally turbulent 1994 election, only one seat in the senate and six seats in the assembly moved from the control of one party to the control of the other.

The balance of power did shift toward the Republican Party and from downstate to upstate in 1994 as Republican state Senator George Pataki defeated Democratic Governor Mario Cuomo, in office since 1982. Upstate interests gained further power following Pataki's election as Joseph Bruno, a Pataki ally representing the Albany area, assumed the post of Senate Majority Leader, dislodging Long Island Senator Ralph Marino.

The Medicaid policy debate centers around the interests of three constituencies: health care recipients, health care providers, and taxpayers. While generalizations often fall prey to the lie of simplification (and this one is no exception), the actions of the assembly, senate, and executive are guided by the wants and needs of these constituencies. The assembly—controlled by urban-based Democrats—has historically defended the interests of Medicaid recipients, thus opposing proposals to limit eligibility and reduce benefits to the indigent. The senate—controlled by suburban Republicans—has historically defended the interests of health care providers, thus opposing proposals to reduce rates of reimbursement to nursing homes, hospitals, and home health care providers. The

Figure 10.1
The Distribution of Power

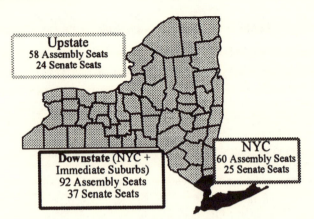

senate has also been wary of restricting eligibility for Medicaid-funded long-term care, services which increasingly support the state's middle class. It falls to the executive to worry about the cost of the entire program, effectively representing the interests of taxpayers.

As the occupant of the governor's mansion is now a Republican, these patterns are shifting. The roles assumed by the two houses of the legislature were influenced by the fact that Mario Cuomo was a Democrat. As the Republican senate was the principal counterweight to Cuomo's executive, its positions partly reflected its opposition role.

The policy debate is driven by the balance of power among the two houses and the executive. Unfortunately, with a politically divided, bicameral legislature, it is difficult for the legislative agenda of any faction to pass intact. One apparent result of New York's political gridlock is that initiatives only pass both houses if they clearly benefit the constituencies of each, thus including benefits for both recipients and providers. New York and federal taxpayers must bear the burden of both generous eligibility rules and liberal access to optional services, along with relatively high rates of reimbursement for the state's medical institutions.[4]

MEDICAID SPENDING IN THE EMPIRE STATE

The Empire State is the nation's leader in both absolute and relative spending on Medicaid. Total federal fiscal year (FY) 1994 spending (including federal, state, and local shares) was $18.7 billion,[5] two-thirds of which was spent in New York City. Total spending in New York exceeded next-highest California by $8.7 billion, despite the fact that California's population exceeds that of New

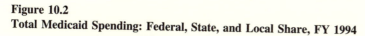

Figure 10.2
Total Medicaid Spending: Federal, State, and Local Share, FY 1994

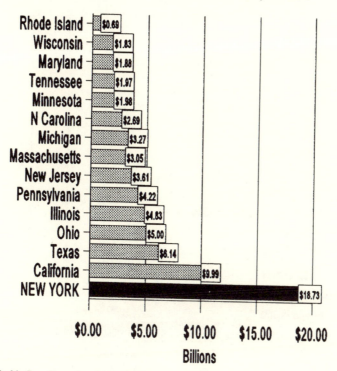

Source: Health Care Financing Administration.

York by 70% (Figure 10.2). In per capita terms, New York spent two and one-half times the average of the rest of the 50 states in FY1994 (Figure 10.3). New York's Medicaid costs are vastly greater than those of other states in virtually all service categories.[6]

Taxes paid by the residents and businesses of the state are dramatically higher as a result of this and other programs. In 1992, state and local taxes per capita in New York were 62% above the average for the rest of the states, second only to Alaska, which effectively "exports" its tax burden to the consumers of oil and gas products.[7]

Both the size and the rate of growth of New York's Medicaid bill are staggering. Between state fiscal years 1983 and 1995, federal, state and county Medicaid expenditures grew from $5.7 billion statewide to over $20 billion. Medicaid spending more than tripled between 1983 and 1995 both in New York City and the rest of the state (Figure 10.4). Half of New York's costs are borne by federal taxpayers (New York's Federal Medicaid Assistance Percentage—FMAP—is 50%), increasing the tax burden on the nation as a whole.

Figure 10.3
Medicaid Spending per Capita, FY 1994

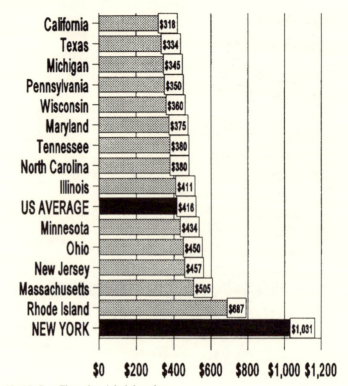

Source: Health Care Financing Administration.

Optional Services

Since Medicaid was enacted in 1965, New York State has endeavored to generate federal matching funds for the health care needs of the poor and elderly. This has resulted in a generous Medicaid plan with a wider variety of optional services provided with fewer restrictions to eligible recipients. It has also resulted in more lenient income requirements than many states. Only one-third of the total New York State Medicaid expenditure was actually required by federal law (Table 10.2). While increasing services and coverage may once have been an affordable strategy for the state to pursue, the dramatic increase in the cost of care has placed an increasing financial burden on federal, state, and county governments.[8]

Only $5.6 billion (32%) of combined federal, state, and county Medicaid spending was federally mandated (Table 10.2). New York State spent $3.7 bil-

Figure 10.4
Total Medicaid Expenditures, 1983–1995

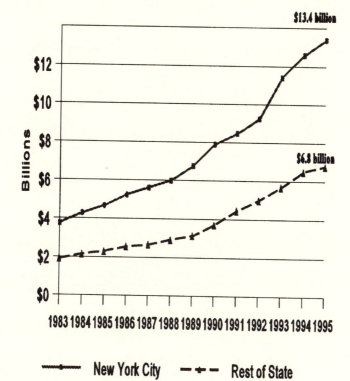

Source: NYS Department of Social Services.

Table 10.2
Medicaid Spending in New York State, FY 1994

	Federally Mandated Spending ($ million)	Percent of Total	N.Y.S. Optional Spending ($ million)	Percent of Total
Categorically Needy	$4,805	25.7	$5,143	27.5
Medically Needy	na	na	$8,783	46.9

Source: Health Care Financing Administration Form 2082, Statistical Report on Medical Care, FY 1994.

lion providing services not required by the federal Medicaid statute to the categorically needy and $8.8 billion on services for the more broadly defined medically needy population. New York also spent $5.1 billion (27% of total Medicaid spending) on long-term care services for the elderly not mandated by the federal government. This included optional services for the categorically needy aged and services for the medically needy aged (see Figure 10.5).

NEW YORK MEDICAID: THE MOST COSTLY PROGRAM IN THE NATION

The Center for Governmental Research (CGR) selected fourteen states for comparison with New York.[9] States selected included most of the nation's major industrial states, states neighboring New York, and selected states known to have implemented a substantially different approach to Medicaid policy (such as Tennessee). The states selected for comparison were California, Illinois, Maryland, Massachusetts, Michigan, Minnesota, New Jersey, North Carolina, Ohio, Pennsylvania, Rhode Island, Tennessee, Texas and Wisconsin. Comparisons are based on the Health Care Financing Administration's Form 2082 for FY 1994 (see Figure 10.6).

Naturally, total spending figures do not tell the whole story. New York State has a larger population than all other states except California and, recently, Texas. Many other demographic features distinguish New York from the comparison states. But if one looks at Medicaid spending by any reasonable standard, New York State is very much out of line. New York spends more than twice the amount per recipient of most other states (Figure 10.7). New York's spending per recipient is almost double that of neighboring Pennsylvania and more than triple that of California.

Median spending on Medicaid per capita in the other states was $416 in FY 1994, while New York spent $1,031 for every state resident (Figure 10.3). Similarly, New York led all states in Medicaid spending as a percent of gross state product (Figure 10.6). New York spent 3.8% of the gross state product of goods and services on Medicaid in 1994 while the median ratio of the other states was only 1.7%. New York's Medicaid expenditure (combined federal, state, and local) was equal to 32% of the total state budget in FY 1994, in contrast to an average of 15.7% for the other states in the comparison (Figure 10.7).

Medicaid Managed Care

In 1991, the New York State legislature passed the statewide Medicaid Managed Care Act, designed to improve the delivery of quality, cost-effective health care through the expansion of managed care. The act encouraged local departments of social services to voluntarily participate in managed care and established participation goals which increase over time. New York State also

Figure 10.5
Medicaid Cost per Recipient, FY 1994

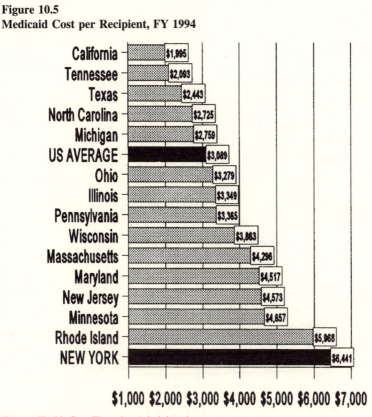

Source: Health Care Financing Administration.

established mandated enrollment in managed care programs in a demonstration project in Southwest Brooklyn established under a federal waiver.

As with many managed care endeavors nationwide, reimbursement at 95% of the estimated fee-for-service cost of care for the enrolled population was sufficient for profitability. Many managed care providers statewide found that enrolling Medicaid eligibles was quite profitable. In New York City, the NYC Health and Hospitals Corporation (HHC)—which traditionally bore much of the burden of indigent care—discovered steadily increasing competition. As of mid-1996, twelve managed care plans (including one operated by HHC) each enroll more than 5,000 eligibles in NYC and many other plans enroll lesser numbers.[10] HHC's Metropolitan Plan is the second largest plan (after Oxford) with just over 12% of Medicaid eligibles enrolled in managed care (48,210). As only 22% of

Figure 10.6
Medicaid Spending, Percent of Gross State Product, FY 1994

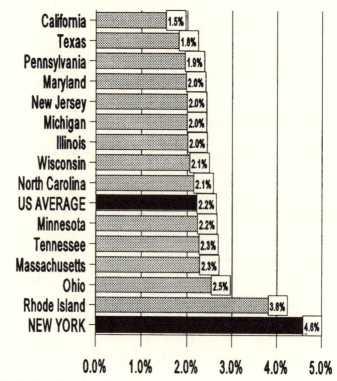

Source: Health Care Financing Administration.

eligibles in NYC are currently covered by managed care, competition for new enrollees has been brisk.[11]

Medicaid Managed Care Penetration in New York State

Use of managed care for Medicaid recipients in New York varies widely within the state. Statewide, about one-quarter of all eligibles are enrolled in managed care plans. In eleven of the state's counties, managed care is virtually invisible with less than 2% of eligibles enrolled in a managed care plan. These are all rural counties, however, and represent only 2% of the state's Medicaid eligibles.

Urban areas are appealing new markets for national and local health care organizations. In thirteen counties, managed care covers over one-third of Medicaid eligibles. All of the state's "Big Five" cities (Yonkers, Albany, Syracuse, Rochester, and Buffalo) are included in this group. Excluding NYC, statewide managed care penetration is about 32%.[12]

Although most of the managed care plans in the state are fully capitated,

Figure 10.7
Medicaid Share of State Spending, Percent of State Spending for FY 1994

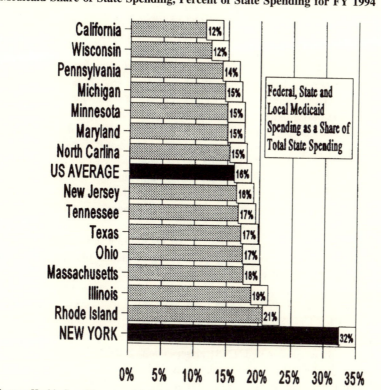

Source: Health Care Financing Administration, *Statistical Abstract of the United States.*

partial capitation plans are common in individual counties. In Erie County (Buffalo), for example, about 14% of managed care enrollees are in a partially capitated plan. Chemung County, the leader in managed care enrollment among Medicaid recipients (with 60% of eligibles covered by a managed care plan), has no fully capitated managed care plan. The Department of Health (DOH) intends to phase out these partial capitation plans within the near future.

Rates for Medicaid Managed Care

Prior to October 1996, rates for Medicaid managed care services were set by reference to estimated fee-for-service (FFS) costs. The NYS DOH set a maximum fee equal to 95% of the predicted FFS expenditure for the population. Not surprisingly, managed care organizations (MCOs) did not choose to set lower rates, although they were invited to do so by the DOH. As a new system for setting rates was in process, capitation rates for 1996 rates were fixed at 1995 levels, subject to an adjustment for the cost of graduate medical education.[13]

The new system for rate determination (part of the state's Partnership Plan, its proposal to institute mandatory managed care for Medicaid recipients) was initiated in the fall of 1995 and took effect October 1, 1996.[14] The New York State Department of Health issued a Request for Proposals (RFP) to MCOs operating statewide. These organizations were invited to bid for the right to provide managed health care services within those counties choosing to participate in the Partnership Plan. In the first phase, 31 of New York's 62 counties were included.[15] Completely voluntary at inception, the state legislature, in summer 1996, made participation mandatory for all counties with a sufficient network of managed care providers. To qualify for participation in the Partnership Plan, counties with more than 350,000 residents must have at least three managed care providers and smaller counties must have at least two managed care providers. According to DOH, twelve counties fail that test. DOH hopes that remaining eligible counties will be phased in during 1997, although the Health Care Financing Administration (HCFA) is urging a more gradual transition to mandatory enrollment in its negotiations with DOH.

The challenge to DOH was to encourage MCOs to bid less than the maximum allowable rate. In cooperation with its consulting actuaries, the department established a set of regionally based rate ranges for each aid category and age/gender cohort. These ranges are based on the expected cost of providing the defined benefit package on an at-risk basis. The rate ranges were not revealed to prospective bidders. MCOs were told that bids above the established range would not be simply reduced to the top of the range, but to a point within the range. After bids were received, DOH either accepted the bid or, in the case of organizations bidding above the band, responded with an offer price equal to the lowest accepted rate within the geographic region. MCOs bidding below the bottom of the range were offered rates equal to the bottom of the rate range.

MANDATORY MANAGED CARE ENROLLMENT FOR MEDICAID RECIPIENTS

New York was not the first state to request a Section 1115 Waiver from the HCFA to require Medicaid recipients to enroll in managed care. Its waiver application may be the most sweeping, however. Originally submitted to HCFA in March of 1995, HCFA approved the waiver in August of 1996, subject to a set of terms and conditions to be negotiated with the state. As of this writing, closure on these conditions had not been reached. HCFA is focusing particular attention on ensuring that the statewide network of providers is sufficient to meet the needs of the Medicaid population and that participants have sufficient protection from possible managed care organization abuses. HCFA is also concerned about the ambitious timetable proposed by New York. A DOH press release indicates that HCFA is seeking a two-year phase-in, while the state wishes to move more quickly.

The scope of the New York waiver proposal sets it apart. Rather than simply excluding individuals with special needs from the managed care population, New York solicited bids from "special needs plans" (SNPs) to manage the care of these individuals. DOH estimates that approximately 100,000 Medicaid recipients are diagnosed with serious mental illnesses or serious behavioral disturbances. The concept proposed by New York DOH includes a "split capitation" scheme in which seriously and persistently mentally ill adults or seriously emotionally disturbed children will be enrolled in both a conventional managed care organization and a mental health SNP. The state will pay a "health only" capitation to the conventional managed care organization and a separate mental health capitation rate to the SNP. Although the SNP assumes all risk for the enrollee's care, the state will establish stop-loss provisions and a reinsurance program for both classes of provider. The SNPs will be permitted to develop the capacity to serve both physical and mental health needs of their enrollees. DOH has proposed a population-based capitation rate (set by estimated incidence of serious mental illness) for rural areas and a more conventional, user-based approach for metropolitan areas where incidence of mental illness is higher.

SNPs will also be established for individuals with HIV, although HIV SNPs will not be at risk for extended nursing home stays. The capitation rates will include nursing home services subject to a 45-day limit, after which the patient reverts to the FFS system. Home care will be included in the capitation rate, subject to stop-loss limitations. DOH reports that twelve proposals from prospective SNPs have been received to date.

The shift to mandatory managed care enrollment was facilitated by passage of wide-ranging managed care legislation in July of 1996. This legislation grew out of an extensive dialogue among stake-holders and the state, and provides numerous protections for enrollees of MCOs. MCOs will now have to provide enrollees information on prior authorization and grievance procedures, provision for 24-hour coverage and emergency services, utilization review mechanisms, and procedures for accessing specialty care. The law also prohibits "gag clauses," adopts a "prudent layperson" approach to defining emergencies, and improves access to specialty care for individuals with life-threatening, degenerative, or disabling conditions.[16]

Long-Term Care

Like many states, New York has participated in demonstrations of managed care vehicles as a means of stabilizing the state's rising expenditure on long-term care. For state fiscal year 1995, total long-term care expenditures approached $8 billion (Figure 10.8). Spending per recipient in New York is substantially higher for both nursing home care and home health care (Figures 10.9 and 10.10).[17]

Figure 10.8
Total Long-Term Care Medicaid Expenditures, 1983–1995

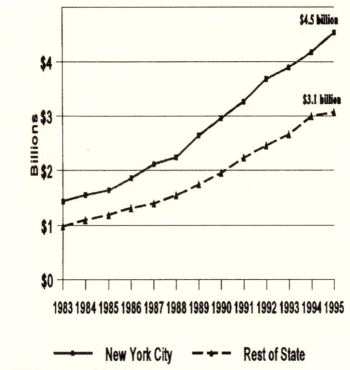

$4.5 billion

$3.1 billion

New York City   — ◆ — Rest of State

Source: NYS Department of Social Services.

The Program of All-Inclusive Care for the Elderly (PACE) is a program with eleven nationwide sites sponsored by the Robert Wood Johnson Foundation. There are two PACE sites in New York, one in the Bronx (Comprehensive Care Management) and one in Rochester (Independent Living for Seniors).[18] While both sites have average costs that are 78% of estimated nursing home costs, researchers suggest that PACE projects often enroll individuals who are more healthy than the general population of nursing home residents.

New York also participates in the Social Health Maintenance Organization (SHMO) demonstration with a site in Brooklyn. Both initiatives include "dual capitation" in which Medicare and Medicaid funds are pooled to provide all acute and long-term care services.[19]

The high cost of NYS home health care (Figure 10.10) has spurred the state to attempt to limit cost in a variety of ways. The Pataki administration proposed limits on the number of eligible hours of home care during the 1995–1996 budget process, but well-organized and well-funded opposition by a combination of home care providers and advocacy groups defeated the initiative. During the

Figure 10.9
Medicaid Nursing Home Costs per Recipient, FY 1994

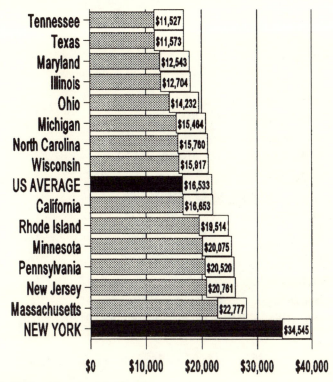

Source: Health Care Financing Administration.

1996–1997 budget deliberations, the administration successfully passed an initiative to establish fourteen pilot projects that will incorporate capitated reimbursement for home care.

CONCLUSION

The disproportionate cost of New York's Medicaid system will not be eliminated simply through mandatory managed care or through an application of managed care to long-term care. Nonetheless, the attempts by the Pataki administration to address needed changes in benefit levels, to eliminate perverse incentives for providers, and to undertake the radical overhaul in delivery of care embodied in various managed care initiatives should begin the process of slowing the rate of increase in local tax rates, reducing already high state taxes, and limiting the share of burden placed on residents of other states by New York's "Medicaid Empire." Even if the cost savings of moving to managed care are only 10% (the savings measured in the Brooklyn managed care pilot

Figure 10.10
Medicaid Home Health Care: Cost per Recipient, FY 1994

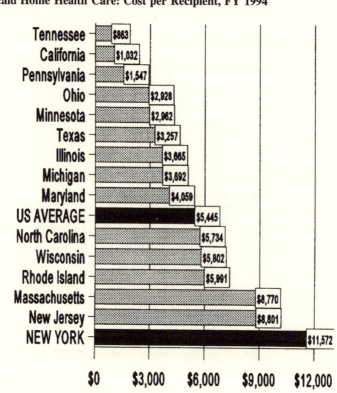

Source: Health Care Financing Administration.

project), the magnitude of New York's Medicaid program guarantees that the absolute savings will be sizeable. Applying the managed care vehicle to "special needs" populations and long-term care is also innovative. As special needs populations and long-term care users represent a disproportionate share of total spending, the inclusion of these populations in managed care could significantly reduce total cost. If the "special needs organizations" and capitated long-term care pilots are properly designed and overseen, individuals requiring more intensive care could receive better care at lower cost.

NOTES

1. New York State (hereafter NYS) Department of Health Bureau of Managed Care, WMS Report, July 1996.

2. NYS Department of Labor, *Employment Review*, April 1996.

3. Kenneth Silber, "New York's Nightmare Legislature," *City Journal* (Spring 1995) (Citing study by National Conference of State Legislators).

4. One exception is physician reimbursement. New York has nearly the lowest physician reimbursement rates in the nation, which had the effect of limiting access to primary care. The response of the state was to establish a network of public health clinics that are reimbursed on the basis of actual costs and are not subject to the restrictive physician reimbursement rate schedule.

5. U.S. Department of Health and Human Services, Health Care Financing Administration, Form 2082.

6. See *Medicaid Cost Containment: Options for New York*, Center for Governmental Research Inc., 1995; and *Medicaid Cost Containment: Statistical Supplement*, Center for Governmental Research Inc., 1996.

7. U.S. Department of Commerce, Bureau of the Census, *State and Local Government Finance 1991–92*.

8. Unlike most states, New York shifts a significant portion of the financial burden for Medicaid onto local government. Counties pay half of the state's share for most acute and ambulatory care expenses, although the local share of long-term care costs and care for the developmentally disabled is much lower.

9. *Medicaid Cost Containment: Options for New York*.

10. NYS Department of Health, Bureau of Managed Care Financing, WMS Report, July 1996.

11. Excesses by overzealous managed care organizations forced the state to place a moratorium on direct enrollment in New York City. Enrollment in managed care plans was delegated to social service district employees. The Health Care Financing Administration has been encouraging the state to contract with an enrollment "broker" to encourage enrollment without the risk of fraudulent practice by managed care organizations.

12. NYS Department of Social Services, Medicaid Management Information System, *Capitation Enrollment Report*, August 1996.

13. Previously bundled into hospital rates, a central pool for compensating hospitals for the cost of graduate medical education was put in place in 1996.

14. A more extended discussion of the waivered portion of the Partnership Plan and the particulars of the Section 1115 Waiver under negotiation between the Health Care Financing Administration and the State of New York appears in the section titled "Mandatory Managed Care Enrollment for Medicaid Recipients." The rate-setting mechanism, while part of the Partnership Plan, is within the powers of the state and is not part of the waiver discussion.

15. Although only half of the counties of the state chose to participate in the first phase of the Partnership Program, all the major population centers of the state are included. Five of the 31 counties are the five boroughs of New York City.

16. NYS Assembly Bill 11328.

17. State officials suggest that the spending in NYS nursing homes reflects the use of an "all-inclusive" reimbursement rate. Direct comparisons with other states are inaccurate as the cost of therapies and treatments are all considered "nursing home" expenditures in New York, but are treated separately in other states.

18. *Independent Living for Seniors: A Longitudinal Evaluation*, Center for Governmental Research Inc., 1994.

19. Brent Gustafson, *Financing Medicaid Long Term Care in New York: An Analysis of the Possibilities and Challenges of Managed Care* (New York State Division of the Budget, April 9, 1996). Cites 1994 Abt Associates study of PACE programs.

11

OhioCare: The Waiver That Wasn't

JAMES BOEX, LAURA C. YANCER, AND TERRY F. BUSS

INTRODUCTION AND BACKGROUND

In 1990, citizens elected George Voinovich, a Republican, Ohio governor, following former Governor Richard Celeste, a Democrat, not noted for his fiscal management skills. Voinovich had previously served as mayor of Cleveland, following Dennis Kucinich, a Democrat, notorious for bankrupting the city. As mayor, Voinovich straightened out Cleveland's finances, and in the process propelled himself into the governorship. He ran, and was elected, as a manager and fiscal conservative whose platform was to reform Ohio's government as he had Cleveland's. He was overwhelmingly reelected in 1994, largely because of his successful first term.

Ohio's Constitution requires government to operate within a balanced budget, even in the face of declining revenues, diminishing resources, and downsizing, while at the same time trying to satisfy increasing demand for education, criminal justice, welfare, and health care, especially Medicaid. In Ohio, from 1988 to 1993, Medicaid recipients grew at a rate of 6% per year, with Medicaid expenditures increasing 16.5% annually,[1] endangering the Voinovich administration's fiscal gains for other programs. On March 2, 1994, the Voinovich administration responded to this pressure by petitioning the Health Care Financing Administration (HCFA) for a Waiver of Section 1115 of the Social Security Act in order to replace its standard Medicaid program with a five-year demonstration project, OhioCare, a program which would have imposed constraints on the existing program, expanded coverage, and enhanced quality. On January 20, 1995, following intense negotiations with the HCFA, the waiver was approved. Enabling legislation to implement OhioCare was never passed by the Ohio legislature. This chapter discusses the waiver that wasn't.

In the following analysis, unless otherwise cited, all data are drawn from the waiver application and from correspondence with the HCFA during the negotiation process prior to OhioCare's approval.

Ohio Medicaid Facts

In FY92, 13% of Ohio's population of 11, 016,388 was on Medicaid, receiving $4.3 billion in health care services. Children in poverty represented 54% of those covered, but received only 20% of funding for services. Adults in poverty constituted 24% of the beneficiaries, but received only 13% of funding. The aged, blind, and disabled, together represented the remaining 22% of participants, while receiving 68% of expenditures.[2] For 1993, this averaged $1,031 per enrollee under age 21, $1,668 per adult, $7,888 for the disabled or blind, and $9,138 for elders. In addition to the 1.4 million beneficiaries under Medicaid, another 1.1 million Ohioans, or 10%, were uninsured in 1992.[3]

OHIO MAKES ITS CASE: THE WAIVER APPLICATION

OhioCare's Goals[4]

Ohio's waiver application listed three goals: (1) Health care services for up to a half million more Ohioans; (2) Better, more affordable care with emphasis on prevention; (3) Controlled state Medicaid spending. The waiver's goals section began with the statement:

Medicaid costs in Ohio are absorbing an increasing proportion of the state's budget. Despite these high costs, almost half a million Ohioans living below the federal poverty level remain uninsured. This is the predominant reason that Ohio requests a research and demonstration waiver.

It then listed the following seven items reiterated throughout the application:

1. Expand Health Care Access Up to 500,000 Individuals
2. Use Managed Care to Contain Growth in Medicaid Costs
3. Use Ohio's Experience in Large-Scale Risk-Based Managed Care
4. Emphasize Preventive Care
5. Extend the Capitated Payment System to State Agencies that Provide Special Health-Related Benefits
6. Improve Both Intra-and Intergovernmental Cooperation
7. Effectively Address Service Delivery Issues that Arise

BENEFITS AND BENEFICIARIES

Basic Benefit Package

OhioCare's basic benefit package did not differ strikingly from the original Ohio Medicaid program. It included most physician services, hospital inpatient services, laboratory and x-ray services, prescription drug coverage, dental services (including orthodontia for children), some vision care, some home health and hospice care, and others. The only major benefit provided in OhioCare, but not covered under Ohio Medicaid, was hospice.

Special Health-Related Services Carve-Out

Ohio Medicaid coverage for mental health and drug/alcohol addiction services was capitated under OhioCare, but singled out in a special "carve-out" section with its own rules and regulations.

Aged, Blind, and Disabled Essentially Excluded

Elderly, blind, and disabled beneficiaries, consumers of two-thirds of Ohio's Medicaid budget, would not be phased into OhioCare until late in the five-year waiver period or would remain in fee-for-service settings. Long-term care patients, consumers of most of Ohio's Medicaid payments, were excluded from OhioCare.

Expanded Access to 100% of Poverty

The proposal offered access to Medicaid coverage of individuals and families with incomes up to 100% of the federal poverty level, while continuing to cover all previously eligible Medicaid participants. An estimated 500,000 previously uninsured Ohioans would be covered. New enrollee application and certification processes were simplified to save administrative overhead.

MANAGED CARE

Mandatory Enrollment

Medicaid recipients under OhioCare enrolled in managed care plans for six months without any possibility of withdrawal except for just cause. Disenrollment possibility from one plan necessitated enrollment in another. Individuals not making a timely selection were assigned, on a rotating basis, to a managed care plan.

Managed Care Providers and Capitation Rates

OhioCare contracted with managed care providers (MCPs) county-by-county (or multi-county for rural areas) on the basis of RFPs for each area. Contract-eligible providers included all licensed Ohio health maintenance organizations (HMOs) and alternative licensing arrangements providing medical service to underserved areas. Capitation rates were set based on historic costs of basic health care in a Medicaid managed care setting.

Managed Care Outreach

Recognizing the need to educate eligible populations about OhioCare changes, outreach efforts, including brochures and personal assistance, were provided. The campaign's goal was to convert existing Medicaid recipients from fee-for-services Medicaid to OhioCare's enrollment in an MCP.

Care for Vulnerable Populations

MCPs would be required to satisfy criteria for Federally Qualified Health Centers (FQHCs) and Title X family planning clinics. Plans were required to contract with providers where they existed, unless they demonstrated capacity to serve vulnerable populations in their area without contracts. Standards and criteria for these determinations were left unspecified.

PREVENTION

Prenatal Care

Existing Medicaid managed care regulations required MCPs to achieve a 70% compliance rate in reporting data on number of prenatal visits, birth weights, and other indicators. Under OhioCare, the Ohio Department of Human Services established a nearly 100% compliance rate, but at an unspecified future date. In addition, specific standards for enrollees with deliveries were established based on recommendations of the American College of Obstetrics and Gynecology, and advice of professional review committees. If standards were not complied with, renewal of MCP's provider status might be affected.

Immunizations

Through MCP, parents were provided with follow-up and assistance to ensure that children received required immunizations and other services. Immunization standards followed the American Academy of Pediatrics. Annual quality assurance surveys established a 70% compliance rate. Ability to assure satisfactory compliance was evaluated at MCP's renewal and actual performance considered in provider agreements.

Early Periodic Screening, Diagnosis, and Treatment (EPSTD) "Healthchek"

Ohio Department of Health Services previously required all Medicaid HMOs to meet federal requirements for federally mandated primary and preventive care for children. In 1995, this required 80% compliance with EPSDT. MCPs not in compliance with utilization and quality assurance requirements completed action plans detailing how future compliance would be met.

COSTS AND COST SAVINGS

Waiver Cost Savings

Waiver approval would reduce Ohio's Medicaid expenditures by $895 million, or 2% of the total projected Ohio Medicaid expenditures over that period. $545 million of those savings would accrue to the federal government, leaving $390 million in savings for Ohio.

Costs Not Affected by Waiver

OhioCare would not affect Medicaid expenditures for long-term institutional care, such as nursing homes. Over the waiver's five-year life, expenditures would continue to represent 56% of all program expenditures, in the pre-waiver period.

ANALYSIS: ASSESSING PRIORITIES AMONG OHIOCARE'S GOALS

Expand Health Care Access up to 500,000 Individuals

According to the waiver application, numbers of new beneficiaries to be added to Ohio's Medicaid rolls without OhioCare would be in excess of 450,000, for a total of 1.65 million. OhioCare's estimates of maximum numbers of individuals covered while maintaining required budget neutrality ranged from 1.75 million to 1.92 million.[5] Numbers of individuals to be added to coverage by OhioCare ranged from as low as 100,000 to as high as 300,000, or 20 to 60% of the stated goal.

Use Managed Care to Contain Growth in Medicaid Costs

Health services literature indicates that moving patients from a fee-for-service to a managed care environment results in approximately 10% lower costs:

through lower utilization rates and cost-shifting to other providers.[6] But OhioCare did not calculate any savings due to this shift. Further, OhioCare only influenced acute care spending, less than half of the state's Medicaid expenditures.

Use Ohio's Experience in Large-Scale Risk-Based Managed Care

At the time of the waiver application, managed care services in Ohio had not reached levels attained in many states. In the state's three largest markets—Cleveland, Cincinnati, Columbus—managed care penetration in 1993 was 20, 18, and 22%, respectively. Coopers & Lybrand, one of the nation's largest management consulting firms, categorizes markets at this level as "emerging." In other major Ohio markets it was lower: in Northeastern Ohio—Akron, Canton, and Youngstown—managed care penetration was at 1, 3, and 3%, respectively.[7]

OhioCare required managed care for over 1,750,000 beneficiaries. Ohio's past experience with Medicaid managed care populations was 43,400 beneficiaries and its total experience with managed care was 170,000, less than 2 to 10%, respectively, of OhioCare's participation. The quality of that experience, too, was called into question in a series of articles which appeared in Ohio's largest newspaper in the summer of 1995.[8]

Emphasize Preventive Care

In Ohio in 1990, rates for births both under 2,500 grams (low birth weight) and under 1,500 grams (very low birth weight) exceeded the national mean: 13.8 versus 12% and 2.9 versus 2.5%, respectively. Percentage of women not receiving care in the first trimester of pregnancy was 18.6%, and 33.8% in the nonwhite population.[9] Ohio's infant mortality rate of 9.1% also exceeded the national mean.[10]

OhioCare's emphasis on quality and preventive care is based on market incentives inherent in managed care, rather than regulation. However, considering prenatal care, for example, health services literature is clear that shifting Medicaid recipients from fee-for-service to managed care results in no improvement in prenatal care and does not affect numbers of low birth weight babies born to Medicaid mothers.[11]

Considering immunizations and child care, with the exception of federally mandated EPSTD programs, MCPs were not required to take part in OhioCare to meet prevention guidelines. These are mentioned only as desirable outcomes, with some thought to be given in the future as to how a given provider's failure to meet standards (yet to be developed) might affect contract renewal.

Capitated Payments and Intergovernmental Cooperation

The OhioCare proposal was developed by an interagency task force headed by the governor's office and Ohio Department of Human Services, the agency of Ohio government with fiscal and structural responsibility for Medicaid. Under the OhioCare proposal, many diverse programs overseen by state agencies would be centralized under Ohio Department of Human Services. This increased efficiency in managing Medicaid programs.

In explaining increased access at reduced costs, Ohio suggested that state programs not previously eligible for federal funding matches would, when combined under OhioCare, result in increased federal matching funds. Currently, the federal government contributes approximately 60% of all Medicaid patient care funds expended in Ohio. OhioCare increased the federal contribution above the 60% level, shifting more costs to the federal partner.

Address Service Delivery Issues

This open-ended goal cannot be analyzed as stated: no information was provided. But, the relative lack of priority given to access, prevention, and quality of care issues, as noted above, casts doubt on OhioCare's capacity to attack these anticipated problems and issues.

SUMMARY

The title page of the OhioCare waiver application contains a map of Ohio and a subtitle "a more rational use of public funds." This subtitle appears to be apt in that it reflected the proposal's high-priority goals of controlling costs as follows:

1. by allowing more of those whose care was previously underwritten completely within Ohio to receive managed care benefits under Medicaid, with federal government providing a majority of the payment;

2. by improving state management and consolidating a number of decentralized programs under leadership of the governor's office and administration of the Ohio Department of Human Services;

3. by obtaining an even higher level of federal matching funds for Medicaid than previously.

OHIOCARE'S FUTURE AND THE REPUBLICAN REVOLUTION

In November 1994, in what has come to be called the "Republican Revolution," national congressional elections put the Republican Party in the majority in both the House of Representatives and the Senate. Among the changes brought about was naming Congressman John Kasich, R-Ohio, chairman of the House Budget Committee. Within six weeks, Ohio became the first state with a Republican administration to receive approval from the Clinton administration for a Medicaid Waiver demonstration project.

At the time of the announcement, the governor's offfice issued a statement, parts of which are quoted below, confirming the analysis in Section III, above:

The centerpiece of OhioCare is a refinancing of the state Medicaid program to extend benefits to tens of thousands of Ohio's low-income working families without requiring new state dollars and without reducing the scope of existing benefits. This will be accomplished by better leveraging and redirecting existing dollars spent on health care. Previous state investments in health care services that received no matching federal dollars such as funds spent on the General Assistance/Disability Assistance program medical components will draw new federal match . . . OhioCare is a fiscally sound approach to expanding care to Ohio's working poor, Voinovich said. Medicaid is currently the single largest item in the state budget and, without reform, will continue to grow beyond our projections and beyond our pocketbooks.

The current Medicaid system operates on what is known as a 60/40 match, meaning that for every $1 the state of Ohio spends on Medicaid services, the federal government contributes 60 cents. OhioCare will maximize the amount of federal matching dollars for which the state is eligible, to cover more people and promote enhanced quality of care. According to Ohio Department of Human Services Director Tompkins:

the same basic medical and dental benefits now offered to Medicaid recipients will be funded with existing state dollars and a combination of existing and new federal dollars. Additional federal dollars will be drawn down when state-only dollars currently used for the general assistance and disability assistance medical program, as well as those funds used in the hospital care assurance program, are allocated for OhioCare's basic benefits package. Special health-related services will be funded with local government dollars including ongoing state subsidies which will be combined and utilized in a way to maximize the amount of matching federal dollars drawn down. . . . We don't want to jeopardize that [community] relationship or the community networks that have developed to serve those needing treatment for mental illness, alcohol or drug addiction, mental retardation or developmental disabilities, said Tompkins. We only want to make as much federal funding available for these services as possible and streamline a system currently plagued by red tape. Persons covered for long-term care facility services and home- and community-based services waiver programs will remain in fee-for-service for basic benefits during the five-year demonstration.[12]

Block Grants Change Assumptions

Ironically, after receiving its Medicaid Waiver, the Voinovich administration questioned its ability to implement OhioCare. Welfare Block Grant proposals for Medicaid, offered by the Republican Congress in its Contract with America, allowed state governments more flexibility in the use of Medicaid funds, while reducing annual increases in the federal Medicaid matching rate from an anticipated 6.5 to 7.3% (as contained in the approved waiver) to only 5%.[13] In addition, "Special Health Related Services," as requested under the waiver, would not draw additional federal matching funds under block grants. The combined effect of these two changes reduced OhioCare's estimated budget by approximately $500 million per year.[14]

The federal shift in Medicaid's funding and control essentially doomed OhioCare. By the spring of 1995, the Ohio Department of Human Services publicly withdrew from its primary goal of increasing Medicaid enrollment. In addition, the Department announced that it might not be able to sustain existing levels of coverage.[15]

On January 26, 1996, more than a year after OhioCare's approval, in his annual State of the State address, Governor Voinovich stated: "OhioCare is great news for Ohio's working poor, and I applaud Speaker Davidson and President Aronoff for appointing a joint House-Senate committee to immediately begin hearings on OhioCare so that we can move forward with implementation."[16] As of October 1996, no hearings on OhioCare have been held or scheduled.

OhioCare's demise has not meant, however, the end of Medicaid managed care in Ohio. Mandatory statewide enrollment of Medicaid acute care patients into managed care plans continues.[17] By July 1, 1996, 14 plans enrolled 38% of Ohio's total eligible Medicaid population into managed care. In the 7 urban counties where managed care is mandatory for ADC Medicaid recipients, 32,897 enrolled, while in 10 counties where enrollment was voluntary, 24,181 participated.[18] The enrollment of Medicaid recipients into managed care has continued, to the point where HCFA, in its February 21 update to its web page (http://www.hcfa.gov) ranks Ohio as 18th among the 50 states in managed care enrollment as of June 30 1996, with 239,306 enrollees. ODHS' own web page (http://www.ohio.gov/ODHS) states that "by the end of 1998, 78% of eligible Medicaid consumers will access care through a managed care system."

Plans to study utilization, cost, and effectiveness of Medicaid managed care exist,[19] and some preliminary data are available. 1994 data, comparing managed care Medicaid and fee-for-service Medicaid recipients' utilization patterns show that managed care groups had fewer inpatient days, shorter lengths of stay, and fewer emergency visits.[20] Policymakers hope that managed care rates, set 6% below those prevailing for fee-for-service, will result in correspondingly lower costs.[21] To date, the only evaluation study undertaken by the Ohio Department of Human Services was an August 1995 telephone survey of recipients in mandatory participation counties.[22] About three-fourths of the sample was found to be invalid, leading survey researchers to speculate: "a significant portion of the population may not have been reached by the survey." On a five-point scale, with "3" as "good," 82% reported receiving good or better quality care, 77% at least good medical care, and 73% at least good access to specialty care. On other measures, 9% reported being unaware that they had enrolled in a manged care plan. Some 17% reported having to wait more than two days for an appointment with their managed care plan for a medical problem, and 40% did not know how to report a medical problem to their plan.[23]

In trying to be innovative in health care, Ohio extended itself beyond other states in developing OhioCare. Considerable public and private resources were expended in preparing for OhioCare, only to see them wasted. Hospitals, in anticipation of OhioCare, hired new staff to compete for contracts which never materialized. Political capital to gain consensus on OhioCare went for naught.

In a rapidly changing policy environment, the lesson for states may be: don't innovate, follow the crowd.

NOTES

1. Diane Rowland et al., *Health Needs and Medicaid Financing: State Facts* (Washington, D.C.: Kaiser Commission on the Future of Medicaid, April 1995.)

2. American Academy of Pediatrics, *Medicaid State Report: Ohio* (Elk Grove Village, Ill.: Division of Health Policy Research, 1994).

3. Rowland et al., *Health Needs*. 1995.

4. Ohio Department of Human Services, *OhioCare: A More Rational Use of Public Resources* (application to HCFA for a waiver of Section 1115, Social Security Act, Columbus, Ohio, 1994).

5. Steven Hoffman, "Medicaid Reformers Make OhioCare Ill," *Akron Beacon Journal* (April 9, 1995).

6. J. Holahan et al., "Explaining the Recent Growth in Medicaid Spending," *Health Affairs* 12, no. 3 (Fall 1993); H. H. Schauffler and T. Rodriguez, "Availability and Utilization of Health Promotion Programs and Satisfaction with Health Plans," *Medical Care* 32, no. 12 (December 1994).

7. Interstudy, Inc., "Metropolitan Market Update," *Interstudy Competitive Edge* (Minneapolis, Minn., April 25, 1994).

8. D. Lane and J. M. Mazzolini, "Emergency Care is Primary Care for Many Poor," *Cleveland Plain Dealer* (June 25, 1995); J. M. Mazzolini and D. Lane, "Medicaid HMO Plan a Loser for Taxpayers," *Cleveland Plain Dealer* (June 25, 1995).

9. American Academy of Pediatrics, 1994.

10. Rowland et al., *Health Needs*.

11. P. A. Beuscher and N. I. Ward, "A Comparison of Low Birth Weight Among Medicaid Patients of Public Health Departments and Other Providers of Prenatal Care in North Carolina and Kentucky," *Public Health Reports* 107, no. 1 (January–February 1992); T. Carey, K. Weiss, and C. Homer, "Prepaid versus Traditional Medicaid Plans: Lack of Effect on Pregnancy Outcomes and Prenatal Care," *HSR: Health Services Research* 26, no. 2 (June 1991); J. W. Krieger, F. A. Connell, and J. P. LoGerfo, "Medicaid Prenatal Care: A Comparison of Use and Outcomes in Fee-for-Service and Managed Care," *American Journal of Public Health* 82 (February 2, 1992); J. Huntington and F. A. Connell, "For Every Dollar Spent—The Cost Savings Argument for Prenatal Care," *New England Journal of Medicine* 331, no. 19 (November 10, 1994); and C. N. Oberg et al., "Prenatal Care Use and Health Insurance Status," *Journal of Health Care for the Poor and Underserved* 2, no. 2 (Fall, 1991).

12. M. Dawson, *Governor Announces Federal Approval of Medicaid Reform Plan* (press release, Office of the Governor, State of Ohio, Columbus Ohio, January 17, 1995).

13. C. Winterbottom, D. W. Lisker, and K. M. Obermaier, *State-Level Databook on Health Care Access and Financing* (Washington, D.C.: The Urban Institute, 1995).

14. Hoffman, ''Medicaid Reformers.''

15. Ibid.; Lane and Mazzolini, ''Emergency Care''; Mazzolini and Lane, ''Medicaid HMO Plan.''

16. G. Voinovich, *State of the State Address* (Office of the Governor, State of Ohio, Columbus, Ohio, January 26, 1996).

17. Hoffman, ''Medicaid Reformers''; Lane and Mazzolini, ''Emergency Care''; Mazzolini and Lane, ''Medicaid HMO Plan.''

18. Burnell, ''Ohio Medicaid Managed Care Program'' (Columbus: Ohio Department of Human Services, memorandum, July 1996).

19. Arnold R. Tompkins, ''Invitation to Participate in Medicaid Related Health Services Research'' (memorandum from Ohio Department of Human Services, December 1995).

20. Burnell, ''Ohio Medicaid.''

21. E. L. Baker et al., ''Health Care Reform and the Health of the Public,'' *Journal of the American Medical Association* 272, no. 16 (October 26, 1994); D. Lipson, ''Public Health Must be a Priority for Reform to Succeed,'' *State Initiatives in Health Care Reform* (Washington, D.C.: Alpha Center/Robert Wood Johnson Foundation, May/June 1994).

22. Strasser, *Quality Assurance Reform Initiative Quantitative Report* (Columbus: Ohio Department of Human Services, August 1995).

23. Ibid.

12

SoonerCare: Reforming Medicaid with Managed Care Oklahoma Style

WILLIAM PARLE AND RON WOOSLEY

This chapter examines the creation and implementation, to date, of SoonerCare, Oklahoma's new managed care program for Medicaid clients. It begins by reviewing the policy debate over health care in Oklahoma that preceded reform and remains ongoing. The major features of SoonerCare and its implementation to date are discussed. Finally, the authors draw on the literature of both political science and managed care in an effort to offer an assessment of the potential of SoonerCare as a vehicle for containing program costs and making efficient use of health resources.

BACKGROUND

In the late 1980s and early 1990s the Oklahoma economy was recovering from the energy crisis of the early and mid-1980s. In 1990, under Governor Henry Bellmon, the state undertook an extensive overhaul of its K-12 educational program. This much needed reform was both controversial and expensive. It committed much of the state's anticipated revenue growth to education and required an increase in taxes. Two years later conservative forces within the state were successful in obtaining passage of a tax limitation initiative. Known as Proposition 640, this initiative required a vote of the people before taxes could be increased.

In 1993, the State Department of Human Services (DHS), at the time the state Medicaid agency, attempted to alleviate a shortfall in Medicaid funding by promoting a tax on health care providers. This was the first issue to arise under Proposition 640. While most providers appeared to go along with this measure as a necessary evil for obtaining federal funds, it was strongly opposed by

nursing homes. In Oklahoma's conservative political climate the measure failed
to obtain popular support. The failure of the provider tax forced the DHS to
embark on a series of cuts and in 1993 the state enacted new limits on Medicaid-
covered services. These included restrictions on hospital days, physician visits,
prescriptions, and diagnostic services for adults.[1] Many physicians responded to
fee schedule cuts and billing difficulties by refusing to see Medicaid patients.

In the meantime, as the newly installed Clinton administration focused national attention on major health care reform, states began to respond to the
possibility of changes in federal policy. Oklahoma was no exception. In February 1992, the Commission on Oklahoma Health Care was created by then
newly elected Democratic Governor David Walters. This Commission, chaired
by Dr. Garth Splinter, was charged with studying Oklahoma's health care system
and making recommendations for improving it. The commission finished its
work and reported to the governor in November 1992.[2]

In its 1992 report the Commission took the position that "all Oklahomans
have a right to basic health services."[3] It identified rising health care costs and
lack of access to health care as the two major problems facing the existing health
care system. It recommended (1) the development of a system of health care
financing based on a regulated market approach, (2) an emphasis on primary
care and prevention, (3) health-related tort reform, and (4) the use of a public
authority model to implement and oversee reform.[4]

While the report indicated an overall direction for reform, it did not make
detailed recommendations because of time and resource constraints and the magnitude of the issues involved. The Oklahoma legislature, however, found merit
in the report and established a Health Care Study Commission in the office of
the governor to continue the work of the previous commission. This action, in
effect, reconstituted the Commission with a legislative mandate.[5] Dr. Garth
Splinter also chaired this new commission.

Following its legislative mandate, the Commission built on the work of its
predecessor. It explored a number of specific reform models. These included
proposed federal reforms, as well as many reform approaches with which other
states were beginning to experiment. The Commission also sought input from
individuals and groups around the state concerned with health care in Oklahoma.
Significantly, the Cost Containment and Finance Sub-Committee of the Commission recommended that the state attempt to control health care costs by implementing a system of managed care.[6] This was the approach ultimately
adopted for Medicaid reform.

Through a grant received from the Robert Wood Johnson foundation, a comprehensive plan for reform, the Oklahoma Family Choice Plan, was proposed.
This plan involved the creation of individual family health accounts, which
could be used to purchase health insurance and other health benefits. Existing
sources would fund these accounts. The plan would require insurance companies
to offer standard basic benefit packages, and would prohibit them from denying
coverage because of preexisting conditions. Accounts would be held and ad-

ministered as a public trust. Income from the accounts could be used to help extend coverage to the uninsured.

Despite the fact that the Commission considered many far-reaching proposals, the reforms that have actually emerged from this debate, to date, are much more limited. In 1994, the legislature rejected a bill supported by health care–oriented legislators and health policy specialists which would have required the legislature to develop a statewide plan for health care reform. Ignoring the fact that there was no specific proposal on the table, the conservative opposition successfully argued that any such plan would be too costly. In the final analysis it was Oklahoma's troubled Medicaid program that provided the impetus for serious health care reform in the state.

In 1992–1993, an Interim Task Force on Medicaid and Welfare Reform, chaired by Representative Bob Benson, was examining the Medicaid program administered by DHS. The task force concluded that DHS was not managing Medicaid money in the most cost-effective manner. Unhappy with what they found, the task force proceeded, with the help of outside consultants, to develop a plan for reforming the state's Medicaid system.[7] The plan which the task force developed was based on a managed care approach to the provision of health services.

At approximately the same time as the task force was developing its recommendation, a second working group of legislators and health policy specialists prepared a proposal to create the Oklahoma Health Care Authority (OHCA). Although creation of the OHCA was proposed in response to the need for a new agency to manage the state's Medicaid program, the design of the agency and the responsibilities ultimately granted to it indicated that the new agency would be in a position to play a central role in all aspects of health care reform in the state.

Both proposals were enacted into law during the 1993 legislative session. The OHCA was created by House Bill 1573 which established the agency and empowered it to purchase health care for all state employees and clients of all state health programs.[8] Senate Bill 76 "authorized conversion of the current fee for service to a managed care system for all Medicaid clients beginning July 1, 1995."[9] The language of the Bill is quite specific as regards managed care: "It is the purpose of the Oklahoma Medicaid Healthcare Options Act to establish a statewide managed care system of comprehensive health care delivery through the Oklahoma Medicaid Program including, but not limited to, prepaid capitated plans and primary case management plans, which shall be offered to all geographic areas of the state."[10]

The OHCA is governed by a seven-member board. The members of this board are appointed by the governor, President Pro Tempore of the Senate, and the Speaker of the House of Representatives. The OHCA is headed by an administrator who is responsible for the overall operation of the Authority. The administrator is appointed by the governor and confirmed by the state senate.[11]

The OHCA is comprised of four divisions, the heads of which are directly responsible to the administrator. The divisions include: (1) Medicaid Operations, which deals with quality assurance, claims adjudication, provider relations, and long-term care; (2) Managed Care, which deals with business and contracts, field operations, and client relations; (3) Health Policy and Planning, which deals with health policy, health care information, and special programs and projects; and (4) Information Services, which deals with systems analysis and planning, MMIS oversight, and data collection and reporting.[12]

The first administrator of the OHCA is Dr. Garth Splinter. Doctor Splinter is a Medical Doctor with a background in family practice. He also holds an MBA from Harvard University. He previously served as Director of the Health Sciences Center Health Affairs and Rural Health Programs at the University of Oklahoma. As noted above, Dr. Splinter chaired both the Commission of Oklahoma Health Care under Governor David Walters, and its successor, the legislatively mandated Health Care Study Commission. Doctor Splinter is not the only carryover from Commission days; the presence of others on the OHCA who worked on or with the Commission suggests that the strong reform-oriented spirit of the Commission is likely to be reflected in the work of the OHCA.

THE CREATION OF SOONERCARE

Upon its creation, the OHCA applied and received permission from the Health Care Financing Administration (HCFA) of the Department of Human Services to develop a Title XIX (Medicaid) managed care demonstration program. The demonstration period was to be five years. The program was to be statewide in scope and to cover all of the state's Title XIX population, including long-term care and chronically mentally ill patients. Following HCFA guidelines, the program was to be revenue-neutral, that is, it would not exceed the costs of the current fee-for-service program of 1995.[13] The name given to the new program was SoonerCare.

Broadly conceived, SoonerCare has both urban and rural components. The urban component of SoonerCare is a typical HMO-based capitated model of health care delivery. It relies heavily on primary care physicians as the gatekeepers or arbiters of more specialized care. HMOs contracting with the OHCA are required to use primary care physicians in this manner. Under this model the state makes a per capita monthly payment to an HMO in exchange for a pre-specified package of basic health services. Most services are included in the prepaid package. Fees for Medicaid-covered services billed by the HMO but not included in the prepaid benefit package are reimbursed by the OHCA in the same way as other fee-for-service providers are reimbursed. The urban component of SoonerCare covers three areas of the state: Oklahoma City, Tulsa, and Lawton.

The remainder of the state is considered rural and has been divided by the OHCA into designated rural areas for management purposes. Implementing managed care in rural Oklahoma requires a different strategy due to small, widely distributed populations and a shortage of primary care physicians in these areas. These conditions make it difficult to spread the risks associated with capitated payments, which in turn makes participation unappealing to providers.

The OHCA's initial reform strategy for rural areas involves the use of three partially capitated models. These include the following:

Primary Care I: This is a model in which capitated payments are made for primary care office visits and case management activities for enrolled patients. It is available to solo practitioners as well as other provider groups.

Primary Care II: In this model capitated payments are made for Primary Care I services, plus selected diagnostic and ancillary services directly linked to a primary care visit. It is also available to solo practitioners and other provider groups.

Outpatient Network: This third model involves capitated payments which cover all or most outpatient services, including specialist visits, diagnostic procedures, and prescriptions. This model is generally available to provider groups with the enrollment, sufficient resources, and medical management expertise to assume a higher degree of risk.[14]

Under all of these partially capitated models, services not covered by the capitated payment would be reimbursed on a fee-for-service basis. The ultimate aim of the OHCA is the development of the Outpatient Network Model as the health care delivery vehicle for rural areas. The OHCA proposes to encourage such development by collaborating in the development of a telemedicine network and promoting other medical and administrative reforms; for example, the use of physicians' assistants and nurse practitioners in rural areas and the creation of a rural medical transportation system. In short, the OHCA hopes to strengthen the infrastructure for health care delivery in rural Oklahoma.

The OHCA also hopes to find some means of integrating its efforts with those of the Indian Health Service operated by the federal government in both rural and urban areas. Eventually, the OHCA would like to see a fully integrated network of health care providers in rural Oklahoma. This would enable the OHCA to more fully extend the managed care approach to rural areas.

The plan to enroll Medicaid clients in SoonerCare was to proceed in three broad phases based on the Medicaid eligibility of different groups of clients as determined by federal law. Groups thought to be most amenable to managed care, such as the relatively young and healthy Aid to Families with Dependent Children (AFDC) population, were to be enrolled first. The first phase began on July 1, 1995, with the enrollment of all AFDC and related clients and was to be completed by July 1, 1996. The second phase was to begin on July 1, 1996, and was to cover the noninstitutional portion of the state's aged, blind, and disabled population. Enrollment of this group was completed July 1, 1997. The third phase is scheduled to begin on July 1, 1999 and will enroll all long-term care and chronically mentally ill Medicaid clients.[15]

IMPLEMENTING SOONERCARE

As the literature on program implementation suggests, legislative approval of a program plan is only the starting point for a solution. What happens to a program during the implementation phase of its life cycle is critical in shaping the final outcome. Few, if any programs are ever implemented as envisioned without compromise, and once implemented, programs continue to change over time.[16]

During implementation many factors both internal and external will operate to influence SoonerCare. Internal factors include such things as the effectiveness of the program's substantive strategy, in this case the managed care approach, the technical skill and competence of program managers, the commitment of program managers to program goals, and to a large extent the political savvy and skill of the program's leadership.

For SoonerCare external factors will include the acceptance of the program by stake-holders such as health care providers, clients and their advocates, elected representatives, and the public. What the federal government chooses to do or not do in the area of Medicaid funding and national health care reform will also affect program outcomes. Other factors more distant from the day-to-day administration of the program, such as developments in the area of medical malpractice law with respect to HMOs, may also influence the program.

Finally, such macro factors as trends in population health, developments in medical technology, and even the performance of the U.S. economy can have both direct and indirect consequences for the program. It should be noted that while some of these factors can be influenced or anticipated by the actions of program officials, many cannot.

Because SoonerCare is still in the early stages of development, it is much too soon to draw broad conclusions about either the overall effectiveness of program implementation or the attainment of program goals. The program is, however, being shaped, and ultimate outcomes will be determined by what is happening now. Thus, the following discussion focuses on the implementation effort to date and what it might imply for the future of SoonerCare.

PROVIDER ISSUES IN IMPLEMENTATION

One key to the successful implementation of SoonerCare lies in obtaining the acceptance of the program by health care providers. If the program is to succeed, provider groups must participate in the program, cooperate with it, and at the very least not effectively oppose it.

Provider acceptance of the SoonerCare program has been and will continue to be influenced by its fairly dramatic re-allocative character, a situation to which program officials have been sensitive. By 1994 the old fee-for-service Title XIX program allocated almost a billion dollars annually for the purchase of health care for Oklahoma's Medicaid population. Thus, a specific group of providers had a direct financial interest in preserving the status quo.

Beyond a financial stake, many providers have a professional and moral commitment to the services they provide and to the groups to which they provide them. For example, those in pediatric medicine are likely to feel that children's health should receive a greater share of the health care dollar because they value it more than other care, not just because they make money by providing it. Such financial and normative commitments can provide powerful incentives for providers to resist changes in the status quo if they regard it as unfavorable.

If the managed care system is implemented as intended, some providers will gain and some will lose as the one-billion-dollar Medicaid budget is re-allocated among health care providers. Under managed care, HMOs and the primary care physicians whom they employ will gain the lion's share of the Medicaid business.

In this climate, those providing more specialized and intensive care, such as specialty physicians and hospitals, will no doubt lose business, as more care is delivered in physicians' offices and outpatient clinics. Furthermore, specialty physicians will depend more on referrals from primary care physicians and hospitals will depend more on primary care physicians for admissions. Since there are also real differences in the medical field about what constitutes an adequate level of care in a given situation, these groups may find both financial and normative incentives for opposing various features of SoonerCare.

So far, provider resistance to SoonerCare appears to be mild. This may be due, in part, to the fact that many providers had already opted out of Medicaid due to low fee schedules and the difficulties of collecting fees for the services they provided. One group that opposed the program in the early stages of implementation were termed traditional Medicaid providers by the OHCA. These were mostly primary care providers that had continued to serve substantial numbers of Medicaid patients and thus had a large financial stake in the existing program.

This group, some of them minority physicians serving minority populations, feared losing their patient base to the large, out-of-state HMOs who were being attracted to Oklahoma by the impending SoonerCare demonstration. Anticipating this development, the OHCA, in its Request For Proposals (RFP) and subsequent contracts, required HMOs to give preference to traditional providers when contracting for medical services, provided that such providers were willing to accept the same reimbursement arrangements as the HMO's other providers.[17] They could continue to serve their patients, but only in a managed care environment. This tactic appears to have eased the situation.

The OHCA also dealt early on with another traditional provider problem. The University of Oklahoma's Health Science Center was a large provider to the state's Title XIX Medicaid population. Due to the research and teaching mission of the university, its fees, which were based on its overhead costs, were very high. In effect, the Medicaid program was helping to fund a substantial part of the university's teaching and research mission. The OHCA handled the situation by allowing the school to participate in the SoonerCare program, with a private hospital company, and receive an additional 5% of the weighted average rate, thus continuing the subsidy.[18] The HMOs complained about the unfair competition and the university complained about what it regarded as a low reimbursement rate.[19]

It should be noted that medical research and teaching have long been subsidized by government health programs, private health plans, and private patients. The introduction of managed care has only served to highlight this cost-shifting. How to fund teaching and research is a special problem that will have to be resolved as managed care becomes more widespread.

By January 1995, OHCA had completed work on the necessary procurement procedures and began to solicit competitive bids from interested HMOs through RFPs. Basically, the RFP spells out the services to be provided by the vendor and specifies, in detail, the rules to be followed in providing them. Under the procurement process, bids must fall within a capitation rate range determined by the OHCA on an actuarial basis. To encourage vendors to submit their best offer the capitation range is not disclosed. Vendors whose bids fall outside this range are excluded from the vendor pool. Vendors whose bids fall within the range are invited to submit a second bid as their final and best offer.[20]

The initial bidding process was successful in attracting managed care organizations. Several out-of-state HMOs participated in the process and a number were successful in obtaining contracts. In addition, the OHCA was successful in encouraging in-state providers, notably the medical college facilities, who had traditionally served Medicaid clients, to form or join HMOs, and to participate in the bidding process.

Because of the difficulties inherent in serving rural areas, progress in incorporating providers has been slower. Rural providers in three counties, however, were persuaded to participate in a demonstration project aimed at encouraging participation by other rural providers. As a result of the successful bidding and contracting process, the OHCA expected to realize an unanticipated cost savings in its first year.[21]

CLIENT ISSUES IN IMPLEMENTATION

In addition to provider participation and cooperation, the success of SoonerCare will depend on the effective use of SoonerCare by program clients. Under managed care, providers should have a strong financial interest in keeping clients healthy; as this reduces costs in the long run. Managed care proponents argue that this can be accomplished through education and prevention programs and by identifying and treating small problems before they become large and expensive emergency room crises.

In order for this strategy to produce benefits, however, clients must cooperate by seeing their primary care physician for check-ups when recommended, by making appointments and going to the doctor when problems first occur, and by complying with medical advice. Unfortunately, there is considerable evidence in the health care literature which suggests that the Medicaid population does not do these things. Research suggests that Medicaid clients do not seek care regularly, do not lead healthy lifestyles, and do not comply very well with medical advice.[22] Also, a number of empirical studies have suggested that health outcomes for Medicaid clients and the poor under managed care systems are little different than under fee-for-service systems.[23]

Some of these problems are no doubt due to past difficulties with access to the health care system, the very problem which SoonerCare proposes to correct. Some problems may be the result of behavioral inertia and lack of understanding of the new system, presumably correctable by education. Other problems may be related to indigent lifestyles; for example, lack of transportation, frequent relocation, or lack of education. These may be more difficult to correct, requiring integration of health care services with other social services.

The enrollment procedure established by the OHCA and DHS for AFDC enrollment involved a face-to-face meeting with a DHS case worker at the time of eligibility application. During this meeting applicants were given literature describing SoonerCare and were informed that they could preselect a provider. If the applicant did not want to make a decision at this time he/she was given a toll-free number to call in order to select a provider. In addition, applicants were also sent a preaddressed, stamped post card on which they could indicate their choice of provider. They were then sent detailed provider information by mail.[24]

Applicants who did not select a plan by one of these methods within ten days were automatically assigned to a plan. Once enrolled, applicants had 30 days in which to change their choice of provider. They were then required to stay with the same provider until recertification. This enrollment plan required considerable cooperation between the OHCA and the DHS, which continues to determine AFDC, and thus Medicaid, eligibility.[25]

An initial and obvious problem was the high turnover of AFDC recipients. The average length of stay on Aid to Families with Dependent Children is eight months.[26] Families can become eligible and ineligible for Medicaid benefits off and on throughout the year, resulting in a continual reenrollment process. This situation had the potential to create significant problems in terms of the provider-patient relationship and the continuity of medical care. The solution arrived at by the OHCA was to guarantee eligibility in SoonerCare for six months even if the beneficiary was to lose AFDC eligibility.[27]

Enrollment has presented SoonerCare and DHS with other difficulties. The enrollment of AFDC applicants in Oklahoma's three urban areas began July 1, 1995, and was not substantially completed until April 1996, three months later than anticipated.[28] Similarly, enrollment periods for other Medicaid groups may have to be extended as well. Only about 30% of AFDC applicants exercised their right to choose a plan; the rest were simply assigned a provider.[29]

Problems with the enrollment method have caused some concern in press reports. The reported problems include the difficulty of explaining the program to applicants effectively, even in face-to-face interviews; the inability of many applicants to understand the enrollment literature and instructions due to literacy problems; and the inability to physically locate many AFDC applicants who tend to be a highly transient group.[30]

These kinds of problems suggest that for many AFDC clients, using the SoonerCare program effectively will require considerable personal attention from both DHS case workers and ultimately HMOs. Furthermore, given high program turnover and the transient nature of the AFDC population, a sustained effort will probably be required. The OHCA is continuing to refine its approach to enrollment as it learns more about client behavior, but it tends to see its role as educating clients rather than hand-holding. Some advocates of the medically indigent feel that a more hands-on approach will be required for many clients if the problems of lack of participation or inefficient participation are to be overcome.

POLICYMAKERS' RESPONSE TO IMPLEMENTATION

If SoonerCare is to proceed successfully it will require continuing support from policymakers and the public. As indicated by press reports and interviews, SoonerCare continues to receive broad support from state policymakers. In fact, the state's newly elected conservative Republican governor has continued to be supportive of the program and personnel put in place by his Democratic predecessor.

Continuing support for SoonerCare appears to be based on several factors. Health reform–minded legislators have continued to stress the potential of improved health care for the medically indigent under SoonerCare, and this has no doubt been an important factor. The very widespread support of policymakers, however, appears to be most strongly linked to the belief or hope that the program will eventually lead to the effective containment of Medicaid costs.

While it is too early to draw concrete conclusions about SoonerCare's ability to contain costs, the first year's experience as reported by the OHCA is optimistic. After the contracting period ended, the OHCA projected an unanticipated $13 million savings over the traditional fee-for-service program. This figure has since been revised downward to $3 million ($1 million in state funds). The spokesperson for the OHCA attributed the downward revision to a decline in the number of Medicaid clients in the state, and delays in enrollment. Nevertheless, given the limited experience of the program and the costs of implementation, any savings at this point can only be seen as a boost for the program. Program officials have been quick to point this out.

Two negative factors also appear to be contributing indirectly to the support of SoonerCare. The first is policymakers' lack of confidence in the DHS, always a popular villain in Oklahoma, due in part to its reputed mishandling of Medicaid under the old fee-for-service system. Second, the perceived lack of other cost containment alternatives to managed care has tended to make SoonerCare the only game in town. Overall, the response of policymakers suggests that the OHCA is doing an effective job of selling the program and maintaining its political base.

SUMMARY AND CONCLUSIONS

Despite some delays, the implementation of SoonerCare appears to be progressing relatively smoothly. During the early phases of implementation the program's leadership has managed to retain the support of policymakers and avoid major controversies with providers and clients. Managed care organizations are in place and the urban AFDC population has been enrolled. Rural implementation has proceeded, albeit more slowly than anticipated, in the form of a demonstration project in three rural counties, Hughes, Okfusgee, and Seminole, which the OHCA regards as successful.

Nevertheless, many hurdles remain. First, the reallocative effects of the program have not been fully felt. Much of Medicaid still remains on a fee-for-service basis at both the OHCA-HMO level and at the HMO-physician level. The latter appears to be part of a strategy to accustom physicians gradually to the managed care setting. As further capitation occurs, physicians will face increased financial incentives to limit the use of health care (or as managed care proponents put it, to use health care resources more efficiently). This is, of course, how managed care proposes to control costs. But, it could lead to opposition from both providers and patients.

On the other hand, continued use of fee-for-service reimbursements has led to the use of traditional "meat ax" cost containment tools by the OHCA. These include limits on services and reduced fee schedules for providers. For example, after a successful gatekeeping program had led to a reduction in inpatient mental health services and a growth in mental health outpatient services, the OHCA proposed severe reductions in fees for outpatient services.[31]

Second, the enrollment experience to date, with its low participation and attendance problems, suggests that a portion of the Medicaid population will be difficult to reach. A strong continuing outreach program on the part of the OHCA, providers, and the DHS will be necessary if the preventative and educational benefits associated with managed care are to be realized for this group. No systematic study of AFDC clients has been initiated either by the OHCA or the DHS to determine if recent enrollees are aware of their benefits under SoonerCare and are taking steps to obtain them. Such a study may be premature at present, but this type of research must eventually be undertaken if the overall impact of SoonerCare on the health of the AFDC population is to be understood.

Finally, bringing the remaining Medicaid population into the system will present major new difficulties. These groups constitute the least healthy, and consequently the most costly to serve segment of the Medicaid population. They are also the least likely to benefit from the basic services and preventive medicine strategies of the managed care approach. These patients often require long-term and costly medical services to achieve even small improvements in their quality of life. Limiting services to these patients, also known as rationing care, as a cost containment strategy can be extremely controversial.

NOTES

1. Dr. Garth Splinter, Chairman of the Oklahoma Health Care Authority, interview with Ron Woosley (March 1, 1996).

2. Ibid.

3. State of Oklahoma, Commission on Oklahoma Health Care, Report to the Legislature and Governor (December 1993).

4. Ibid.

5. Interview with Dr. Garth Splinter, 1996.

6. Commission on Oklahoma Health Care, 1993.

7. Interview with Dr. Garth Splinter, 1996.

8. State of Oklahoma, House Bill Number 1573 (May 1993).

9. State of Oklahoma, Senate Bill Number 76 (August 1993).

10. Ibid.

11. State of Oklahoma, Oklahoma Health Care Authority, Application to the Department of Health and Human Services for the Development of SoonerCare (December 1994).

12. Ibid.

13. State of Oklahoma, Health Care Financing Administration, SoonerCare—Terms and Conditions (October 12, 1995).

14. Oklahoma Health Care Authority, 1994.

15. State of Oklahoma, Oklahoma Health Care Authority, Report on State-Purchased Health Care (January 1, 1996).

16. William N. Dunn, *Public Policy Analysis* (Englewood Cliffs, N.J.: Prentice-Hall, 1994).

17. Dr. Jerry Brickner, Member of Board of Directors for the Oklahoma Health Care Authority, telephone interview with Ron Woosley (April 9, 1996).

18. Ms. Rhonda Peters, Public Information Officer for Oklahoma Health Care Authority, telephone interview with Ron Woosley (July 29, 1996).

19. Interview with Dr. Jerry Brickner, 1996.

20. Oklahoma Health Care Authority, 1994.

21. Interview with Dr. Garth Splinter, 1996.

22. Ibid.

23. Claine Kohrman, James Hughes, and Ronald Andersen, "Medicaid Enrollees in HMOs: A Comparative Analysis of Perinatal Outcomes for Mothers and Newborns in a Large Chicago HMO," *Health Care Reform Links* (August 1990).

24. Oklahoma Health Care Authority, 1994.

25. Ibid.

26. Interview with Dr. Garth Splinter, 1996.

27. Ibid.

28. Interview with Ms. Rhonda Peters, 1996.

29. Interview with Dr. Jerry Brickner, 1996.

30. Laurie Winslow, "Managed Switch Is Confusing for Recipients," *Tulsa World* (January 14, 1996).

31. State of Oklahoma, Oklahoma Health Care Authority, Presentation to Committee on Rates and Standards Proposed Outpatient Mental Health Rates, 1996.

13

Medicaid Reform in Oregon: A Case of Intellectual Honesty

LEONARD H. FRIEDMAN AND BRENDA GOLDSTEIN

Like virtually every other state in the country, Oregon has wrestled with how to meet the need to provide health services to an ever-growing number of Medicaid recipients yet, at the same time, manage to control the costs of the program which were increasing at a rate that began to threaten both quality and access. In addition to spiraling costs, there had been a small number of highly publicized cases that highlighted the dilemma faced by those Medicaid patients whose conditions were not covered and subsequently died as a result.

While these few dramatic cases focused the public's attention on the issue of access to services for Medicaid patients, there was a more mundane but perhaps equally significant problem. Oregon, in the past 25 years, has been a state whose economic base has shifted from timber to service industries and high technology and has seen a resultant increase in the creation of new jobs and increased prosperity. In combination with this economic growth there has been a continued focus on environmental protection and the maintenance of a lifestyle that many individuals viewed as ideal. The economic shift resulted in two simultaneous events. The first was a growth in the number of people moving to Oregon in search of jobs and a fresh start for themselves and their families. This growth is most evident in the population increase for the tri-county area containing Portland (the largest city in Oregon) and its suburbs. The three counties (Multnomah, Clackamas, and Washington) grew in population from 1,050,418 in 1980 to 1,285,000 in 1994, a 22% increase.[1] At the same time that the population was expanding, a more fundamental transformation was taking place. The economy of Oregon, particularly in the smaller communities in the southern, central, and eastern parts of the state, had depended upon the timber industry as the primary source of jobs and of tax revenue for local government operations. A gradual shift had been underway since the early 1970s away from timber and wood products to an economic base that was highlighted by high technology industries including Intel, Tektronix, Hewlett-Packard, and many others. Former timber workers found themselves retraining for new jobs. Many of the new jobs were with small firms that could not afford to provide health insurance to their employees so that by 1989, it was estimated that of a total population of approximately 2.8 million, there were almost 400,000 persons (under age 65) in Oregon without health insurance, the majority of whom were working full-time.[2]

Oregon was not immune to the budgetary shortfall created by rising costs associated with providing health services to the persons eligible for Medicaid under the rules in effect at that time. Rather than simply resign itself to having to pay ever-increasing costs for those most needy under the eligibility structure in place at that time, the state legislature embarked upon one of the most dramatic and provocative plans ever designed to restructure the payment and delivery of health services for persons without employer-sponsored health insurance and for those on Medicaid. Thus, the foundation for the Oregon Health Plan was laid in the latter half of the 1980s.

This chapter is designed to tell the story of a work in progress. We attempt to describe how the Oregon Health Plan evolved, how it was designed, and what the prospects are for its future. The story is one of a cold, economic calculus tempered by optimism and compassion. This is a story of visionary leadership, building community consensus, and simply being in the right place at the right time. It is a story of the politics of reality and of the compromise between what is ideal and what is possible. As much as anything, the Oregon Health Plan is a lesson in honesty, and recognizes that government plays an important role in the lives of everyday people.

PRELUDE TO THE PLAN

In order to understand the economics of Medicaid in Oregon and how the Oregon Health Plan was developed in order to address this issue, it is necessary to provide some grounding on the legislative process in the state. Oregon's legislature is made up of a 60-member House of Representatives and a 30-member Senate. Both houses convene beginning the second Monday of each odd-numbered year. While there is no length of time the legislature can meet, most sessions are completed within six months. The legislature approves two-year budgets. In the case of state agencies that require additional funds between legislative sessions, an Emergency Board (consisting of seventeen House and Senate members) can authorize additional expenditures out of a special fund or can move allocated funding from one appropriation to another.

Our story begins in the 1987 session of the Oregon legislature. The president of the Senate at that time was John Kitzhaber, M.D. Then Senator Kitzhaber had practiced emergency medicine in Roseburg, Oregon for thirteen years while at the same time serving in the House and then the Senate. In addition to Senator

Kitzhaber, the remainder of both the House and Senate were dominated by Democrats. The Speaker of the House, Vera Katz, was closely aligned politically with Senator Kitzhaber. A Democratic governor, Neil Goldschmidt, had just been elected the previous November.

Oregon had been participating in the federal Medicaid program since its inception in 1966 with the same sorts of fiscal and access problems encountered by all other states. An obvious difficulty faced in the 1987–1988 legislative session was inflationary pressure and increased utilization that together forced a reexamination of the types of medical procedures the state would fund under its Medicaid program. As it stood in 1987, Oregon could afford to provide Medicaid to those persons at 67% of the federal poverty level or below. Given the need to control Medicaid spending, two unrelated but equally important decisions were made. The first was to allocate additional state Medicaid funding into providing coverage for pregnant women and young children. The second decision was the elimination of most transplants (with the exception of kidneys and corneas) as a covered benefit under Medicaid.

While these two decisions were made independent of one another, the public perception was less than favorable. Galvanizing this response was the death of seven-year-old Coby Howard, a leukemia patient whose bone marrow transplant was denied when his parents could not raise the additional $30,000 needed to complete funding of the $100,000 procedure. While he had to agree with the fiscal necessity to discontinue funding transplants, Senator Kitzhaber realized that the state could not go on with this type of de facto rationing of health services and piecemeal provision of care to only a small segment of those persons who needed medical services. Data was available, both nationally and in Oregon, that the emergency departments of local hospitals were for many people their primary care providers. Not only was treatment extremely costly but there was neither continuity of care nor the availability of follow-up.

The solution, to Senator Kitzhaber, was obvious. Simply creating a "fix" for Oregon's Medicaid problem was both insufficient and inadequate. Following the 1987 legislative session and while meeting informally with a number of both Senate and House colleagues, Kitzhaber posed the question of what could be done to institute a program that would ensure access to health services for all Oregonians and not just for a small number of Medicaid patients. While there were a number of persons at that meeting who were quick to say why a plan of this magnitude would not work, the vision of Senator Kitzhaber was ultimately to prevail.

The first step in the process involved funding a small pilot study titled the Oregon Medicaid Prioritization Project. The result of the study demonstrated that health services could be prioritized via broad scales using a 1–10 ranking.[3] Another important development took place when Oregon Health Decisions authored "Quality of Life in Allocating Health Care Resources." Oregon Health Decisions was a community-based, nonprofit organization which, since 1983, had been actively involved in health policy issues. The combination of the reports from Oregon Health Decisions and Oregon Medicaid Prioritization project, when coupled with community, business, and labor support and combined with the persuasive vision put forth by Senator Kitzhaber, was enough to gain the bipartisan consensus necessary to lay the legislative foundation for the Oregon Health Plan.

FOUNDATION FOR THE PLAN

More than simply an expansion of Medicaid, the Oregon Health Plan (OHP) was envisioned as a means to ensure that a basic level of health services would be made available to all Oregonians. Beyond expanding Medicaid to cover all recipients below the federal poverty level, additional needs were identified in the 1989 legislative session that included development of a high risk pool, and a small employer incentive program with an employer mandate to follow if necessary.

Three pieces of legislation, enacted in the 1989 session, formed the basis of the Oregon Health Plan. The first law (titled Senate Bill 27) extended Medicaid coverage to most Oregonians living at or below the federal poverty level and guaranteed them a basic benefit package based on a prioritized list of health services. Services were to be delivered through managed care plans in order to coordinate treatment and reduce costs. In order to help end cost-shifting, managed care capitation rates were to be set by an independent actuary based on "reasonable costs." In order to implement the program, Oregon would have to receive a waiver from the Health Care Financing Administration (HCFA), a task that policymakers in state government thought could be done.[4] Senate Bill 27 also created the Oregon Health Services Commission to "rank medical services from the most important to the least important to the entire population."[5] In addition, once implemented and in a period of budgetary shortfall, the legislature would not have the authority to limit the number of recipients but would have to either decrease the number of services available or increase the level of funding for existing programs.[6] Furthermore, reimbursement to providers and plans would be contractually agreed upon and could not be reduced at a time of insufficient resources. During the first phase of implementation, Medicaid services provided to the elderly, blind, persons with disabilities, or children in foster care were to continue without prioritization.[7]

The additional laws passed in the 1989 session were Senate Bills 534 and 935. The former funded the Oregon Medical Insurance Pool (OMIP). Senator Kitzhaber and other health policy experts recognized that there were a large number of Oregonians (approximately 150,000) who were unable to purchase conventional health insurance as a result of preexisting medical problems. Insurance companies doing business in Oregon would be "taxed" in order to create a pool of funds that would be used to help these persons obtain insurance.

Senate Bill 935 would ultimately prove to be the most contentious part of all the measures connected with OHP. This law "required employers to [provide health insurance] coverage to all permanent employees (working 17.5 hours or more per week) and their dependents by July 1, 1995 or pay into a special state fund that would offer coverage to those employees."[8] Implementation of the employer mandate part of OHP was contingent on obtaining an exemption from the Employee Retirement Income and Security Act (ERISA), a task that would prove to be quite formidable.

While the high risk pool and the employer mandate were seen as extremely important to the success of OHP, the Medicaid expansion would initially be the most visible and controversial part of the program. In order to create the prioritized list of services, the Oregon Health Services Commission was charged with the responsibility of "reporting . . . a list of health services ranked by priority from the most important to the least important, representing the comparative benefits of each service to the entire population to be served."[9] More than simply coming up with a ranked list of services, the Commission was instructed to "actively solicit public involvement in a meeting process to build a consensus on the values to be used to guide health resource allocation decisions."[10]

The Health Services Commission was made up of eleven persons, including five primary care physicians (three family practitioners, one obstetrician, and one pediatrician), one public health nurse, one social worker, and four laypersons. The inclusion of primary care physicians exclusively was intended to decrease pressure from special interests and increase chances of acceptance of the final plan. The commissioners wanted to receive as much public input and participation as possible and specifically targeted advocates for seniors, persons with disabilities, mental health service consumers, low-income persons, and providers of care. Between August 1989 and May 1990, twelve public hearings were held throughout the state with an average of 45 formal testimonies given at each hearing.[11] In addition, Oregon Health Decisions conducted 47 "town hall" meetings during the same time and along with the Commission, met with over 1,000 persons who expressed their views on health values and services.[12]

Emerging from those public hearings were two main themes. The first of those was philosophical in nature. The public viewed health care as a right and recognized the need to guarantee adequate health care for all persons. Simultaneous with this viewpoint was the desire to ensure personal choice among delivery systems and providers. The second theme focused on the relative importance of specific health services. Transplant services, family planning, reproductive services, maternity care, and reimbursement for midwifery were given high value, whereas "unnecessary surgery" was not valued highly. The highest rated values coming out of the public hearings were prevention, quality of life, cost-effectiveness, ability to function, and equity.[13]

At the completion of public hearings, the Health Services Commission (HSC) developed a list of more than 1,600 "condition-treatment" (CT) pairs that linked a specific medical condition with its appropriate treatment. Each CT pair appeared on a line on the prioritized list that would ultimately have to be considered for funding by the legislature. A cost-utility ratio was then developed for each of the CT pairs based on input from several sources, including 54 provider groups and over 200 individual providers. Virtually all licensed practitioner associations in Oregon were represented including chiropractors, acupuncturists, and massage therapists.[14] In addition, the Office of Technology Assessment independently evaluated the draft priority list and found it acceptable. Work on the priority list continued through May 1991 when the HSC presented its final report to the governor and legislature.

ROADBLOCKS TO THE PLAN

At the start of the 1991 legislative session, the Oregon Health Plan waiver request had been drafted and efforts began to move into the implementation planning phase. One key hurdle needed to be crossed prior to launching the Plan. In August 1991, the Oregon legislature, with the strong support of both United States Senators Mark Hatfield and Bob Packwood, in addition to the five House members, formally petitioned HCFA for a waiver of Medicaid regulations. Almost immediately, a firestorm of protest arose over the Plan, and in particular the construction of the priority list. Two reasons were cited as the primary problem areas. They included the concern that OHP rationed care to women and children and that the plan did not adequately address administrative waste and duplication of services in the health system.[15]

Problematic in both arguments was that the critics were fundamentally wrong and their denunciations of OHP were based on trying to gain political advantage rather than attempting to correct any actual deficiencies. In the first instance, the benefit package provided to women and children was not only extremely "rich" but access as a result of increasing eligibility to 100% of federal poverty level would have added many more beneficiaries to the Medicaid rolls. While the second criticism dealing with program costs was grounded in a greater degree of veracity, legislation enacted in the 1991 session addressed the areas of cost containment, technology assessment, and clinical guidelines.[16]

Coupled with these criticisms were influential voices raised about the perception that OHP unfairly denied or limited services to the disabled (in violation of the Americans with Disabilities Act), low birth weight babies, and could result in more women seeking abortion services. These arguments were highlighted during the March 1, 1992, broadcast of the CBS News program, *60 Minutes*.[17] While Senate President Kitzhaber made a strong case for the Plan, Representative Henry Waxman of California, then Chair of the House Health and Human Services Subcommittee, denounced the Plan as rationing care to the poor. A final observation is that the Oregon Medicaid waiver was submitted during the final year of the George Bush presidency and the potential existed for a conservative president and executive branch to deny the waiver to a relatively liberal state legislature and governor. All of these examples illustrate the likelihood that public policy is created not only from sound analysis and appropriate social/ethical values, but from sound bites, special interest pressure, and political expediency.

The waiver was officially denied by HCFA on August 3, 1992, at which time the Oregon Health Services Commission went "back to the drawing board" in order to address the specific criticisms raised by HCFA. At the same time that the waiver application was under consideration, three additional pieces of legislation were enacted. Senate Bill 44 began the process of expanding OHP coverage to seniors and persons with disabilities. Senate Bill 1076 had two objectives. The first intent was to include chemical dependency and mental health services into future priority lists. The second piece of SB 1076 created a Small Carrier Advisory Committee charged with making health insurance affordable to businesses with between 3 and 25 employees. The benefit package would be similar to the OHP standard benefit set. The third law, Senate Bill 1077, established a Health Resources Commission to examine the impact of capital expenditures in medical technology.[18]

The priority list was modified to include 696 CT pairs that were ranked in a way to recognize both the important values expressed during the public hearings, and took into account their cost-effectiveness. Given the changes in both style and substance to the priority list, the Office of Medical Assistance Programs resubmitted the waiver request to HCFA and on March 19, 1993, Donna Shalala, Secretary of the Department of Health and Human Services, approved the request. The terms of the waiver approval established a five-year Medicaid expansion demonstration project with a start date of February 1, 1994. After six years of analysis, planning, public hearings, withering criticism, and renewal, the Plan was ready to be put into action. Only one question remained unanswered—how to pay for an estimated 120,000 new Medicaid enrollees.

IMPLEMENTATION OF THE PLAN

The Oregon legislature had less than one year to develop and roll out the implementation plan for OHP. Given the terms of the Medicaid Waiver granted in March, the legislature passed House Bill 5530 that set forth the mechanism to implement the Plan. There were six provisions to this important law and they included:

1. Finance the Medicaid expansion from general fund revenues coupled with a $0.10 per pack increase in the cigarette tax;

2. Fund the Basic Benefit Package to cover 565 of 696 CT pairs on the priority list;

3. Fund the inclusion of seniors and persons with disabilities to begin January 1, 1995;

4. Approve the expansion of services for mental health and chemical dependency

(and the concurrent growth in the total CT pairs on the priority list and number of services covered) beginning January 1, 1995 with full phase-in by July 1, 1996;

5. Move the start of the employer mandate for medium and large employers to March 31, 1997, and for small employers to January 1, 1998; and

6. Create the position of Oregon Health Plan Administrator to oversee the Plan and coordinate health care reform.

Two items in HB 5530 are particularly noteworthy for students of public policy. The first point centers around funding of the first 565 items on the priority list. In order to determine the costs of each of the 696 CT pairs, an actuarial report was prepared by the firm of Coopers & Lybrand. Their report collected data from a variety of public and private health payers in Oregon and provided to the legislature a per capita cost estimate for the list as a whole and down to selected lines. Using the Coopers & Lybrand pricing as the basis for the program costs, the legislature determined that there were sufficient funds to set the cut-off point at line 565.

The second item of interest is with respect to the employer mandate. As was noted earlier, the original language of SB 935 required all employers to either provide health insurance to their employees or pay into a state fund that would offer health coverage as part of OHP. The scheduled date of implementation for the employer mandate was to be July 1, 1995. With the passage of HB 5530, phase-in of the mandate would be pushed back almost two years. There are at least two compelling reasons for the delay (and ultimate demise) of the employer mandate. The first reason centered around opposition from both large and small businesses. Traditionally, large and mid-sized businesses had provided employer-sponsored health insurance for their employees. The Oregon Health Plan was never intended to be exclusively an expansion of Medicaid but instead a mechanism to provide health services to all Oregonians and as such, was originally supported by business groups. However, when HCFA granted the waiver in 1993, small businesses realized that they only had a two-year window before the "play or pay" provision of OHP began. At this point the National Federation of Independent Businessmen (NFIB), a group representing small businesses, began to object more strenuously. Forcing small businesses to either purchase health insurance or pay into the state-run system would, according to their representatives, force businesses to either dramatically increase their prices or close altogether. The hope and expectation of NFIB was that the required ERISA exemption would fail, thereby negating the employer mandate. At the same time, large businesses felt that if small businesses were allowed to purchase health insurance through OHP, then they (the large businesses) would be at a competitive disadvantage.

The second reason for the delay in the mandate centered around a change in the political makeup of the Oregon legislature that was not unlike similar changes occurring in other states and at the federal level. John Kitzhaber announced his retirement from the Oregon Senate at the end of the 1991 session. In addition, during the 1992 election, the majority party in the Oregon House switched from Democrat to Republican and Vera Katz was replaced by Larry Campbell. Governor Barbara Roberts, a Democrat, was in the middle of her one and only term in office. The effect of the loss of Senator Kitzhaber and the election of a Republican majority in the House was to create a split legislature, one of whose houses was much more likely to be sympathetic to the needs and concerns of the business community. In addition, it should be remembered that for all intents and purposes, the bipartisan spirit that helped shape the OHP began to evaporate during the 1993 session, creating a legislature that took a harder view toward the role of government in providing health services.

LAUNCHING THE PLAN

Given the passage of HB 5530, planning for initial launching of the Oregon Health Plan could take place. The Office of Medical Assistance Programs (OMAP) was the state agency in charge of the details involved in the implementation, enrollment, and operationalization of the Oregon Health Plan. The first hurdle to overcome was contracting with the managed care organizations through which health services would be provided. In fact, Oregon had been providing Medicaid managed care to some recipients since 1985. Given the experience of both the state and recipients with managed care (fully and partially capitated health plans), 20 insurers offering managed care products signed up to accept OHP participants. In addition, OMAP began an intensive, community-based educational program designed to provide current and potential OHP participants with the information needed to sign up with a managed care plan and begin receiving care through their primary care provider.

Phase I of the Medicaid expansion of OHP began as scheduled on February 1, 1994. Within one year, 112,000 of the 120,000 new eligibles (resulting from the inclusion of persons at 100% or below the federal poverty level) had signed up with OHP. In addition to the managed care plans, there were five dental care organizations that provided dental benefits to OHP recipients. Depending on the population served, the system had both fully and partially capitated plans, dental care organizations, and primary care case managers (PCCMs).

Virtually any entity that met OMAP's standards could participate in the OHP. The standards include rules relative to provision of health care services, emergent and urgent care medical services, continuity of care, medical record keeping, quality assurance, access, complaint procedures, informational requirements, member education, member rights and responsibilities, financial solvency, chemical dependency (as of January 1, 1995), and exceptional needs care coordination. The last standard referred to the ability to coordinate services for persons with multiple physical, economic, and social problems. In every case, participating managed care plans received a preset and nonnegotiable capitation rate that represents the funding provided to the plan per OHP member per month. The rate varies depending on the county in which the recipient resides and the eligibility category of each person. In addition, a 6% administrative cost is included in the capitation rate. Participating managed care plans are also required to undergo two levels of evaluation that include a site visit review and desk audit of all policies and procedures and an external review by a professional review organization. In addition to these reviews, on a monthly basis, medical directors from the participating health plans meet with OMAP's medical director and staff and managed care plan administrators meet with OMAP staff.

Phase I of the OHP began with the expected number of complaints and minor snafus that were dutifully recorded in newspapers from Portland to Medford. However, given the size and scope of the Plan, the Phase I implementation was remarkable because, for the most part, it worked exactly as expected. It should be noted that far more people than were initially expected requested applications and filed those materials in the first few months of the Plan. New Medicaid recipients signed up for one of the managed care plans in their community and began seeing their primary care provider. Anecdotal reports declared that emergency department utilization by Medicaid patients had dropped significantly. The complaints by both providers and patients were comparatively small in number. Although there was a definite "learning curve" for persons who were unfamiliar with managed care, OHP recipients soon adapted to the provisions and requirements of the health plans. The one service that gave OMAP the most difficulty was dental services, for at least two reasons. The first was that the managed care plans that offered dental benefits found themselves with far more OHP participants than they had expected. The second problem area centered around the very high demand for dental services and providers simply could not keep pace. Difficulties with dental benefits continue to plague OHP, although there appear to be fewer problems than in months past.

PHASE II

There were several key events and difficulties that marked the second phase of the Plan. On January 1, 1995, several new groups of people became eligible for the OHP basic benefit package. These groups included Medicaid-eligible elderly, blind and disabled, and children in foster care. In order to meet the special needs of these populations, the state created the Ombudsman Program and included in the capitation payment funding for exceptional needs care coordinators to be provided by the managed care plans. In addition to increasing the number of eligibles, mental health and chemical dependency services became part of the Plan. When these new services were added, the number of CT pairs in the priority list expanded. The most recent version of the list, adopted February 1, 1997, ranked 745 lines with the top-ranked diagnosis as severe/moderate head injury and disorders of refraction and accommodation, treated by radial keratotomy listed as number 745 with the cut-off line at number 606.[19]

There were almost immediately a number of problems arising with mental health and chemical dependency services. First and most important was the dichotomy that existed from day one. The managed care plans were responsible for chemical dependency. However, the decision was made to create a parallel system for mental health. Mental health services were provided by county mental health departments who have the option to contract with local providers. This system did not lend itself to effective coordination of services between the primary care provider and mental health practitioner.

At the same time that new eligibles were being added and services were expanded, OMAP became aware that the Plan was becoming a victim of its own success in that the combination of services and total eligibles created a large projected budget overrun for the coming 1995–1997 biennium. In an effort to shave costs from the Plan, OMAP proposed a variety of measures. The first was designed to provide fewer services by moving the cut-off line from number 606 to 581. The second step was the imposition of premiums for the newly eligible groups of OHP participants. The level of premiums was capped at $28 per month and floated, depending on income level and family size. Premiums could not be charged to Native Americans, pregnant women, children under thirteen years of age and any other categorically eligible recipient. Another step was applying a $5,000 asset test and a three-month income averaging test to new applicants. Finally, full-time college students were unable to receive OHP benefits effective October 1, 1995.

Despite all of these cuts, OHP is currently facing an $18 million revenue shortfall. The reasons for the shortfall can be traced to four primary factors. The first resulted from the expanded number of eligibles having come on board during Phase II who were already part of a fee-for-service system. The second problem resulted from the policy of OHP to pay for emergency hospitalizations prior to the person enrolling in a managed care plan. The third factor came from an improvement in Oregon's economy that resulted in a $4 million reduction in federal Medicaid matching funds. The final problem stemmed from a delay in federal approval for imposition of the premiums on new eligibles and the federal requirement that the state make significant exceptions to the premium requirement.

January 1, 1995, also meant a new legislative session and the creation of a particularly interesting dichotomy. John Kitzhaber was inaugurated Oregon's governor as a result of his victory in the previous November's election. Both houses of the Oregon legislature mirrored the changes occurring on the federal level and Republicans gained control in the House and Senate. The result of the shift of control of the legislature sealed the fate of the employer mandate and put additional pressure on the Medicaid part of the Plan. Earlier, we noted that an ERISA exemption was required in order to implement the employer mandate. The governor vetoed an attempt to rescind the employer mandate that the 1995 legislature passed. However, the legislature assumed that the federal government would not approve the exemption, thereby obviating the need for the House and

Senate to take any direct action to eliminate the mandate themselves. Any action on the part of the legislature would be contingent on congressional authorization of an exemption no later than January 1, 1996. It should be noted that only one other state, Hawaii, has an ERISA exemption for its health plan. Despite attempts to introduce the exemption, Congress never voted on the request. On January 2, 1996, Oregon's ERISA exemption request was rescinded and only then did the employer mandate officially go off the books. Although Governor Kitzhaber vetoed the bill passed by the legislature, elimination of the mandate was a "done deal."

The second outcome in the 1995 legislative session was a growing dissatisfaction with the Plan as expressed by a number of conservative House and Senate members. Reports appearing in state and local newspapers suggested that perhaps the state would be better off without the Plan given the $18 million cost overrun and isolated reports of consumer and provider dissatisfaction. Concurrent with the legislative rumblings were the effects of ballot initiatives passed in November 1994. As written, these ballot measures mandated an increased funding emphasis on prisons and corrections with no increase in general fund revenue. Coupled with a property tax reduction approved by the voters in 1990, multiple state agencies and services found themselves competing with one another for scarce general fund revenues. The desire to shrink the size of government, increase spending on corrections, yet continue to provide essential services including education, transportation, parks, and health services placed the legislature and governor at odds with one another with respect to prioritizing which items to fund and at what level.

PERSPECTIVES

The Oregon Health Plan, and in particular the Medicaid expansion, has proved by all accounts to be a tremendous success. By June 1996, there were 373,000 people enrolled with OHP and of that number, 115,000 were new eligibles. Over 81% of all OHP recipients were enrolled in one of seventeen managed care plans. Data collected by the Oregon Association of Hospitals shows that emergency room visits by Medicaid patients had dropped by almost 5% and that charity care had decreased by 30% since the Oregon Health Plan began February 1, 1994.[20] Overall, consumers and providers appeared to be satisfied with OHP and the services made available under the Plan. Evaluation studies are currently underway to determine the actual effects of the Plan. OMAP staff have been invited to talk with state health policy personnel from across the country about the design and results of the OHP.

Ordinarily, the results seen by OMAP and the Oregon legislature would be enough to convince all parties that the Plan was a success and it should be continued in both form and substance. However, at the present time, considerable uncertainty hangs over the future of the Oregon Health Plan. The possible problem areas take many forms but they are all scenarios that represent the thinking of people closest to the Plan. The most immediate question is the outcome of the 1996 elections. The general assumption is that a Democratic legislature in both federal and state governments and a Democratic president would be much more receptive to the provisions of the Plan and the desire to provide universal health coverage. This shift in legislative control is particularly important in Oregon where all state government appears to be locked in competition with corrections for general fund revenue. In this context of scarce resources and competing demands, several members of the Republican-controlled Oregon legislature have publicly complained that OHP benefits are too rich and that the program is too difficult to control.

Further clouding the fate of the Plan are the effects of a term limit measure passed by the voters in 1992. While the voters of Oregon seemed to be expressing their desire to limit the amount of time legislators could stay in office, the "law of unintended consequences" appears to have proved itself true once again. In this case, a turnover of "incumbent" legislators assures that virtually no one in the House or Senate has the historical context of how OHP was shaped or the original intent of the framers of the Plan. This knowledge vacuum allows special interests to shape the debate to meet their own agendas rather than with a view toward what is best for the large majority of the people of Oregon.

In November 1996 the State of Oregon passed a 30 cent cigarette tax to maintain and expand the Oregon Health Plan. This will bring in approximately $200 million new dollars to support and expand the OHP. The Tobacco Tax revenue is estimated to bring in 10% of the funding for the Oregon Health Plan.

The Legislature funded expansion of the Poverty Level Medical Program for pregnant women and young children up to 170% of poverty and coverage of some full-time college students. Funding was also set aside to help stabilize "safety net clinics" (such as FQHCs and Rural Health Centers). Funding was also provided to help subsidize health care insurance costs for working people with income under 150% of poverty. This will enable the OHP to now cover approximately 50,000 additional people in 1997–1999.

CONCLUSIONS

As it was designed, the Oregon Health Plan represented a four-pronged (Medicaid reform, employer mandate, small market reform, and high risk pool) approach to providing universal health coverage for all the people of the state. The forces that shaped the Plan came from a variety of sources and collectively served to bring about meaningful change. If Coby Howard had not tragically died because of having been denied a bone marrow transplant in 1987, public opinion in support of Medicaid reform would probably not have taken shape as it did. If the Plan were to simply have focused on Medicaid eligibles, there would have been little chance for the Plan to have achieved the legislative and citizen support that it has gathered. If the opinions and values expressed by hundreds of ordinary citizens not been taken into account and a legitimate effort not made to gain across-the-board consensus, the Plan would have never been accepted. If not for the vision and energy of Governor John Kitzhaber, then president of the Oregon Senate, there would be no Oregon Health Plan.

During a speech given to several local community groups, Kitzhaber spoke about the "intellectual honesty" that formed the foundation for the Plan. The State of Oregon recognized two simultaneous duties. First, it was the duty of state government to provide health services for the poor and disabled. Second, there were only a limited number of dollars available to fund state services and health services had to be as cost-effective as possible. The state could not afford to provide everything to everybody so it had to address a fundamental question: do you allow a small number of people access to all services or increase access but limit that which people can receive?

The decision to pursue the latter option, while fraught with controversy, will prove ultimately to be the right choice. This is in our opinion the greatest strength of the Plan and is the foundation for its continued utility as the means by which low-income residents receive health coverage in Oregon.

NOTES

1. Phil Keisling, *Oregon Blue Book 1995–96* (Salem, Ore.: Secretary of State's Office, 1995).

2. Harvey D. Klevit, Alan C. Bates, Tina Castanares, E. Paul Kirk, Page R. Sipes-Metzler, and Richard Wopat, "Prioritization of Health Care Services: A Progress Report by the Oregon Health Services Commission," *Archives of Internal Medicine* 151 (May 1991): 912–916.

3. Paige R. Sipes-Metzler, "Oregon Health Plan: Ration or Reason," *Journal of Medicine and Philosophy* 19 (1994): 305–314.

4. Oregon Medical Assistance Programs (OMAP), *The Oregon Health Plan* (Salem, Ore.: Oregon Department of Human Resources, 1993).

5. Ibid.

6. Klevit et al., "Prioritization."

7. Ibid.

8. OMAP, *The Oregon Health Plan.*

9. Klevit et al., "Prioritization."

10. Ibid.

11. Ibid.

12. Robert M. Kaplan, "Value Judgement in the Oregon Medicaid Experiment," *Medical Care* 32 (November 1994): 975–988.

13. Klevit et al., "Prioritization."

14. Kaplan, "Value Judgement."

15. Sipes-Metzler, "Oregon Health Plan."

16. Ibid.

17. Frank, Coffey, *60 Minutes: 25 Years of Television's Finest Hour* (Santa Monica, Calif.: General Publishing Group, Inc., 1993).

18. OMAP, *The Oregon Health Plan*.

19. Oregon Association of Hospitals and Health Systems (OAHHS), *Oregon Databank Program* (Lake Oswego, Ore.: Oregon Association of Hospitals and Health Systems, 1996).

20. Ibid.

14

Medicaid Reform in South Dakota: Managed Care in a Rural Environment

DAVID L. ARONSON

THE ECONOMIC AND POLITICAL CLIMATE IN SOUTH DAKOTA

Health care has emerged as one of the most important public policy topics in South Dakota. As a public policy, health care in South Dakota is affected by the conservative political views of the state legislature and a poor economy. Included among South Dakota's many unique health care variables are inflation, the American Indian community which constitutes almost 35% of Medicaid clients, rural medical care, small hospitals, nursing homes, assisted-living facilities, access to health care, quality of care, and cost. Managed health care is currently the most intensely debated issue and is the subject of this chapter.

Affordable and accessible health services are particularly problematic in a state where there is an average of fewer than ten people per square mile. South Dakota is largely populated by rural residents. Only five communities in South Dakota have a population of more than 15,000 residents. Geographically, the state covers 77,615 square miles encompassing 66 counties. There are more than 300 municipalities, and nearly 1,000 townships, many of which do not have the benefit of nearby medical facilities. Its largest community, Sioux Falls, had a population count of 100,281 in the 1990 census. In 1994, the census bureau estimated the population at 721,000, which identifies it as 45th in size.

The South Dakota death rate is higher in rural areas than in urban areas, where most of the physicians practice and where the three largest hospitals are located. This suggests that the health care of residents in rural areas is less than satisfactory. These limited population bases impede the capacity of these areas to support health care providers. South Dakota, the Mount Rushmore state, is one of the poorer states in the nation. According to the U.S. Census Bureau estimates for 1994,[1] average disposable personal income per person amounted to $17,751, which ranks it 29th among the states. Median household income for the same period was $29,733, which places it 36th among the states.

Today, there are 52 hospitals in South Dakota, 49 in rural communities, that "are truly becoming more than hospitals. They've become health care centers,"[2] involved in home health, hospice care, wellness care, and health education. South Dakota in 1995 had the first hospital in the nation certified in the Primary Rural Care Hospital Program under the Essential Access Community Hospital Program. South Dakota was also recognized in 1995 as being the nation's most improved health system by Reliastar life and health rating system. Nurses and dentists have volunteered their services to provide care for the citizens of the state. In addition, South Dakota is "the only state in the Union where Telemedicine has moved from the academic setting into the real world setting."[3] Telemedicine provides for health care by electronically transmitting medical information to less accessible areas, such as in South Dakota. This is aimed at improving quality and reducing costs. The three largest hospitals in South Dakota have come together in a demonstration program, and other hospitals in the state are linking together electronically. Nevertheless, the number of hospitals is inadequate to serve a scattered population.

MEDICAID

The State of South Dakota is not unique in its operation of the Medicaid program. Medicaid is a jointly funded federal–state program provided through Title XIX of the Social Security Act. The Medicaid program provides financial assistance to the states to improve access and to provide adequate medical care for eligible low-income and needy individuals: those with no health insurance or means to pay for health care. In South Dakota the federal–state dollar match in 1994 was approximately 70%—30%, based on a formula that weighs each state's economic condition and per capita income. The state must comply with the federal regulations regarding eligibility and mandatory services which affect the state's fiscal share of the program.

Overall prudent management of the program is being augmented in South Dakota by promoting managed care and case-mix reimbursement policies. There is a State Managed Care Task Force, but as yet it has not completed its work, and its members are having difficulty reaching agreement. It is a large body with members representing the health care providers, health systems, the insurance industry, the business community, and one member representing consumers. Its hope is to involve more consumers at a later time in the process.[4]

The Medicaid population has steadily increased in South Dakota from 33,693 in 1986 to almost 60,000 in 1994 and to an estimated 66,000 in 1996[5] (see Table 14.1) Categorical numbers, however, can be deceiving. The largest share of the dollars is expended on the aged and for nursing home care. In addition,

Table 14.1
Department of Social Services: Medicaid Eligible Comparisons

1990	39,718
1991	45,862
1992	52,138
1993	56,551
1994	58,755
1995	59,739
1996, ESTIMATED	66,226

Medicaid program costs are increasing as individuals' direct burdens are lessened by the use of third-party payers, such as health insurers and government programs. The availability of new technology and increasing labor costs are also a contributing factor. These all encourage health care use and contribute to health care cost increases.

David M. Christensen, of the South Dakota Department of Social Services, is the Medical Services Program Administrator and is responsible for processing claims and reimbursing payments to providers of the program. Despite budgetary shortfalls in South Dakota that have resulted in staffing cuts, approximately two million Medicaid claims each year are paid within seven working days of submission, a notable achievement.

According to Mr. Christensen,[6] saving money is the key motivator in employing strategies and incentives to provide dependable and reliable health care, but there are other motivators and objectives for the health care system as well. A secondary mission is to improve recipient access to services and increase the number of participating providers in all areas of health care. Another objective is to enhance client responsibility so that beneficiaries become more independent and self-sufficient. As clients find employment and obtain employer-provided health care coverage, they will often be directed to particular providers or limited to specific health care plans. This training, through the managed care program, helps prepare clients for later employment responsibilities.

MANAGED CARE

In an attempt to better manage the Medicaid program and control costs, South Dakota has initiated a program of managed care. In the Medicaid program, reimbursement should be made at a rate that encourages economic and efficient providers to participate in the program while meeting their incurred costs. Managed care functions under the theory of medical care on a wholesale basis for large groups of people by negotiating care at lower rates. The intent is to organize and centralize health care. By using the group concept, various factors, such as dollars and access, can be controlled.

The South Dakota Medicaid Managed Care program was initially set up July 1, 1993, under a two-year waiver granted pursuant to 1915(b)(1) of the Social Security Act. It is being incrementally carried out statewide at this time. This is a Medicaid managed health care system for primary care services including the following: inpatient/outpatient care; general medical care (pregnancy services); surgery; community mental health centers; psychiatrist/psychologist; specialists such as ophthalmologists, neurologists, and allergists; prescription drugs; durable medical equipment/prosthetic; home health; chemical dependency treatment; healthy Kids Klub doctors' visits, and school district services. For not-managed care services, recipients do not need to go to a primary care provider nor do they need to have a referral card. Medicaid-covered nonmanaged care services included: emergency; family planning; dental/orthodontic/oral surgery; optical (basic vision and eyeglasses); podiatrist care; chiropractic care; ambulance/transportation; independent lab/x-ray services; and radiology/anesthesiology services.

The Primary Care Provider Program is intended to furnish recipients access to and the availability of better health care in a manner that is efficiently achieved. By choosing one health care provider from a list of those who have agreed to serve (family and general practitioners, pediatricians, internists, OB/GYN, clinics certified as Rural Health Clinics, clinics certified as Federally Qualified Health Centers, clinics designated as Indian Health Clinics), it creates a one-on-one "partnership" between that primary care contact and the Medicaid-eligible recipient. Recipients must go to that provider and are responsible to call for, keep, or cancel appointments. At the time of service, clients must present their Medicaid-managed care identification card. This is as important to them as their driver's license or a credit card. It is the client's responsibility, not the clinic's, the doctor's, nor the caseworker's, to present this card to all providers at the time each service is rendered. Unless this identification card is presented at each time of service, the provider can refuse service or the client will be responsible to pay. If the card should be lost, it cannot be replaced by the caseworker. The caseworker or the Medicaid office in Pierre must be notified and a new card will be prepared and mailed the next working day.

Other than for emergencies, a recipient must first consult the primary care provider either for treatment or for referral to a specialist. It is also the responsibility of the client to have a referral card to see another doctor or hospital. It is important for them to obtain this from the primary care provider and see that it is given to specialty providers. Medicaid will not pay for managed care services without this referral card. Without it, the client is responsible to pay for services.

It is also emphasized to the clients in the managed care training sessions that the hospital emergency room is not a clinic and is not to be used for routine care. The hospital emergency room is more costly and is to be used only for true emergency care. Again the clients are warned that if they choose to go to the emergency room, the hospital will not refuse to see them. But if they do obtain nonemergency services, Medicaid will not pay the bill and they will be responsible to pay.

Recipients are matched to primary care providers based on their prior medical history. Some clients are matched to previous providers of record. If there is no prior provider, the recipient is required to select one. If this is not done, a provider is designated and assigned by the Medicaid office. Recipients may change their primary care provider at their annual eligibility redetermination or if the provider to whom they are assigned is not acceptable, as long as they show good cause for such a change. These are state management efforts intended to control, but not restrict, access.

The managed care program is required for low-income children and pregnant women, SSI-blind/disabled, and those receiving Aid to Families with Dependent Children (AFDC). These make up approximately two-thirds of the South Dakota Medicaid population. These Medicaid-eligible recipients are required to receive managed care–covered services from their primary care provider and/or have medically necessary managed care specialty services authorized by their primary care provider.

Medicaid recipients diagnosed as severely emotionally disturbed (SED) or severely and persistently mentally ill (SPMI) are excluded from the Medicaid managed care program for mental health services only. These clients still need authorization from the primary care provider for all other health care services. In addition, some services are also exempt. These include the following: emergency care, family planning, dental-orthodontic, podiatry, optometric-optical, chiropractic, immunizations, ambulance-transportation, and independent lab.[7]

In the past, Medicaid recipients had a choice regarding health care. Today, if a patient needs care, one must contact a specific physician. In the past, there was physician and clinic hopping. No one physician or clinic managed a patient's needs. Medicaid recipients had difficulties with access to physicians and clinics. Facilities would set quotas for themselves, over which the state had no control. With the primary care physician concept, there is more continuity of care for the individual. The state also hopes to encounter less abuse of emergency room care. The state is experiencing a decrease in emergency room charges (although the state has yet to release information in support of this fact).

With special reference to pregnant women, it was the case that Medicaid recipients were more at risk because they were more prone to wait for prenatal care. Those children then placed very expensive medical burdens on the state as many of them were premature and needed neonatal care. That situation has now changed; pregnancies are now managed. Patients are more apt to maintain prenatal care with a willing physician. Pregnancies have a better outcome (again, the state has not released any hard figures in support of this).

Managed care is intended to better utilize different treatment levels of the health system.[8] In the past, recipients have used emergency facilities as a primary care provider for routine care at their convenience. Under the managed care system, a cooperating medical practitioner agrees to be the primary care provider for a block of patients. The State of South Dakota pays each provider $3 per patient each month for administrative expenses, regardless of care. The state also reimburses for the cost of treatment on a fee-for-service basis as determined by the Medicaid program. At the present time, there is no capitation in the state program.

Capitation is a relatively new concept and is not used at the present time in South Dakota. A capitation program is workable in areas where Health Maintenance Organization Programs (HMOs) are available and operating. South Dakota, with its small population, does not have a large HMO community or experience to draw on. In a capitated system, there is a calculated risk, and it works best when many people who have low medical expenses paid are offset by the few who have high medical expenses. The population in South Dakota is not seen as large enough to manage this risk. Additionally, waivers are necessary from the Health Care Finance Administration (HCFA) and this has been a very difficult and time-consuming process for other states, such as Minnesota and Utah. Currently, there have been no studies made in South Dakota as to common services provided and fees charged. Therefore, it would be difficult to determine what fair capitation payments should be.

State officials have chosen to go to the fee-for-service route. Because the state has chosen the managed care concept, it has been easier to work with providers making only this one change, rather than implementing both a managed care and a capitated fee structure at the same time. State officials believe this has also increased the group of providers to clients. Another factor which made the initiation of the managed care program in South Dakota go so smoothly was its slow implementation. It was initiated in only three to five counties at any one time. Both recipients and providers were trained in face-to-face sessions. These were held in various locations to give ample opportunity for all to attend. Ample opportunities were also given to ask questions and overcome any misgivings they might have.

One of the problems seen with the managed care system, as with HMOs, is that in this age of specialization, which also contributes to the high cost of health care, the primary care provider does more diagnosing and referring than beneficial treatment of disease. Under the managed care program, there is no payment guaranteed to a specialist without an approved referral. Access to health care becomes a function of ability to pay and location. The needy and uninsured have limited access to specialized health care. Rural residents have less access than urban citizens. Urban citizens with health care insurance or who are able to pay for their health care have access to immediate, specialized health care while others must first access their primary care provider to enter the system. Quality of health care also is an issue because of the possible delay in proper and knowledgeable treatment of the disease or illness. While a managed care system may be perceived as efficient and effective for those not knowledgeable about health care providers, the process of having specialists cleared through primary care physicians can add to the expense and lead to delay in proper treatment.

In the future, a flat or capitated amount might be paid to the primary care provider to cover both administrative and medical costs per patient on a monthly basis. The fees due specialists from referrals might also be deducted from this amount. This would affect the primary care provider's income and would further affect the client's access to quality health care. As this data is collected, diagnostic profiles will be established and exceptions noted for atypical treatment processes. The providers' actions may come under state surveillance and peer review when too many referrals are made. This could bring adverse reactions to the primary care provider from state officials. Despite concerns about reducing costs, the managed care system in South Dakota has not yet advanced to this situation, and access to quality health care is not now affected by these factors.

At the present time, state officials are working on focused studies asking both clients and providers their opinions on health care and the process. It is a real struggle to coordinate these broadly spread-out, statewide studies with state budget and operating personnel and systems in order to determine the effectiveness and efficiency of this state program. Nevertheless, the Department of Social Services is satisfied that the results of the program to date have shown cost savings and have increased control over the utilization of services: over-utilization and duplication of services have decreased.[9] This is giving clients more continuity of health care and better health results.

The managed care system has been very well accepted in South Dakota. Every county is now covered with managed care. Even though the managed care system was implemented slowly, the process did not take an extraordinary amount of time to implement. It is, after all, a state where people work closely and well together which makes it easier to work out many problems. The state is now starting to consider managed care for long-term care of the elderly and prescription drug utilization.[10]

South Dakota must also deal with other difficult problems—the rural aspect and the American Indian health care system. There are many small rural hospitals with no competition—competition being a major aspect of managed care. American Indians have serious health problems and cultural differences that make compliance difficult.

REFORM

There is a squeeze in dollars at both the federal and state levels. Reluctance on the part of taxpayers to increase their tax burden puts pressure on government executives and legislative bodies to look for ways to satisfy constituents and economize rather than meet rising costs.

President Clinton, in his budget proposal, has recommended cutting $59 bil-

lion from the Medicaid budget over a seven-year period. The Republican proposal would cut $184 billion out of the Medicaid budget over the same
seven-year period. Cuts will likely occur somewhere between these two figures.
To date, there has been no change in the funding of these programs. Without a
current budget, the Medicaid program has been operating under a continuing
resolution, but large changes are anticipated. Once a budget is passed, it will
surely mean fewer dollars.

In South Dakota, it has been made clear that the state is unwilling to spend
any more money for the Medicaid program. The governor's budget this year
was reduced by $1.7 million earmarked for inflation. The federal government
would have supplemented this amount. Providers lost not only state dollars but
the matching funds from the federal government as well. These are dollars that
will be shifted to the private-pay patients.

Another political issue that is now facing the states is the block grant concept
that is under discussion in Washington. Governor Janklow stated that:

we've got block grants coming . . . whether it is going to be the House version, the Senate
version, the Clinton version or some new version. . . . We've run too many different
scenarios, . . . so we'll just take whatever they give us from Washington and I'll trust
that they can't treat us any different than they treat all the rest of the states in the Union.
But the net result will be a dramatic difference in how we are doing business in South
Dakota. It will be a dramatic difference.[11]

If the federal government would give grants to the states with few or very
few mandates attached, it might be advantageous to the states. This would give
the states the power to decide eligibility and benefits. This would affect access
and quality of care, however that might be defined, but the states would be able
to deal with the Medicaid health care issue based on their own financial capa-
bilities. It would be disadvantageous if the present mandates and regulations
were to remain. Another disadvantage for the poorer states is the comparison
between the amount of dollars received from the federal government and the
revenues the federal government receives from those states. In South Dakota,
for example, this imbalance amounts to $800 million per year in the state's
favor. In other states, this imbalance is reversed. States such as California and
New York do not receive federal dollars greater than what is paid in federal
revenues. Another issue for those states is the proportion of Medicaid dollars
received. Again there is disparity among the states. This is another key issue
going on currently in the Medicaid debates in Congress. Some states are on a
50–50 basis, whereas other states may enjoy a three-fourths–one-fourth split.
South Dakota sustains an approximate two-thirds–one-third split. Larger states
receiving a smaller proportional share of Medicaid dollars and other federal
funds, however, have more political power given the number of their congressional delegates. South Dakota has only three members in Congress, and that is
very little power. Smaller states run the risk of losing not only their proportional

share of present Medicaid funding but a decrease caused by any adjustments in the way of calculating the distribution to the states. This will be compounded if federal legislation continues to maintain such tight control over the eligibility and benefit requirements of the Medicaid system.

Block grants will also have an effect on the State of South Dakota and the American Indian community's participation in the Medicaid program. Governor Janklow has said:

> If there is a federal block grant, we must make sure that in the Medicaid area they carve out special exceptions for ways they're going to deal with the [American Indian] reservation community, because to dump that onto the state would bankrupt the State of South Dakota in a very short period of time. Because, now for everybody who carries a Title XIX card, including all the AFDC population, where they choose to go . . . we at state government still get the bill. We pay it, but the federal government reimburses us under the program at 100 cents on the dollar. We needn't put up the match rate. If, under the new program, we got a block grant that included that without 100 percent reimbursement, it would break us.[12]

Another aspect compounding the problem is capping the amount of growth allowed over the seven-year period. It has been suggested in the Republican plan that growth be capped between 3 and 5% despite the numbers of citizens eligible and despite the amount of inflation. President Clinton's alternative to this would be to cap costs on a per recipient basis. On what basis this will be done is unknown, a fact which opens the distinct possibility of equalization among the states. This would be catastrophic for states like South Dakota.

With continued federal control but with fewer federal dollars, states such as South Dakota are going to have insurmountable problems. With no change in control and fewer dollars, who can predict what the result would be in terms of access and quality of health care for the Medicaid recipients? When one looks at where cuts might be possible in the Medicaid program and considering the eligible clientele, government is hard put to decide where cuts might be made. Considering that the average working family pays more each year for a health care protection policy than a Medicaid family spends on actual health care, it becomes even more of a question how Medicaid costs can be cut. There are very few places left other than to refuse services for some clients—which ones?—or discontinue certain selected services—which ones?—for all. Already, hospitals, nursing homes, pharmacists, and other providers are receiving less than their actual costs to provide medical care. Asking providers to receive even less is not feasible or equitable, which would mean even more cost-shifting to individuals having health insurance and private pay patients—or lose participating providers. Further cost-cutting could force providers into a position of refusing to participate in government programs, thus decreasing the availability of health care services to Medicaid clients.

Competition for federal aid is intensifying as government resources are diminishing. This financial crunch demands that the benefits of social programs be reexamined. As expenditures increase, there must be benefit contractions. States have limited resources, unstable economies, and competition for economic development. Growth and expanding revenues are difficult to maintain. Yet the needs of citizens must continue to be met. State leadership is important. States, not being financial equals, need to organize politically through organizations such as the National Governors Association and the Council of State Governments to negotiate arbitrary federal mandates in order to provide the health care needs of Medicaid clients as efficiently and effectively as possible within their means.

NOTES

1. U.S. Department of Commerce, Bureau of the Census, *Statistical Abstract of the United States* (Washington, D.C., 1995).

2. Governor William J. Janklow's State-of-the-State Address (January 9, 1996).

3. Ibid.

4. Governor William J. Janklow's Budget Address to the South Dakota Legislature (November 30, 1995).

5. Jeff Bostic, Fiscal Analyst for the South Dakota Legislative Research Council, Issue Memorandum 94–18 (August 2, 1994).

6. Interview with David Christensen, South Dakota Department of Social Services, Medicaid Administrator.

7. This information was provided by the South Dakota Department of Social Services.

8. Interview with Michael C. Rost, M.D., President: Health Care Medical Solutions, L.L.C., Sioux Falls, South Dakota.

9. Interview with David Christensen.

10. This information was provided by the South Dakota Department of Social Services: Sara Green and Carol Job.

11. Governor William J. Janklow's Budget Address (November 30, 1995).

12. Governor William J. Janklow's State-of-the-State Address (January 9, 1996).

15

Medicaid Reform from the Executive Branch: Tennessee's TennCare Program

MARK R. DANIELS

INTRODUCTION

Frustrated by yearly revisions of Medicaid, faced with over 1.5 million citizens with no medical coverage, and grappling with skyrocketing costs, Tennessee lawmakers decided in 1993 to create a new health care system that would provide medical insurance for virtually every Tennessean: TennCare.

During the five-year period from 1987 to 1992, Medicaid expenditures in Tennessee increased 500%, from $500 million to $2.5 billion. This increase was due, in part, to the reasons associated with the overall rising cost of health care. These included the use of expensive, sophisticated technology; innovative but costly treatment of illnesses such as heart disease; the increasing incidence of AIDS and cancer; the increasing number and longevity of the elderly population who have a great need for health care; and the treatment of illnesses and injuries caused by alcohol and drug abuse.[1] In addition, the increase was due to the spiraling numbers of individuals eligible for Medicaid. During the period from 1987 to 1992, a report issued by the Tennessee Department of Finance and Administration (DFA) estimated that the number of Medicaid-eligible individuals increased by over 70%, from 507,934 to 878,981 individuals, close to 20% of all Tennesseans.[2]

Tennessee's DFA estimated that Medicaid's five-year trend from 1987 to 1992 would result in a 220% increase in cost by 1997, or approximately $5.5 billion. Based on the assumption that the federal share of Medicaid would remain constant, this $3.0 billion increase would be met by a $851 million tax increase and health care benefit cuts of $2.6 billion. The most significant consequences of such massive benefit cuts would be the loss of coverage for thousands of Medicaid recipients, reductions in the rates of reimbursement for providers of health services, and additional cost-shifts to insured patients.

While Medicaid costs were spiraling, the cost of providing health care for Tennessee's 250,000 public employees actually declined by 1.2%. Democratic Governor Ned McWherter and Finance Commissioner David Manning attributed this cost containment to the system of managed health care available for state employees since 1988. Tennessee's state employees receive managed care through Blue Cross/Blue Shield of Tennessee, Inc., and have a choice of managed care programs. McWherter and Manning decided that managed care might also be the answer to the state's Medicaid dilemma.

In June 1993, Governor McWherter announced his solution for the Medicaid crisis: the termination of Medicaid in Tennessee and the creation of TennCare, a managed care program that would cover virtually every uninsured Tennessean. In order to use Medicaid funding for the new TennCare plan, McWherter had to apply for a Section 1115 Demonstration Waiver for review and approval by Donna E. Shalala, Secretary of the U.S. Department of Health and Human Services, and the Health Care Financing Administration (HCFA). The waiver would be good for one year, and would require reapproval.

Financed primarily with federal funds, TennCare delivers health services through Managed Care Organizations (MCOs) such as Health Maintenance Organizations (HMOs) and Preferred Provider Organizations (PPOs). As proposed, all Medicaid-eligible and uninsured citizens would be eligible for TennCare, and participants would share the costs of the program through premiums, deductibles, and co-payments, depending upon their ability to pay.

TennCare incorporated many aspects of health care reform that are being discussed currently on a national level.[3] First, Medicaid was a fee-for-service–based program, and the budget was essentially the amount billed by health care providers. Unlike Medicaid, TennCare uses cost containment and competitive marketplace contracting as part of the budget process. This approach is called global budgeting.

Second, because of the cost containment features of managed care, TennCare's projected savings are used to extend coverage to 500,000 uninsured Tennesseans, including the working poor. In addition, all health care providers who wish to treat the 250,000 state employees under the Blue Cross/Blue Shield program must also contract for TennCare patients. The combined purchasing power of these groups of potential patients (the pooled purchasing power of approximately 1.75 million people) provides lower-cost pricing of health care services.

Third, unlike Medicaid, TennCare provides preventive care at low or no cost. This feature will keep TennCare's pool of people healthier and assist in earlier diagnosis of serious illness, both of which help control health care costs.

Fourth, TennCare is available at no cost for individuals with income below an established "poverty level." For those above the poverty level, there is a sliding deductible, co-payment, and monthly premium, based on percentile above the poverty level. Unlike Medicaid, if a family lifts itself out of poverty its members will still be eligible for health insurance coverage. Approximately 33% of all families below the poverty line leave poverty each year. In the past, these families would have lost their Medicaid eligibility. If their employer did not offer a group health insurance program, then they would have to purchase health insurance on the open marketplace. Nongroup health insurance can cost as much as $750 per month for a family with two adults and two dependents. Under Medicaid, leaving poverty meant losing health coverage. TennCare allows families to continue health insurance coverage, with premiums based upon income level.

TennCare places Tennessee among a few states that have conducted a comprehensive reform of state-funded and -administered health care. The manner in which such an innovative health reform program was formulated and implemented provides insight into Tennessee's unique political characteristics.

THE POLITICS OF TENNCARE'S IMPLEMENTATION

TennCare was from the start a policy initiative of the executive branch of government. McWherter received legislative permission to apply for a Medicaid Waiver; however, the content of the TennCare plan was developed by officials in the Department of Health and the Department of Finance and Administration. On June 16, 1993, Governor McWherter and DFA Commissioner Manning released the application for the Medicaid Waiver with a start-up date of January 1, 1994. Within just six months, McWherter planned to: obtain the waiver from HCFA; negotiate managed care contracts with MCOs; inform all eligible citizens about the new program; enroll participants and obtain their initial MCO choices; and inform health care providers about the administrative and financial changes brought about by TennCare. The reason for such speed was the anticipated opposition from one of the state's most powerful interest groups: the Tennessee Medical Association (TMA).

McWherter talked more about the approval of TennCare than he did about the termination of Medicaid. Most of TennCare is a MCO type of Medicaid, and the majority of revenue that funds TennCare is supplied by the federal government and would be spent through a Medicaid program if TennCare did not exist. If McWherter had focused attention on the termination of Medicaid, TennCare's opponents would have had an easier target. By focusing on health care reform and the beginning of a new program, McWherter forced his opponents to argue against a new health care reform program instead of arguing against the elimination of the established program of Medicaid.

The TMA felt that TennCare's reimbursement rates would be inadequate because of below-cost fee schedules and "overzealous MCO withholding."[4] Mark Green, Executive Director of the TMA, cynically observed that "the governor couldn't afford 1 million people on Medicaid, so he handed it over to providers through TennCare and now 1.5 million people will be covered with the same revenue.''[5] The state contacted Medicaid recipients in October 1993, informed them about the proposed changes, and requested that they return an enclosed ballot to state Medicaid officials by November 1 and identify which new provider they had selected. This ''ballot'' resulted in a deluge of calls to physicians by patients asking for advice about enrollment. According to Mark Greene, ''in some places the volume of calls to physicians' offices has just about ground business to a halt.''[6]

TMA asked each of its 6,700 members to contribute $200 each toward the cost of a lawsuit against the state, for a total of $1,340,000, and eventually was able to raise over $1 million. The filing of the lawsuit was planned for January 1, 1994, the same date as the start-up of TennCare. The TMA claimed that TennCare was unconstitutional because it gave too much administrative power to the executive branch of government and took power away from the legislature, which is the appropriate branch of government to initiate health care reform. TMA also claimed that the governor was behind TennCare's ''secret development'' which ''provided no advance notice or opportunity to comment on the proposed rules governing TennCare,'' and which TMA therefore felt violated the Tennessee Administrative Procedures Act.[7]

The officials at HCFA were not initially supportive of a waiver. An associate administrator of HCFA observed that 1,220 faxes were received in one week's time from Tennessee physicians and about 200 letters from Medicaid recipients opposing the waiver.[8] HCFA also questioned $595 million claimed by the governor's application as state-provided revenue which was actually the estimated amount of charity care traditionally offered by physicians and hospitals.[9] Governor McWherter blamed the delay on heavy lobbying by Tennessee doctors of HCFA officials in Washington.[10] The governor, a land mine engineer in the U.S. Army Reserves, dismissed the delay by saying, ''We're in a minefield and we're laying bridges to get out.''[11]

Governor McWherter responded by contacting fellow Democrat President Clinton about the prospects of bypassing HCFA's waiver procedures and receiving an executive order to have the waiver issued.[12] The TMA charged that bypassing HCFA would be unconstitutional, and threatened a federal lawsuit if an executive order was issued.

The original TennCare plan included the elimination of a special hospital tax which brought in over $202 million yearly.[13] This tax reduction was an inducement to hospitals across the state which together form a major health care interest group. Once opposition began to the plan, McWherter threatened to reimpose the tax, and expand it to include physicians' practices. Eliminating this tax from TennCare served two purposes: it was a buy-off of potential opposition groups, and also served to undermine opposition when McWherter threatened to reimpose and expand the tax.

The cost savings from the termination of Tennessee's Medicaid depended upon TennCare's managed care services operating in a way similar to the Blue

Cross/Blue Shield of Tennessee (BCBS) plan offered for one million state employees. However, TennCare would pay less for certain services than BCBS. Why would providers contract with TennCare if they will subsequently receive comparatively lower payments for services? Governor McWherter had the answer: require all providers who want to contract with BCBS of Tennessee to also contract with TennCare. The TMA called this requirement "a big stick" to force doctors to join TennCare and accept lower payments for some of their patients.[14] In a letter to HCFA, TMA's General Counsel wrote that "the phrase 'cram down' which physicians are using to describe the BCBS TennCare contract is appropriate since it so effectively symbolizes how the state is trying to enlist physician support."[15] The TMA encouraged all 8,000 Tennessee doctors to boycott BCBS of Tennessee, of which 7,000 were members, and most doctors announced plans to end their contract with BCBS of Tennessee on January 1, 1994, the start-up date for TennCare.

DFA Commissioner Manning responded by saying that the BCBS requirement allowed the state to use the leverage it has in the marketplace to "ensure the best price and access."[16] The TMA requested HCFA to increase the level of payments for certain treatments before granting a waiver.

McWherter refused to compromise. Finally, he agreed to cut $300 million out of the estimated amount of charity care, lowered the number of covered participants from 1.8 million to 1.5 million with a cap of 1.3 million until June 30, 1994, and received the waiver from HCFA.[17] TennCare received approval only five months after requested, in large part because it was one step ahead of organized opposition.

Only days after HCFA granted the waiver, a senior vice president of Blue Cross/Blue Shield of Tennessee announced that doctors were coming back to the plan and renewing their contracts for the next year. Even Dr. Charles White, President of the Tennessee Medical Association, finally agreed to sign contracts with Managed Care Organizations to treat TennCare patients.[18]

Months after the January 1 starting date of TennCare, more than two dozen bills were still pending in the legislature to change certain parts of the program. Some of the bills were intended to weaken the so-called "cram down" provision that required providers for the state employees' Blue Cross/Blue Shield plan to also accept TennCare patients. Others dealt with fears that MCOs would shortchange the needs of the seriously mentally ill now that TennCare would be delivering mental health services to patients previously served by the state through Medicaid.

Acknowledging the legal right of legislators to change the TennCare program, McWherter "begged" them to defeat the pending bills. He explained, "I'm not opposed to them, I just don't want them to pass. The members of the legislature brought those bills because they're concerned and I respect them."[19] Recognizing that there were problems to be solved, McWherter urged legislators to give his office a chance to improve the administration of the program without resorting to legislation.

The last legislation to be defeated was the so-called "anti–cram down" bill: it died quietly in subcommittee. The sponsor of the bill lamented the legislature's unwillingness to address constituents' problems with legislation.[20] Governor McWherter responded to opposition legislation by correcting the glitches in TennCare addressed by the bills, and not by opposing the legislation itself. By avoiding a heavy-handed approach to opposition bills, McWherter also avoided any appearance of encroaching upon legislative prerogatives.

TENNCARE'S QUALITY OF SERVICE AND PATIENT ACCESS

TennCare's clientele were not only former Medicaid patients, but also impoverished individuals who for some reason did not qualify for Medicaid, the working poor, and all other uninsured individuals. Ironically, a recent survey by the American Medical Association revealed that during 1992, about one-third of the nation's physicians did not offer health insurance to their employees.[21] Many of the uninsured who work for physicians will now be able to have insurance coverage. The enlarged clientele of TennCare provided a new constituency who supported the end of Medicaid. Governor McWherter tied the end of Medicaid to the expanded coverage of TennCare.

"I think they should have left Medicaid alone. All this was jumped into before they thought it through," said Debbie Armstrong, mother of a blind 20-year-old in a wheelchair with the mental functioning of a toddler.[22] She had just found out that the pediatrician who is familiar with her son's medical history was not an authorized TennCare provider, and that she must now search for a new doctor. One cost of TennCare's rapid implementation—it started just eight months after the governor unveiled his creation—was that there were numerous operational problems resulting from such an early start-up date.

Confusion reigned at local emergency rooms as patients arrived unsure of what MCO plan they were in and hospitals tried to learn if their services were covered under TennCare.[23] State officials investigated the death of a baby whose mother said she was denied health care by area hospitals.[24] The mother claimed that hospital emergency rooms would not see her and that she was unable to get an appointment at clinics that contract with TennCare. Former Medicaid patients are accustomed to receiving care through emergency rooms, but TennCare limits payment for emergency room treatment of anything less than critical illness or trauma-type injuries.

TennCare also affected special services such as dental and vision care services. Without Medicaid's level of reimbursement, some high-volume vision operations went out of business, leaving patients to search for optometrists who participated in TennCare.[25]

During the first six months of TennCare, the Regional Medical Center at Memphis dismissed 250 employees in what was described as a response to declining business. The Chief Operating Officer of "the Med" explained that over $9 million was lost during the first six months of TennCare due primarily to incentives that keep patients out of the hospital and emergency room. The Med plans to market ambulatory and outpatient services in response to declining hospital admissions.

Annie Dickens went a week without the prescription medicine she needed to combat insomnia because her TennCare provider would not pay for it, and she could not afford to spend the $20.99 plus tax for a one-month supply. Her monthly income was $446.[26] TennCare coverage does not automatically mean a patient's MCO will purchase prescribed drugs. MCOs do not pay for about 15% of prescribed medication, according to W. R. C. Smith of Whitehaven Mental Health Center. Patients unable to obtain prescription medicine for psychiatric illnesses from MCOs can obtain the medicine from community mental health centers. The Whitehaven Center, which served about 1,200 people in 1993, spent $25,000 during the first half of 1994 on medication not covered by MCOs.[27]

The MCOs received about $100 a month from the state for each enrollee, and they competed fiercely with one another in order to maintain sufficient cash flow for operations. One MCO in search of increased enrollments went so far as to enroll county jail inmates in TennCare, even though inmates are prohibited by federal law from participation.[28] Because inmates' health care is paid for directly by the county, state, or federal government, an MCO could pocket the $100 a month for each inmate enrolled and use it to inflate cash flow and increase profit margin. The Attorney General's office is prosecuting the accused MCO for consumer fraud.

There are currently twelve MCOs participating in TennCare out of an original eighteen, and only two of them cover the entire state. An independent health care consultant, who wishes to remain anonymous, confides that more of these MCOs will probably drop out, leaving only four MCOs remaining. These "dropouts" will occur because of low enrollment, poor utilization review, and a lack of adequate cash flow. MCOs must be able to operate with a very small profit margin, making high enrollments essential for adequate fund balances. Good utilization review results in optimal cost control, also providing important cash reserves. Low enrollment and poor utilization review results in a lack of adequate cash flow to operate. Once MCOs begin to drop out as TennCare providers, participants will have to choose from the remaining MCOs.

Jim Moss, President of Jackson-Madison County General Hospital, repeated his call for the implementation of TennCare to be slowed.[29] The rapid implementation of TennCare was necessary to keep one step ahead of opposition groups, and to inhibit compromise. But its intended long-term savings resulted in programmatic and, in some cases, human short-term costs.

Republican Governor Don Sundquist, elected in 1994, faced numerous compaints from health care providers about low reimbursement rates. With the help of Republican Congressman Ed Bryant, Sundquist obtained an extra $182 million in federal funds for TennCare in 1995. In addition, Sundquist increased the state payments to MCOs from $100 per enrollee per month to $128.20 in order to provide higher reimbursement amounts for providers. Sundquist also tightened collection procedures for those enrollees who were paying part or all of their TennCare premiums, and for the first time began to require a small monthly premium from those enrollees with family income below the poverty line. Governor Sundquist's success at increasing TennCare's funding has so far received a favorable response from health care providers.

Most recently, TennCare has been expanded to include state Mental Health and Retardation programs and has been moved from the Department of Finance and Administration to the state's new superagency, the Department of Human Services. TennCare not only adds to the state's largest bureaucracy but it is also the state's most expensive program, costing over $3.5 billion in fiscal year 1997.

CONCLUSION

What implications are there from Tennessee's experience at health care reform for other states faced with ever-increasing health care costs and underfunded Medicaid programs? First, Tennessee's experience demonstrates that the politics of health care reform is just as important as its content or structure. The speed of TennCare's implementation was intended to keep reform one step ahead of opposition from the Tennessee Medical Association. Once the TMA mounted an opposition campaign, Governor McWherter required physicians participating in the state's Blue Cross/Blue Shield plan to also participate in TennCare. This "cram down" provision of TennCare was a coercive incentive for physician participation in TennCare. McWherter also eliminated the hospital tax in order to gain support for TennCare from major health care organizations, but threatened to reimpose and expand the tax to physicians' practices if TennCare wasn't adopted. Other states contemplating health care reform should keep in mind the strong executive leadership, the check on opposition groups, and the hang-tough politics that characterized Tennessee's reform efforts.

Second, employing a managed care approach for state health care reform affects the access and quality of health care. Confusion about which doctors and hospitals were participating in TennCare was accompanied by some Medicaid specialty providers (for example, vision care centers) going out of business. By changing reimbursement rates and providers, Tennessee made it more difficult for some former Medicaid patients to obtain services they were accustomed to receiving.

However, TennCare also made it possible for some of those previously without coverage (the working poor) to purchase health benefits. Although some participants experienced limited access and a reduction in quality of health services, TennCare enabled other participants to finally obtain health care coverage for themselves and their families. Legislators contemplating health care reform should keep in mind that there are winners and losers in any reform program.

Leaders of Tennessee's statehouse felt that more restrictive access and a some-what lower quality of health services was acceptable in order to control the costs of health care and to expand health care coverage to a greater number of citizens. Ultimately, the access and quality of health services provided to citizens by the state depends upon the amount of money the state decides to spend on public health services.

Another lesson for other states contemplating a managed care system is that marketplace competition will eventually eliminate all but the best-funded, best-managed MCOs. The marketplace submits MCOs to a process of natural selection that forces the weaker MCOs—those with lower enrollments, poor utilization review, and less cash flow—to go out of business. Individuals and families covered by the managed care system become confused, frustrated, and discouraged when their MCO closes its doors. Perhaps the State of Tennessee should have accepted bids from MCOs, and then selected the best three to be the MCO vendors for TennCare. Although this would be an intrusion by government into the marketplace, it would result in stable MCOs, and less enrollment confusion.

For the present, increases in the cost of health care provided by Tennessee have been stabilized. Despite protests from some participants about the access and quality of health services, and complaints from providers about low reimbursement rates, TennCare has operated closer to its budget and has not experienced the severe underfunding of the previous Medicaid plan. Issues surrounding access, quality of services, and reimbursement rates will doubtlessly continue to be addressed as TennCare establishes its financial operating record. If nothing else, TennCare has demonstrated how managed care can better control costs when compared to the previous Medicaid plan.

NOTES

1. James M. Hoefler and Khi V. Thai, "Introduction to the Politics and Economics of Health Care Finance: A Symposium," *Journal of Health and Human Resources Administration* 16, no. 2 (1993): 116, 117.

2. Tennessee Department of Finance and Administration, *TennCare: A New Direction in Health Care* (Nashville: State of Tennessee, 1993): 95.

3. Department of Finance and Administration, *Medicaid: Tennessee's Health Care Problem* (Nashville: State of Tennessee, 1993): 3, 4.

4. Tennessee Medical Association, *TennCare Alert* VIII (January 26, 1994).

5. Personal interview with Mark Greene, Executive Director, Tennessee Medical Association (January 10, 1994).

6. Ed Cromer, and Bill Snyder, "Doctors Deluged by TennCare Calls," *Nashville Banner* (October 8, 1993).

7. Tennessee Medical Association.

8. Jeff Woods, "TennCare: Banner Publisher Thinks Blue Cross Abusing Its Power," *Nashville Banner* (November 9, 1993).

9. Ed Cromer, "McWherter Says It's Time Feds Decide on TennCare," *Nashville Banner* (November 10, 1993).

10. Rebecca Ferrar, "Governor Says U.S. Delay in OK for TennCare Nears Critical Point," *Knoxville News-Sentinel* (October 13, 1993).

11. Reed Branson, "State to Play Politics for TennCare Waiver," *Commercial Appeal* (Memphis, Tenn., October 13, 1993).

12. Ed Cromer and Bill Snyder, "McWherter Takes Case for TennCare to Clinton," *Nashville Banner* (November 9, 1993).

13. Unlike federal income tax which is based upon net profit, the hospital gross-receipts tax is based upon the amount of income received through billing. Under the gross-receipts tax, it is possible for a hospital to owe tax even though it earns no profit.

14. Rebecca Ferrar, "Is TennCare Bully Stick or Cash Carrot?" *Knoxville News-Sentinel* (November 14, 1993).

15. Michael Finn, "Governor Warned on Waiver Tactics," *Chattanooga News-Free Press* (November 9, 1993).

16. Ed Cromer and Bill Snyder, "McWherter Takes Case for TennCare to Clinton," *Nashville Banner* (November 9, 1993).

17. Reed Branson and James W. Brosnan, "Reduced TennCare Gets Federal OK," *Commercial Appeal* (Memphis, Tenn., November 19, 1993).

18. Duren Cheek, "Health-Plan Summit Slated," *The Tennessean* (Nashville, Tenn., February 3, 1994).

19. Paula Wade, "Leave TennCare Alone, McWherter Implores Bill-Happy Lawmakers," *Commercial Appeal* (Memphis, Tenn., April, 1, 1994).

20. Nashville Bureau, "TennCare Reform Sponsor Decries Death of Last Bill," *Commercial Appeal* (Memphis, Tenn., April 1, 1994).

21. Natalie Sleeth, "AMA Cools to Employer Health Rule," *Commercial Appeal* (Memphis, Tenn., December 8, 1993): A1.

22. Samuel Galant, "Confusion Surrounds TennCare," *Commercial Appeal* (Memphis, Tenn., January 11, 1994): A1.

23. Kilgore Trout, "TennCare Gets off to a Shaky Start at City's Hospitals," *Commercial Appeal* (Memphis, Tenn., January 5, 1994): B1.

24. John Adams, "Baby Death, TennCare Link Probed," *Commercial Appeal* (Memphis, Tenn., February 19, 1994): A8.

25. Memphis Bureau, "Move to TennCare Reduced Eye, Dental Services to Poor," *Commercial Appeal* (Memphis, Tenn., March 17, 1994): A1.

26. Ibid.

27. Ibid.

28. Kenneth W. Hollman and Robert D. Hayes, "TennCare: Many Problems Unresolved," *Tennessee's Business* 6, no. 3 (1995): 8, 9.

29. Ibid.

16

Medicaid Reform in the Lone Star State: State of Texas Access Reform *Star

CAROL WATERS AND AARON KNIGHT

INTRODUCTION

Texas policymakers are scrambling to find solutions to the daunting problems generated by its complex, burdensome, and controversial Medicaid program. In this state of vast diversity, extensive land mass, and strongly voiced interest groups, many potential reform measures are launched with great optimism only to be shot down in the crossfire of competing interests. The dust is beginning to settle, leaving Texas citizens with a hazy, but somewhat clearer view of the future of Medicaid reform. The unique geographic, demographic, societal, and political characteristics of the state have made the path to reform steep and rocky; the convoluted, inefficient health care delivery system and increasing costs have made reform essential.

DIVERSITY AND CONTRAST

The population of Texas is 80.3%[1] urban but the land mass is approximately 80% rural.[2] The majority of Texas residents live in urbanized areas where medical facilities are abundant and modern. In contrast, the rural areas of the state have scattered, often poor inhabitants with high levels of medical needs but limited access to medical facilities. Sixty-one of the 254 Texas counties are designated medically underserved, having only one to three physicians. There are 20 Texas counties with no physicians at all.[3]

Texas has its share of millionaires and of prosperous middle-class citizenry with adequate access to the most innovative health care facilities and procedures, but there are many poor Texans as well. In this relatively prosperous state, 18.1% of the population live in poverty.[4] Among ethnic groups, 28% of the state's African-American citizens (including 40% of African-American children) and 30% of Hispanic Texans (including 39% of Hispanic children) live in poverty. Approximately 50% of Medicaid eligibles are very poor, living below the federal poverty line. Statewide, the Medicaid program itself pays for 47% of all births in the state. In some regions, the proportion of Medicaid-paid births is as high as 75% of all births.[5]

In addition, the number of potential recipients is increasing rapidly. Texas has the highest number of residents under age eighteen of any state. The birth rate in 1992 was 18.4/100,000, above the national average of 16.0/100,000.[6] The relatively young population portends high birth rates and high demands on the Medicaid system in the future. Implications for the growth of the Medicaid program are reflected in state data that indicate that the cost of two eligible groups, children and disabled adults, is three times that for other covered groups.[7]

HEALTH STATUS OF TEXANS

Despite intensive efforts of providers to include all eligible pregnant women and all eligible children in preventative health care services, the immunization rate for children under two years of age is 55%. Other evidence of low utilization of preventative care is the above-average rate of deaths from diabetes (20.2/ 100,000). The rate of death from cervical cancer, highly curable with early detection, is increasing among Hispanic women at a rate twice that of the increase among the white population.[8] Almost one-fourth (21.1%) of the Texas population lacks any type of health insurance, giving the state the dubious distinction of ranking last among the states and the District of Columbia.[9] Residents without health insurance do not have private insurance nor do they qualify for government programs.

Reasons for the high number of uninsured Texas residents include the high number of jobs in service industries and small firms which offer low rates of health benefits. Almost 45% of Texas jobs are in retail and service industries, while 65% of jobs in rural areas and 43% of jobs in urban areas are provided by small businesses. Many of those who work in these low-paying jobs are simply unable to afford health insurance. Furthermore, the changing circumstances of Medicaid recipients results in an "on again off again" cycle in which clients lose and regain eligibility with such frequency that continuity of care is disrupted. Currently, job growth is expected to continue in low-paying service industries.[10] The situation is somewhat alleviated along the Texas-Mexico border because many Texas residents obtain health care in Mexico. According to a recent study, even though 52% of Texas border residents are completely lacking any health insurance, 25% gain access to health care through this route.[11] Obviously, that is not a remedy convenient, or even available, to all Texans.

POLITICAL CLIMATE OF TEXAS

Republican Governor George Bush, Jr., and Democratic Lieutenant Governor Bob Bullock, have both expressed a commitment to "budget neutrality" in reforming Medicaid.[12] In other words, no new taxes to support the growing demand on the program can be expected. The Texas legislature is not permitted, according to the State Constitution, to run a budget deficit. This creates tremendous pressure to cut spending for social programs during tough economic times. With unorganized political constituencies, programs designed for the poor would seem likely targets for cuts. Considering increasing state costs, the 1995 legislature attached a rider to an appropriations bill requiring Texas state agencies to cut expenditures by $200 million in fiscal year 1996–1997. The agencies responsible for administering Medicaid, Human Services, and the Texas Department of Health will find stretching dollars even more difficult. The Texas Department of Health, which operates or administers a large number of clinics with heavy Medicaid use, has recently cut 600 people from its staff and closed 60 public health clinics. The remaining clinics are largely being moved toward privatization, with a view to fee-for-service charges to clients, whether Medicaid-paid or privately paid.[13]

Furthermore, local and community health clinics which have historically filled in gaps in the health care delivery system have been reduced or even eliminated in many jurisdictions to compensate for budget constraints among local governments.[14] These factors compel more emphasis on Medicaid efficiency in service delivery if access is not to be reduced for many Texans. The efficiencies of managed care are attractive in an environment of increasing need, decreasing alternative sources of care, and public unwillingness to support tax increases.

STATE RESOURCES

Texas remains one of only five states without a personal or corporate state income tax. Instead, it relies heavily on sales taxes, drawing 31% of its indigenous revenues from general sales tax, making it the fifth highest among states in sales tax assessment. In comparison with other states, the overall tax burden is relatively light, ranked 44th among states, but the burden on local jurisdictions is 31st, indicating limited state aid to localities.[15] Local government derives 39% of its revenue from the highly unpopular property tax. While oil and gas severance taxes once produced substantial revenues for Texas, that source has been declining steadily since the mid-1980s. Although the state lottery and other, miscellaneous sources provide some state money, few alternative sources of revenue are available in the conservative political climate of Texas.

The conservative, business-friendly political culture is reluctant, at best, to support "welfare" programs. Texas spends $2,500 a year per Medicaid recipient compared with a national average of $3,900.[16] It ranks 48th among the states in average per recipient spending on Medicaid and 47th in overall health spending.[17] The same study found that Texas ranks 26th in the number of public health workers per 1,000 population. The annual growth rate for Medicaid enrollment between 1988 and 1992 was 8.6% nationally. The growth rate in Texas was twice that.[18] The Kaiser Foundation projects that growth rates on health spending will increase 33% in Texas from 1996 to 2000, compared with growth rates of 28% in California and 41% in New York.[19] With already extremely low benefits and strict qualifying criteria, Texas can do little to shrink Medicaid enrollment. Texas is constrained by federal legislation and judicial activity regarding just how austere its Medicaid payments can be and how limited in scope the program can get. Indeed, the lack of support for local public health agencies has been attributed to the public perception that these programs primarily benefit the poor.[20] The large number of residents without health insurance severely strains the resources of counties, and draws from the state treasury large sums of money for the most expensive form of care for the uninsured.

HEALTH CARE FOR THE POOR IN TEXAS

Medicaid provides the primary source of access to health care for poor and near-poor Texans. In 1994, 16% of the Texas population were 1115 Waiver Proposal–enrolled in Medicaid. A large percentage of the income-eligible population has not enrolled in the program, though some of those may be undocumented aliens who are not actually eligible because of citizen status.[21] Others may be unaware of their eligibility, may lack transportation to health care facilities, or may face other access barriers such as the inability to find a participating physician in the current fee-for-service reimbursement system.[22]

Those low-income Texans who are not eligible for Medicaid rely on other, somewhat uncoordinated, sources for care. Hospital districts, public hospitals, hospital authorities, medical schools, state-operated teaching hospitals, and counties that have no hospital district or public hospital bear much of the burden for providing care for uninsured residents. Municipal health departments and charitable clinics also provide screening and some types of care for those ineligible for other programs.

Funding for indigent care in hospital districts and public hospitals is derived from property tax revenues and from state reimbursement through the County Indigent Health Care Program (CIHCP). CIHCP requires hospital districts and public hospitals to be fully responsible for care for needy inhabitants. Counties without public hospitals or hospital districts must provide care to the limit of $30,000 or 30 days' hospitalization per year. The state pays 80% of the expenditures after the county has spent 10% of its general tax levy for the fiscal year on indigent clients.[23]

The indigent health care programs result in millions of dollars of uncompensated medical care, often incurred through inappropriate use of emergency room services or because of delay in treatment. Primary care, particularly preventative programs, is underused by the uninsured population so that the overall costs, per patient, are high in terms of money and suffering. Costs to local governments are high, but have been offset by the Disproportionate Share Hospital program (DSH). DSH funds originated to compensate hospitals that serve a high number of Medicaid recipients and other poor clients through augmented reimbursement of hospital "donations" to the state's Medicaid funds to attract federal matching dollars. Originally, the program set no ceiling on money spent or restrictions on fund-raising sources so that it became a source of unlimited funding for participating hospitals, and drove up Medicaid expenditures substantially. Nationally, 14% of Medicaid spending from the federal government is for disproportionate share hospital payments. These payments go to assisted hospitals with large proportions of uninsured and indigent patient populations.[24] In 1994, DSH funds were capped at $1.5 billion, but still provide a significant source of revenue for many Texas hospitals.

THE MOVEMENT TOWARD REFORM

The Medicaid program in Texas, always costly and lacking broad-based political support, severely stressed the state's coffers when rolls increased with expansion of federally mandated eligibility criteria in the early 1990s. The U.S. Supreme Court decision in *Sullivan v. Zebley* (1990) meant substantial growth for the number of children brought into the program. From 1988 to 1995, total nationwide spending on Medicaid more than tripled from $51 billion to $158 billion.[25] Since the program is jointly financed by the federal and state governments, the explosion in cost had a dramatic impact in Texas where, surpassing the 50-state average by 6%, Medicaid spending makes up 26% of the state's budget.[26] While Washington contemplates reforms, which seem almost sure to mean a reduction in the per recipient federal commitment to Medicaid, Austin has been scrambling to restructure its indigent public health delivery system in such a way as to cope with the evolving crisis. Trying to cope with the phenomenal growth in Medicaid enrollments and costs without overhauling the system, substantially cutting the scope of the program, or increasing the burden on the state's budget occupied Texas throughout the 1980s. Costs of the program rose from $7.5 billion in 1990–1991 to a projected $17 billion in 1996–1997. A projected $2.9 million shortfall in 1994 kindled efforts of state officials to institute reform measures, culminating in 1995 Senate Bill 10, approving a proposed Medicaid 1115 Waiver that details a Texas-designed Medicaid delivery system with a major emphasis on managed care.

In 1991, Texas passed limited legislation enabling the state to experiment with the concept of managed care for Medicaid recipients. House Bill 7 passed by the 72nd legislature created the Bureau of Managed Care within the Texas Department of Health. This enabling legislation charged the Bureau with establishment and oversight of the state's first Medicaid managed care pilot projects. Utilizing already proven approaches for comprehensive managed care, the program pursued five key goals; through the use of the primary provider model (PCP), managed care in Texas seeks to improve access to care, quality of care, client and provider satisfaction, cost-effectiveness, and recipient health status.[27] Managed care pilot projects were initiated in two areas in Texas beginning in 1993. The Travis County (Austin) area in central Texas implemented a combination of Health Maintenance Organization (HMO) and partially capitated, prepaid health plan enrolling approximately 30,000 eligibles. The tri-county Gulf Coast area including Jefferson, Chambers, and Galveston counties instituted an enhanced PCCM plan, with 32,000 clients. The evaluation of those programs was positive in terms of reducing costs and improving access, quality of care, and provider and client satisfaction.[28]

TEXAS 1115 WAIVER PROPOSAL

On March 15, 1994, Lieutenant Governor Bob Bullock, the leader of the Texas State Senate, directed the Texas Senate Health and Human Services Committee (SHHSC) to recommend changes to the state's Medicaid program aimed at saving state money. With the legislature in recess, as it always is during even-numbered years, the staff of the SHHSC, together with the State Medicaid Office (SMO) worked throughout the remainder of 1994 to hammer out what became the Medicaid reform bills which passed both the House and Senate during the 1995 74th meeting of the Texas legislature. By the close of the legislative session, ten separate reform measures had passed. The most significant of the reforms was contained in Senate Bill 10, authorizing the Texas Health and Human Services Commission (THHSC) to seek a section 1115 Waiver from HFCA to allow a comprehensive overhaul of the state's Medicaid system.[29] This restructuring was aimed at bringing as much of the state's program as possible into the managed care model, expanding the population covered by Medicaid, and giving local providers a greater role in administration and financing of managed care in their areas. A key component of the waiver request was the implementation of managed care via a major reorganization which would maximize use of available funds by creation of state-local partnerships, using local money formerly used for indigent care and DSH funds to "draw down" federal matching dollars, increasing state coordination of local delivery systems, and applying additional moneys realized to expansion of Medicaid eligibility criteria within the state. The plan was to invite local entities such as counties, multiple counties, hospital districts, medical schools, and state teaching hospitals to form nonprofit corporations called Intergovernmental Initiatives (IGIs or "iggys") which would select and administer the locally preferred managed care model. The plan included state-implemented managed care in local areas choosing not to form IGIs.

The concept of IGIs was founded on recognition of the importance of local control and flexibility in order to meet the unique needs of diverse communities. Contributions from county tax revenue and other local public health care funds to the Medicaid fund would attract more federal money which could then be used to finance extension of eligibility to certain currently ineligible groups. Current levels of federal funding for DSH would be included, converting DSH into an expanded Medicaid program. Local entities would be guaranteed to receive back at least as much as the amount they originally made available. The state government, of course, would oversee IGIs. With the additional federal money made available through IGIs, Medicaid coverage would be extended to: certain low-income children and adults currently ineligible, including children through age eighteen with incomes at or below 133% of federal poverty level (FPL) and adults with income at or below 45% of FPL with a goal of 75% FPL. Much to the distress of those who constructed the waiver, IGIs were universally rejected by local jurisdictions, particularly the larger hospital districts and teaching hospitals, who were fearful of losing control to the state.

Other significant provisions in the waiver proposal to encourage physician participation included: high-volume payments to facilities which serve unusually large numbers of Medicaid recipients; value-added reimbursement to providers for services that are valued by the state but that are not rewarded or reimbursed by the market; and, establishment of a special $20 million fund for rural hospitals that are sole community providers for a significant number of Medicaid and charity care patients, and that are part of an IGI. The state also assured three-year continuing participation in Medicaid to those providers who have a history of Medicaid participation.

INTEREST GROUP CONFLICTS AND CONCERNS

The many interest groups involved in health care delivery in Texas were instrumental in altering the direction of the state in its movement toward Medicaid reform. Even the concept of managed care itself has generated controversy among health care providers in Texas. Lack of cooperation with state officials in modifying the method of care delivery stems from conflicting interests which vary from region to region. Primary care physicians in lucrative markets may be reluctant to participate in managed care with its overwhelming paperwork and myriad of restrictions; in areas with heavy Medicaid usage, Medicaid patients may make up a large percentage of the patients in all primary providers' caseloads. In the latter markets, primary care physicians who have been traditional Medicaid providers are concerned with the prospect of being left out if they do not choose to participate in a managed care organization. Other, very conservative physicians object to any form of coverage which does not "engage patients as payers and, thus, in collaboration with their physicians, . . . become more economical, responsible decision-makers in the direction of their own care."[30] In his article in *Texas Medicine*, Dr. Rappaport insists that effective reform should: educate people about the importance of preventive services and of budgeting for those services; include means-testing for Medicare coverage; and encourage medical savings accounts to help people prepare for increasing medical needs.

Some specialists who do not offer primary care object to the managed care provision that requires referral for special treatment. They recognize that continuity of care is crucial to reduce unnecessary duplication and inappropriate or conflicting treatments, but see the dependency on primary care physicians (who have incentives to cut costs of treatment) as threatening to minimize referrals in marginal cases. They argue that such reluctance is likely to have a deleterious effect on the health outcomes of patients. Implementation of managed care in pilot projects has required intensive communication between state officials and local interests. The selection of the particular managed care model or combination of models best fitted for each region continues to be heavily dependent on local input. Regional hearings to facilitate dialogue between officials, citizens, and providers are planned in all targeted managed care sites.

Additional controversy arose because of disagreements between the state and some hospital administrators over the level of matching funds provided to hospitals by the state. Administrators insisted that the language of the section 1115 Waiver proposal be amended to clearly state that money in the transition pool be first used to make additional high-volume payments and then, to the extent that funds remain, be used to expand Medicaid eligibility. Commissioner of Health and Human Services, Dr. Michael D. McKinney, argued that such change would violate the intent of the legislature, expressed in Senate Bill 10, to eventually extend eligibility to adults at 75% FPL.[31] Reimbursement rates and compensation for inequities in caseloads for treatment of Medicaid patients continues to be a source of debate. Texas physicians are still smarting from the 1994 freeze on Medicaid reimbursement fees imposed by Governor Bush. The announcement of the freeze in 1993 elicited strong reaction among providers who argued that such government action reduces the number of providers who are willing to participate in Medicaid.[32]

Physicians from Texas have traveled to Washington to lobby Congress concerning reforms to protect health care providers in the changing environment of service delivery. Among the demands of Texas physicians are liability reform and antitrust relief to enable primary care physicians to compete with MCOs. On the other hand, conservative business persons, hospitals, and managed care interests oppose antitrust reform.[33] Those entities support Patient Protection Laws similar to those that have been passed in 33 other states and are pending in others. Such laws limit the right of MCOs to restrict patient choice by requiring payment of fees to physicians outside the HMO or other MCO. They also generally contain provisions which will require payment of emergency room fees outside the system as long as the emergency was reasonably believed to have been bona fide.

The Texas legislature passed a Patient Protection Law in 1995 only to have the legislation vetoed by Governor Bush.[34] Other managed care legislation did become law in 1995. HB 3111 requires that nonprofit corporations which intend to provide or arrange for a health care plan on a capitated basis separate from a HMO receive a certificate of authority from the Texas Department of Insurance as if they were HMOs. SB 1407 clarifies who can contract with HMOs. These new laws allow physicians to contract to provide or arrange for medical care through other physicians and other providers for ancillary services. Providers can contract for services they are not licensed to provide so long as those services do not exceed 15% of its total services. The Texas Department of Insurance, the licensing authority for MCOs, has recently issued new regulations to implement some of the areas addressed in the vetoed patient protection act.[35]

The great concern with liability reform stems, in part, from the misconception that Medicaid clients are more likely than others to file malpractice claims. Studies have indicated that those patients, in reality, file fewer claims, but the average award is higher for Medicaid clients. That may be a result of the limitations in access to legal remedies among Medicaid recipients which leads to only those most seriously injured filing suits.

Participation in Medicaid by providers varies according to the market. In some areas, Medicaid recipients have difficulty finding willing providers. Reimbursement rates set by the state, controlled by the Boren Amendment, may affect willingness of physicians to participate. In an attempt to stem costs, Governor Bush froze Medicaid reimbursements in 1994. The number of participating physicians did not increase during that year, whereas an increase in reimbursement fees resulted, in 1990, in an 11% increase in participation.

Other providers, including home health services, nurse practitioners, and therapists have expressed lack of support for managed care systems which may limit the participation of independent services in Medicaid-paid cases. For example, Heather Vasek, Research and Policy Specialist for the Texas Association for Home Care (TAHC), in testimony before the SHHSC during public hearings in March of 1995, expressed concerns about the creation of IGIs and about the movement to mandatory MCO provision of Medicaid-paid services. Representing over 700 provider companies, TAHC is the largest organized voice of home care interests in the state.

Vasek expressed two major fears regarding the move toward managed care in Texas. First, she feared that the interests of home care providers would not be adequately represented on the IGI governing boards as described in SB 10. Second, because at least 25% of all home health care providers are connected with hospitals, the providers, after expiration of the three-year grace period which assures that current providers will continue to serve Medicaid clients, Vasek was concerned that IGI governing boards would develop managed care contracts using only one selected home care provider. This would effectively end competition in a contracted area and would limit patient choice. This would be especially troublesome for the populations who are the heaviest users of home

care, the elderly and the disabled, as they tend to be the populations least able
to move to areas where superior care is available.[36]

In a related, cost-saving move, Texas attempted to install a market-based
reimbursement formula for Medicaid-paid pharmaceuticals in 1995. The pharmacists were able to obtain injunctive relief restraining the state from reducing
reimbursement rates per prescription. According to pharmacists, the reimbursement rate under the new system would have fallen from $4.55 per prescription
to $3.00 per prescription, an untenable cut for a product that costs an average
of $5.01 to fill.

The Vendor Drug Program, administered by the Texas Department of Health,
affects approximately 3,500 pharmacies which fill close to 2 million prescriptions each year. The savings realized by the reduction in reimbursement would
be substantial; however, 70% of Texas pharmacies participate in the program
and are likely to form a strong interest group in opposition to reduction. Especially ardent are the pharmacists on the Texas-Mexico border who compete, in
best of times, with pharmaceutical sales by Mexican drug companies and sup-
pliers. A Laredo pharmacist, Francisco Rodriquez, indicated that 80% of prescriptions he fills are Medicaid-paid. He charged that "This fee cut would have
been devastating to local independent pharmacies, possibly forcing some of them
to close their doors which would deprive the Medicaid recipient of needed pharmacy services and hurt the very people the Texas Department of Health is
supposed to be helping: the Medicaid recipient."[37] In 1997, during the 75th
Texas Legislature, the Board of Pharmacy avoided both selective contracting
with individual pharmacies and inclusion of the Vendor Drug Program in managed care. The result is a compromise that maintains reimbursement rates within
the limits of costs to pharmacists, and increases dispensing fees up to a maximum cap.

MANAGED CARE

Pilot projects are expected to begin in Bexar County (San Antonio) and its
contiguous surrounding counties on August 1, 1996; Lubbock County and its
surrounding counties as well as Tarrant (Fort Worth) and contiguous counties,
and an expansion of the Travis County program to include surrounding counties
will begin September 1. Other managed care sites are planned throughout the
state. All metropolitan statistical areas (MSAs) of the state are projected to be
included by 1999. Because participation rates in newly established MCOs take
approximately three years to grow to include all eligible recipients, the maximum enrollment of Medicaid recipients in managed care is not expected until
2001. As that potential source of increased funding has faded into the horizon,
the emphasis has become introducing state-implemented managed care statewide. The waiver request will be modified, with a hope of greater success, for

presentation to the upcoming state legislature. Managed care pilot projects have offered encouraging results, but the unique conditions within Texas create a challenging environment to implementation of MCOs for all Medicaid recipients.

In spite of the vast, sparsely populated regions of Texas, a 1995 study indicated that only 4% of Medicaid recipients live outside an area which could support a managed care system. For Medicaid clients in those areas, a traditional fee-for-service system is likely to continue for some time. Nationally, MCOs are beginning to penetrate markets formerly thought to be inappropriate for managed care because of sparse population distribution.[38] Following the failure of local jurisdictions to accept IGIs, and recognizing that implementation is "stalled" until matching fund agreements can be arranged, Health and Human Services Commissioner Michael McKinney has vowed to incorporate as many aspects of the Medicaid reform bill enacted by the 74th legislature as possible. McKinney expressed concern that the vetoed balanced budget bill provides clues to the eventual changes in Medicaid at a national level. Changes, particularly any movement toward capping federal expenditures would, naturally, have a severe impact on state capacity.[39] The projected expansion of eligibility criteria in the 1995 waiver proposal was dependent on contributions of funds from IGIs. With that idea rendered politically unfeasible, the possibility of expanding eligibility becomes more remote. The conservative political climate of Texas is unlikely to support increased taxation for Medicaid expansion.

CONCLUSION

For now, Texas will continue to gradually institute managed care delivery systems throughout the state in order to cover as much of the state's Medicaid eligible population as possible. While the impact of such systems will no doubt vary throughout the state's demographically diverse regions, preliminary evidence produced in pilot programs suggests that some net savings for the state will be realized, at least in the short run.

Unfortunately, comprehensive and inclusive reform, capable of better serving the poorest and most medically underserved Texas residents, seems, for now, unlikely. This is troubling given the rapid growth that is expected in the near future for these populations. As Donald Lee, Executive Director of the Conference of Urban Counties puts it, "we don't have a Medicaid population in Texas, we have an indigent population that at times is Medicaid-eligible."[40] Lee is voicing what many people in Texas are coming to realize: as long as Medicaid and indigent care continue as uncoordinated programs, often in competition for the same local funding dollars, the move toward managed care will be only a partial solution to a growing problem.

NOTES

1. U.S. Department of Health and Human Services, National Center for Health Statistics, "Live Births and Birth Rates by State," Compuserve: Online Groliers' Encyclopedia.

2. Texas Health and Human Services Commission, *Texas 1115 Medicaid Waiver: State of Texas Access Reform* (Austin, Texas, 1995). Unless otherwise noted, data in this chapter are derived from the text of that document.

3. U.S. Department of Health and Human Services, *Texas Map of Underserved Counties*, prepared by the Center for Rural Health Initiatives (Washington, D.C., 1995).

4. Susan Coleman, James V. Calvi, and Fred L. Marsh, *Texas Government* (Upper Saddle River, N.J.: Prentice-Hall, 1996).

5. Adolfo Cardenas, "Proposed Medicare, Medicaid Cuts Will Affect Everyone in Laredo," *Laredo Morning Times* (December 9, 1995).

6. U.S. Dept. H.H.S., National Center for Health Statistics.

7. Current eligibles in Texas: the three principal groups included in Medicaid in Texas are: recipients of Aid to Families with Dependent Children (AFDC); pregnant women and children; and the aged, blind, and disabled. Mandatory eligibles also include AFDC families whose benefits are denied because of employment or child support collections; children aged one to five with family income up to 133% federal poverty level (FPL); children ages 6 and older with family income up to 100% FPL; children receiving Title IV-E foster care; individuals receiving SSI; certain aged, blind, and disabled persons who lose SSI eligibility because of Title II income; qualified Medicare beneficiaries, qualified disabled and working individuals, and specified low-income Medicare beneficiaries whose benefits are limited to Medicare cost-sharing. Optional eligibles are: pregnant women and infants with family income between 133% and 185% FPL; children born before October 1, 1983 who are not in a single, disabled, or unemployed parent household, but whose family income meets the state-established income eligibility standards for AFDC; children in foster care in conservatorship of the Department of Protective and Regulatory Services; children in custody of the Texas Youth Commission; aged, blind, disabled persons who qualify for Medicaid at the institutional income cap (300% SSI) in nursing facility care; individuals in ICF-MR facilities or state schools for the mentally retarded who qualify at the institutional cap; medically needy children under eighteen, pregnant women, and caretaker relatives of dependent children. The "medically needy" are persons who would qualify under one of the listed groups but whose family income is too high. They can qualify for Medicaid if: their income is between the AFDC payment standard and up to 133.3% of AFDC standard; or, through spending down (whereby medical expenses are subtracted from family income). Benefits for the optional eligibles can be discontinued in the case of state budgetary insufficiency. Entitled eligibles must be covered regardless of the state's fiscal condition.

8. Antonio Rene et al., "Mortality Preventable by Medical Intervention: Ethnic and Regional Differences in Texas," *Journal of the National Medical Association* 11 (1987): 820–825.

9. David U. Himmelstein, Steffie Wollhandler, and Sidney M. Wolfe, "The Vanishing Health Care Safety Net: New Data on Uninsured Americans," The Center for National Health Program Studies (Harvard Medical School, The Cambridge Hospital, 1994). Accessed via Compuserve Online.

10. Richard H. Kraemer, Charldean Newell, and David F. Prindle, *Texas Politics*, 6th ed. (Minneapolis/St. Paul: West Publishing Co., 1996), 416.

11. Rene et al., "Mortality Preventable."

12. *Texas Family Physician*, "TAFP Talks with Texas' Lieutenant Governor Bob Bullock" (March 1995): 10–11.

13. Texas Department of Health, Press Release (August 25, 1995).

14. Laura, Beil, *The Dallas Morning News* (May 5, 1996).

15. Kraemer, Newell, and Prindle, *Texas Politics*.

16. Vermeer Medical Association, *Medicaid Managed Care: Implications for Texas* (May 1996), Internet via Texas Department of Health.

17. Leiyu Shi, "Public Health, Medical Care, and Mortality Rates," *Journal of Health Care for the Poor and Underserved* 6 (1995): 307–321.

18. Teresa Coughlin et al., "State Responses to the Medicaid Spending Crisis: 1988 to 1992," *Journal of Health Politics, Policy and Law* 19 (1994): 837–864.

19. Vermeer Medical Association, *Medicaid Managed Care: Implications for Texas*.

20. Laura Beil, *The Dallas Morning News* (May 5, 1996). Comments by Health Commissioner Dr. David Smith.

21. T.H.H.S.C., *Texas 1115 Medicaid Waiver*.

22. Ibid.

23. Ibid.

24. Kaiser Commission on the Future of Medicaid, *Health Needs and Medicaid Financing: State Facts* (Washington, D.C.: Kaiser Commission on the Future of Medicaid, 1995).

25. D. Checkett, Medicaid Restructuring. Testimony before the Senate Finance Committee, U.S. Senate (July 12, 1995).

26. Texas Department of Health, "Texas Medicaid Facts," (1995) Internet: http://www.hhsc.texas.gov/medfacts.htm.

27. T.H.H.S.C., *Texas 1115 Medicaid Waiver*.

28. Dwayne Keeran, Bureau of Managed Care's Director of Operations, telephone interview by Aaron Knight, May 1996. Mr. Keeran reported that at this time there is no definitive evidence to suggest the superiority of any model of managed care in Texas with regard to efficiency or effectiveness.

29. Texas Department of Health, "Medicaid Reform in Texas," and "Texas Medicaid Legislation," (1995), Internet.

30. Norman H. Rappaport, M.D., "Commentary: Meaningful Reform Demands Individual Responsibility for Health-Care Expenditures," *Texas Medicine* 91 (1995): 46–47.

31. Michael D. McKinney, M.D., Statement in November 21, 1995 letter from Dr. McKinney to the Senate Health and Human Services Committee, November 29, 1995 (Courtesy of S.H.H. S.C. Chair Judith Zafferini, Texas State Senator, District 21).

32. Troy Alexander, "Legislative Bulletin," *Texas Family Physician* 45 (1993): 14–15.

33. Ken Ortolon, "Sqeeze Play," *Texas Medicine* 91 (1995): 12–15.

34. Locke Purnell Rain Harrell: A Professional Corporation, "Managed Care Legislation Presents New Issues for Texas Health Care Providers . . ." (Winter 1995), Internet access at http://www.lprh.com/hcare.htm.

35. Ibid.

36. Heather Vasek, telephone interview by Aaron Knight (May 1996).

37. Mark Peterson, "Local Pharmacists Get Reprieve," *Laredo Morning Times* (March 15, 1996).

38. Locke Purnell Rain Harrell, "Managed Care Legislation Presents New Issues for Texas Health Care Providers."

39. Michael D. McKinney, M.D., Statement by Michael McKinney before the Senate Health and Human Services Committee (Courtesy of Judith Zafferini, Texas State Senator, District 21, November 29, 1995).

40. Donald Lee, Executive Director of the Conference of Urban Counties, telephone interview by Aaron Knight (May 1996). The Conference of Urban Counties represents the 30 most populous counties in Texas.

17

Uncertain Prospects: West Virginia and Medicaid Reform

L. CHRISTOPHER PLEIN

INTRODUCTION

During the course of 1997, the State of West Virginia sought to move Medicaid recipients in twelve of its 55 countries into a managed care pilot project called Mountain Health Trust.[1] Under the program, those receiving Aid to Families with Dependent Children, or what is now referred to as Temporary Assistance to Needy Families (TANF), will be the first to be enrolled. Next, those receiving Supplemental Security Income will be transferred to Medicaid managed care arrangements. By April of 1997, 46,453 people had been enrolled in the program.[2] Like many other states, West Virginia is seeking to achieve Medicaid program cost-efficiencies by moving eligible participants under the aegis of managed care organizations. This chapter seeks to recount how and why West Virginia has embraced this approach to Medicaid reform. After providing background on the Medicaid experience in West Virginia and the managed care demonstration project now underway, the focus of discussion turns to evolution of Medicaid reform during the early and mid-1990s, to reveal how changing political, economic, and social conditions and priorities influenced policy design and formulation. Analysis reveals that two paths of reform emerged during this time, the first embraced community-based health care networks that relied on public-private partnerships between the state and providers. The second, and more recent, favors service delivery by HMOs and relies on private firms to administer and implement the effort.

Seen in context of changing conditions and events, the state's move toward a private model of managed care is not surprising. The popularity of social service privatization nationwide, the move toward managed care arrangements across the states, and the pressing concerns of budget shortfalls all contributed to the state's decision to rely on private HMOs to deliver Medicaid services. But the pending adoption of this program statewide has created a climate of uncertainty among established players in the health care sector. At stake are issues which are distributive in nature, but will require regulatory action to resolve. This paper argues that while there are obvious reasons for conflict among those who stand to "gain" or "lose" in the face of program transition, there are even more powerful incentives for long-term cooperation among the various institutional and individual providers who make up the state's health care community.

WEST VIRGINIA: A LEGACY OF PROGRAM IMPLEMENTATION CHALLENGES

Demographic and economic factors have conspired to create serious difficulties for Medicaid program implementation in West Virginia. A demographic profile of West Virginia illustrates some of the challenges in providing adequate medical treatment to the poor. Currently, 368,000 West Virginians are covered by Medicaid.[3] This translates into approximately 20% of the state's population. In addition, approximately 200,000 West Virginians lack health insurance, placing additional burdens on health care service delivery costs.[4] Other demographic factors present challenges as well. For example, West Virginia has one of the largest populations of elderly, relative to population base. This creates a high demand for long-term care arrangements that are among the most expensive of Medicaid expenditures. The health of West Virginians is frequently cited as below national averages. For instance, one study found that the state ranked highest in incidences of smoking, heart disease, and disabled workers. Added to this, there are considerable "at risk" populations relating to such factors as poverty, nutrition, and high rates of teenage pregnancies.[5] Then there are the difficulties associated with delivering health care in a predominantly rural state. A good illustration of this is that 19 of the state's 55 counties lack hospitals.

Like many other states, West Virginia's Medicaid program provides services and assists a population that is broader than mandated by federal law. Eligibility has been extended to those classified as "medically needy." These individuals represent those who may not necessarily qualify for AFDC/TANF or SSI programs, but whose income is so limited as to make access to health care difficult. Another significant feature of the state Medicaid program is the disproportionate share hospital payment program. Through these payments to hospitals, the burden of uncompensated costs of caring for the indigent is shared under the Medicaid program.[6] As in many other states, West Virginia also provides numerous services not required under federal guidelines. Prior to 1996, optional programs accounted for approximately 26% of West Virginia's Medicaid costs. These services include prescription drug coverage, physical and occupational therapy, psychological care, and various clinical services. In all, sixteen optional services are provided under West Virginia's Medicaid program.[7]

West Virginia has long had a limited revenue base due to one of the lowest rates of gross state product in the nation and a political and policy tradition that favors low tax rates. Frequent periods of fiscal stress have often made funding programs, such as Medicaid, daunting. The poor financial conditions are reflected in the state's Medicaid funding match rate, which is one of the most generous in the nation—averaging approximately 76% federal support to 24% state-contributed. The state raises funds for match rates through both general revenues and through a special tax levied on health care providers. In the past, the state has had difficulty in meeting its match.

Unfortunately, for West Virginia, in recent years the federal share of matching funds has been decreasing incrementally but significantly. Recent policy initiatives at the federal level hold the prospect of accelerating cutbacks over the course of the next seven years. While it is uncertain how the budget battles between the Democrats and Republicans at the federal level will play out in the years to come, it seems clear that Medicaid expenditures will be one of the targeted areas. By 1996, leading members of Congress had signaled an intent to reduce the growth of federal spending on Medicaid by $180 billion by 2002. If such a plan is implemented, it would cut unevenly across the states due to disparities in match rates. According to one study, West Virginia would be hardest hit in proportional terms by enduring a 37% decrease in federal funding by 2002 from 1995 levels.[8] As of the summer of 1997, the dangers of systematic reform of Medicaid through block-granting and other fundamental cost-cutting practices seem to have diminished in the face of bipartisan efforts to achieve a balanced budget agreement that preserves the Medicaid program in its general form.

For West Virginia, cuts in federal funding are particularly daunting given the explosive growth in the state's Medicaid program spending since the early 1990s. For fiscal year 1995, the state's Medicaid budget stood at approximately $1.2 billion. Six years earlier, the annual Medicaid budget was approximately $300 million.[9] Indeed, since 1975, West Virginia has experienced one of the highest rates of annual increase in Medicaid spending.[10] In fiscal year 1994, the state was not able to cover program costs within budget, and was forced to withdraw $35.6 million from a special Medicaid trust fund to cover expenses. At the end of fiscal year 1995, the state carried over $31 million in debts to the new fiscal year. A shortfall of $161 million was projected for fiscal year 1996.[11] For the 1996 fiscal year, the legislature prohibited additional state monies to be used for federal matching purposes. This amounts to what one policy analyst has called a "no more growth" position where $110 million in federal dollars will be foregone.[12]

In 1995, the chronic Medicaid funding shortfalls led Governor Gaston Caperton to establish a special Medicaid Crisis Panel to assess and recommend policy actions aimed at cutting $200 million from the state's Medicaid budget. After months of deliberation, the panel identified $157 million in recommended cuts which, in turn, were accepted by the governor. The cuts were aimed at both health care providers and Medicaid recipients. For providers, reductions were ordered in reimbursement for lab services, behavioral health and psychiatric services, and standard payments provided for under Diagnosis Related Group Systems (DRGs). For Medicaid clients, restrictions were placed on the number of visits made to physicians without prior approval and requirements that clients pay a portion of the health care costs.[13]

The Medicaid program has become a major feature in the state's political landscape, with funding problems often being at the source of controversy and debate. Throughout the 1990s, debates have flared within the state house and between the governor and the legislature as to what direction the program should take. Some have lobbied for cutting back services to save money, others for reform efforts aimed at greater efficiencies in program management and administration. Still others have advocated expanding the program to needy populations and groups. Given its salience and visibility, the Medicaid reform debate in West Virginia has also provided a convenient vehicle for those seeking to gain agenda access for issues ranging from the general merits of welfare policies to the need for privatization of government services, to the appropriate balance of federal and state responsibilities and obligations under intergovernmental programs and policies. Out of this mix of politics, economics, and social concerns have come calls to "fix" the Medicaid program. West Virginia has responded by pursuing strategies that first emphasized access issues, but more recently have concentrated on cost containment priorities. This is reflected in West Virginia's most recent experiment with Medicaid managed care reform.

WEST VIRGINIA'S "MOUNTAIN HEALTH TRUST" PROGRAM

In the mid-1990s, pressure for cost-savings–oriented reform, encouragement from federal authorities for states to develop innovative approaches to program delivery, and a wealth of experiences and models to borrow from other states converged to help give shape to West Virginia's Medicaid managed care program. The idea for the program originated within the West Virginia Department of Health and Human Resources, gained support from the governor, and was embraced by key interest groups and policy players. After a lengthy application process, the state was granted a formal waiver from the Health Care Financing Administration in April 1996 to conduct a two-year demonstration program which will terminate in June 1998. Under the program, all AFDC/TANF and SSI recipients in twelve West Virginia counties will be required to enroll in the Mountain Health Trust program.

The move to Medicaid managed care parallels a general transition to managed care arrangements for the state as a whole, for West Virginia is a relative newcomer to managed care. For example, as of September 1995, managed care represented merely 2% of the state's health care market. By December of 1996, this figure had grown to 6% with 128,000 West Virginians enrolled in managed care organizations.[14] A small population base (1.79 million in 1990; 1.83 million in 1996), a limited pool of service providers, and large numbers of uninsured have delayed the development of managed care operations in West Virginia. Added to this has been a sentiment among many in the health care field that the state's regulatory structure is inhospitable to managed care arrangements. But in the last two years, interest in providing managed care services has grown. This stems from the state's decision to modify its public employee insurance program to allow managed care enrollment. By this action, the state literally created a managed care market in West Virginia. Because the state is the largest insurer in West Virginia, this decision sparked a flurry of activity as established out-of-state and new in-state managed care organizations sought licensure. As of 1997, there were seven HMOs licensed in the state. Allowing public employees to join HMOs is a critical first step toward managed care Medicaid. It allows the state to have maximum leverage in the marketplace. This lesson was drawn from the experience of other states, such as Tennessee, which converted indemnity programs to a managed care approach prior to adopting managed care Medicaid programs. As the director of West Virginia's Medicaid office commented, "In terms of luring HMOs to the state, it would be very hard to start with Medicaid," noting, "We're not known as the best payer in the world."[15]

Under the Mountain Health Trust program, HMOs will be paid 5% less per patient than the standard fee-for-service approach of Medicaid. A set fee will be provided to participating HMOs under this capitation plan. In this way, the state hopes to garner cost savings.[16] It is anticipated that these savings will be achieved through the prevention of unnecessary utilization, the reduction of inappropriate utilization, and the reduction of costs associated with administration. Due to the lack of availability of medical services in a predominantly rural state, improving access is also an important component of the program. The state expects to realize $26.67 million in savings over the two-year period, which translates into a 6% savings on program implementation.[17]

Under the Mountain Health Trust demonstration project, only AFDC/TANF and SSI recipients in twelve targeted counties will be enrolled in the program.[18] With the capitation rates provided to HMOs, services ranging from primary care to emergency hospital services, to prevention and screening services will be provided. In all, 25 services will be required under the program. Excluded from the program will be services related to dental care, nonemergency transportation, outpatient prescription drugs, and behavioral health care. Behavioral health care was specifically excluded because of the state's intent to create a separate managed care system for this area. Moving on parallel paths with the Medicaid managed care initiative, the state petitioned HCFA for waivers to create a managed care organization (MCO) system for Medicaid recipients needing behavioral health services. Under this plan, the state would contract with a single MCO to provide services statewide.[19] However, the state failed to win HCFA approval for the plan, and efforts to further pursue the initiative are now on hold.

In order to remain within federal guidelines, participating HMOs will be required to enter into contracts with rural health clinics and federally qualified health centers in developing primary care provider resources. In addition, the state is considering incentives to encourage HMOs to contract with local health departments.[20] It is clear that the state expects the *Mountain Health Trust* program to provide a significant incentive for HMOs to locate and operate in West Virginia. For example, the program follows the rather liberal federal ceiling on enrollment, allowing for up to 75% of an HMO's patient base to be Medicaid recipients.[21]

One of the distinguishing characteristics of the Mountain Health Trust program is that it constitutes an experiment in what might be termed vertical privatization. In this sense, not only will private firms be detailed with the responsibility of client administration under the managed care program, but other dimensions of the program such as enrollment and general administration will rely, to a great degree, on private firms. Under the program, the state has contracted with a "neutral" broker to provide services to enroll Medicaid clients in managed care organizations. The broker will use "health benefits managers" to provide marketing materials and other information regarding specific managed care organizations.

The role of the broker will extend beyond the enrollment function. The broker's health benefits managers will also be responsible for educating local welfare organizations about the Mountain Health Trust program, encouraging community-based advocacy groups to take part in "education and outreach" efforts, and to serve as a liaison for the health and human resources department among participating HMOs in the managed care program. The West Virginia Department of Health and Human Resources acknowledges that the complexities and time-intensity of brokering activities make contracting an attractive option. Referring to the experiences of other states, the department also claims that "the use of a health benefits manager can minimize the sometimes unsavory tactics undertaken by HMOs when they are allowed to market directly to Medicaid recipients."[22] However, these arrangements do not preclude HMOs from engaging in general marketing and advertising activities on their own.[23]

Apart from direct service delivery, enrollment functions, and coordination in the field, the Mountain Health Trust program also features two other privatized elements. First, the program has relied on private consultants to assist in policy formulation. In developing the state's managed care plan, the Department of Health and Human Resources contracted with consultants to devise the plan and prepare the waiver application for the Health Care Financing Administration (HCFA).[24] As the demonstration program now moves to implementation, the state has contracted with a management firm to provide in-house assistance in administering the initiative.

If the Mountain Health Trust program is successful, the state will seek to expand the program across West Virginia.[25] This may prove problematic because there are substantial impediments to successful managed care operations in West Virginia. For example, the lack of a large health care market may mean that HMOs will face lean times as they compete to become established in the state. Such conditions have led to speculation that there may be a shake-out among managed care providers in the state. This will result in relatively few organizations retaining operations in the state. Apart from these economic constraints, antitrust regulations stand in the way of establishing managed care operations in areas which cannot sustain two or more plans. Some argue that special exceptions may be needed so that integrated health care networks can be developed.[26] Thus, for at least the near term, West Virginia's Medicaid managed care program will be limited to those counties in the state which can sustain a competitive managed care environment. Currently, three of the state's seven managed care organizations are under contract to provide services under the Mountain Health Trust program.[27] Since its implementation in the fall of 1996, there have been difficulties with the Mountain Trust Program. In three of the twelve demonstration program counties, the lack of health care providers willing to enter into managed care contracts has prevented program enrollment. In those counties where the program has been implemented, assessments have been mixed. There have been complaints about paperwork burdens, difficulties in processing billings, and confusion among patients regarding enrollment procedures. On the other hand, there are those who argue that the problems associated with transition to managed care are minor and are to be expected.[28]

THE EVOLUTION OF A MANAGED CARE APPROACH TO MEDICAID IN WEST VIRGINIA

For almost a decade, West Virginia's search for improved Medicaid service delivery has centered on two themes: health care service access and cost management. Since the early 1990s emphasis has increasingly shifted from access to cost issues. This shift in priorities mirrors developments on the national scene, but also reflects the deepening and chronic difficulties associated with West Virginia's ability to fund its portion of the Medicaid program. This transition can be clearly seen in the state's move toward a Medicaid managed care approach that will rely largely on private HMOs. The move toward this approach represents a departure from an earlier managed care strategy that focused more on the development of a community and regional managed care system that placed emphasis on public-private partnerships.

West Virginia's first experiment in a managed care approach to Medicaid case administration started in September of 1989 with a demonstration project called the Physician Assured Access System (PAAS). The PAAS program was patterned along efforts taken in other states, such as Kentucky, to develop regional health care systems. Ideally, physicians, acting as case managers, could more effectively coordinate the medical services that the poor received, thus improving service access. Further, the program would strengthen informal networks among care providers. Expansion of the program to other regions of the state followed and by June of 1992, the program was implemented throughout the state. Enrollment in the program eventually reached 45 to 50% of the state's AFDC population.[29] However, the program did not achieve the level of desired success because of implementation challenges. The incentives provided to physicians for enrolling Medicaid recipients into their operations were limited to small cash awards for each new participant. Physicians were also paid a small monthly fee for patient management. The state also found the administrative burdens of information management and compliance daunting.[30] In addition, the program was not uniformly embraced by primary care physicians.

While the PAAS program focused on both access and cost-effectiveness issues relating to Medicaid, other complementary state initiatives were afoot that focused on health care access issues in the state on more general terms. During the early 1990s such issues as disease and injury prevention, community-based health care arrangements, integrated service delivery, and the needs of delivering health care in remote rural areas gained prominence. Particular attention was given to rural and community-based health care initiatives. This emphasis was reflected in policy actions which saw the creation of an Office of Community and Rural Health and Office of Rural Health Policy in the state's Bureau of Public Health. The Bureau of Public Health was also mandated to establish community-based programs aimed at facilitating wellness and prevention and to coordinate health education activities among public health professionals.[31] Federal and philanthropic funding provided the opportunity for various demonstration projects to be carried out across the state. Indeed, many of these initiatives were funded under the Medicaid program. In 1991, the Rural Health Initiative was established to enhance coordination of medical and public health services, encourage future health professionals to go into rural practice and service, and attract primary care physicians to rural areas. Important to these efforts were partnerships forged with the state's universities and health care industry. With the former, emphasis was placed on providing resources and expertise to address rural health issues and foster programs aimed at encouraging medical students to plan for careers in rural primary practice. For the latter, their involvement concentrated on identifying areas of primary care need and facilitating the development of integrated care networks in rural areas.[32]

Within this climate of reform, Governor Gaster Caperton established the West Virginia Health Care Planning Commission. The Commission was charged with assessing West Virginia health needs and developing policy recommendations to address these needs. Borrowing from the reform experiences of other states, such as Kentucky, and embracing principles of public-private partnerships, the Commission called for fundamental reforms in the manner in which health care services were delivered in West Virginia. Among the suggestions of the panel were the creation of community-based managed care networks where primary care physicians would serve as the hub for referring patients to more specialized services, an overhaul of the state public employee insurance system to allow coverage under community networks, integration of services provided by local health departments into the managed care system of community networks, reorganization of local public health functions on a regional level, and the establishment of a permanent health care commission to implement and assess reforms.[33]

The sweeping changes advocated by the Commission reflect the tenor of times in which the group deliberated. For instance, the final recommendations of the Commission, offered after the November 1992 elections, assumed that the Clinton agenda of universal access and cost controls would be realized as law in 1993.[34] Second, the Commission assumed that federal funding for Medicaid would continue to grow. Thus, the Commission recommended that Medicaid eligibility be expanded in order to "reduce the number of uninsured as inexpensively as possible." Doing so would allow the state to benefit from its generous federal match ratio.[35]

The Commission's efforts helped to focus attention on issues dealing with health care costs and access issues. However, the recommendations of the Commission, delivered in December 1992, were not fully embraced by state policymakers. By early 1993, reform priorities had clearly shifted from access concerns to cost-effectiveness and cost containment. Furthermore, Medicaid became a central focus of discussion for reform. In an environment dominated by a pervading sense of fiscal crisis, the recommendations of the health care reform Commission were seen as expansive and expensive. Orientation shifted from expanding to minimizing the role of the state in Medicaid service delivery. Governor Caperton decided to incorporate some aspects of the Commission's suggestions in legislative proposals offered to the state house in 1993, but the efforts died in session. In subsequent sessions Caperton sought to advance bills aimed at health care reform planning and improving rural health care partnerships between hospitals and health providers, but these too failed to be passed.[36] Indeed, the governor encountered considerable resistance in the legislature toward his health care reform agenda. The legislature was also critical of state Medicaid management. Depictions of runaway program costs, the provision of inappropriate optional services, and bureaucratic bungling were common. Debates over Medicaid funding, administration, and program services led to contentious legislative hearings, veto threats, and lawsuits.[37] Since West Virginia is a one-party state, the Medicaid debate helped reveal the rifts and factions within the state's Democratic Party.

The crisis dimensions of funding difficulties and program deficiencies provided a powerful impetus for the creation of a managed care "solution" to West Virginia's Medicaid program shortcomings. Such a solution played well to prevailing policy prescriptions that market-oriented approaches to public service delivery might be more efficient than those relying on government agencies. The availability of other state models to borrow from meant that designing a managed care system would not have to be a *de novo* process. Further, the broader intent of the state to move toward managed care for its public employees meant that there would be the HMO presence necessary to transfer Medicaid recipients under a new program. In short, the approach achieved the level of political attractiveness and economic feasibility necessary to be put into action.

Originating within the Department of Health and Human Resources, the managed care approach had the backing of key policymakers—including the governor. Although at times skeptical over the efficacy of moving toward managed care, the legislature did not stand in the way of the initiative. In the interest group arena, the managed care initiative enjoyed the backing of major players in the health care market. For example, in outlining its 1996 legislative goals, the West Virginia Hospital Association encouraged expeditious implementation of the demonstration program.[38] And as early as January 1994, the West Virginia State Medical Association was pushing for an HMO managed care approach to Medicaid service delivery.[39] Indeed, in the desire to secure backing and prevent opposition and conflict, the proposed program called for the establishment of a Medicaid Managed Care Advisory Group comprising provider and consumer advocacy groups. The West Virginia Department of Health and Human Resources held that in addition to providing insights on the development and implementation process, enlisting such groups would enable these groups to be "participants and assistants in the process, rather than creating an environment that pitches the Department against these groups."[40]

The support of key stake-holders in the health industry has been seen as critical to the success of the Medicaid managed care program. Obviously, securing the support of institutional and individual health care providers is central to program success. Politically, these actors have substantial influence in the policy process and their support has been key to advancing managed care reforms in the state, for both Medicaid and as a general model of health care delivery. Such backing and cooperation could not be taken for granted given the often contentious relationship between providers and the state. For example, in 1993 the West Virginia Hospital Association lobbied hard to secure legislative opposition to the governor's proposal for hospitals to increase their share of a tax aimed at funding the Medicaid program. In these efforts they were successful in reaching a compromise which increased the hospitals' share of Medicaid DSH funds.[41] In 1994, the West Virginia State Medical Association filed suit petitioning for a court-appointed monitor which would take over administration of Medicaid from the state. The association's complaint cited poor administration, an unfair provider tax system, and poor reimbursement rates and management.[42] In 1995, the speaker of the West Virginia House of Delegates laid blame for much of the state's problems on the seeming inability of the West Virginia Department of Health and Human Resources and the health care industry to cooperate on issues relating to the Medicaid program.[43]

The evolution of Medicaid reform in West Virginia displays the dynamics of policy design and experimentation. Both the community-based network and private managed care approaches to Medicaid reform have been shaped by current events, economic factors, political environment, and the participation of key stake-holders in the policy process. The network approach was indeed the product of a short-lived perspective at the state and federal levels that government could be a positive force for change in health care reform. The private managed care approach reflects a rejection of such a perspective, holding instead that markets and free enterprise are the most effective vehicles for stemming the growth of public funding in health care. But because elements of community network approaches have already been put into place, the first effort at reform was more than a paper exercise. The outcome has been to strengthen a set of stake-holders who have an interest in continuing community-based initiatives and who are concerned about the implications that a private managed care system may have for their welfare. In the same vein, the Mountain Health Trust program stands to mobilize those interested in expansion of managed care throughout the state.

PROSPECTS FOR THE FUTURE: THE UNCERTAINTIES OF REFORM

As a policy issue, Medicaid is often framed in redistributive terms. In this depiction, the issue turns on the balance of health access for the poor and the costs borne by the taxpayer to underwrite the program. This element of issue debate has made Medicaid emotive and value-laden, lending to its intractability and enduring presence in the political arena. In an era where cost consciousness prevails, attention has increasingly turned to regulatory policy matters. In these issue framings, regulation and administrative arrangements are often portrayed as impediments to efficiency and effectiveness. It is in this context that private models of service delivery have gained popularity, for in such depictions the discipline of the market is seen as much stronger than that of the bureaucracy. Reform of the regulations that guide Medicaid have become a focal point of policy activity at the state and federal levels. The outcomes of regulatory decisions will have considerable bearing on the *distributive* aspects of Medicaid policy.

Medicaid reform in West Virginia may best be understood from a distributive policy perspective. Medicaid and other health care programs have provided a funding base that has allocated benefits across the health care community in West Virginia. Regulatory arrangements have helped to maintain and sustain these arrangements. The prospects of reform now create a set of uncertain conditions which pose challenges, opportunities, and risks for established players in the health care sector. These interests have benefited from Medicaid and other programs that have compensated care for the uninsured, reimbursed physicians for services, initiated prevention programs, supported screening and diagnostic services, and carried out direct health care services in local departments of health. In the early 1990s, the expansion of Medicaid and the priorities placed on prevention and access issues afforded greater resources to these interests. Physicians, group practices, hospitals, nonprofit agencies, and local health departments all had a stake in these arrangements. Now that the state appears to be willing to withdraw significant program funding in the face of federal cutbacks and the adoption of a private HMO managed care system, these interests must adapt to new conditions. In the face of such change, there is the temptation to claim that these interests stand to "lose" in light of the reforms underway. But, as we shall see, this judgement is premature and may be misinformed.

Ostensibly, those who stand to gain the most from a transition to the Mountain Trust Health program are managed care organizations. By regulatory fiat, the state has created a managed care market by allowing public employees to enroll in HMOs and signaling the intent to convert the state Medicaid program to managed care. However, the fortunes of these interests are not secure. The ability of HMOs to expand to other parts of the state are currently checked by federal antitrust regulations. Given the limited prospects for rural areas to sustain two or more competing managed care operations, regulatory relief will be needed to enter into these markets. This has led to efforts to gain legislative backing for antitrust exemptions, but this has not been forthcoming from the statehouse. Nationwide, some 20 states have adopted statutes supporting antitrust immunity.[44]

In reviewing the Medicaid reform experience in West Virginia, one can tender the observation that expansion of the Mountain Health Trust program will depend on cooperation between those who have benefited under past arrangements and those eager to make the most of the state's transition to managed care. In the short term, the risks and uncertainties involved in this transformation may lead to retrenchment and conflict. This tension is bound to be amplified by pending cuts in the Medicaid budget which are not tied directly to the managed care initative. But the tide of change and conditions will necessitate cooperative efforts. Indeed, this is the character of distributive policy debate, where conflict is reconciled through compromise based on the reallocation of program benefits. Because the transition to managed care in West Virginia includes not only Medicaid, but health care delivery as a whole, the pressure for compromise will be great.

Compromise will likely be needed to break impasses regarding antitrust regulation, to heal rifts within the health care community, and to make managed care a viable approach to health care delivery in West Virginia. For example, advocates of both private and community-network approaches have already expressed interest in securing antitrust exemptions and other regulatory arrangements that will facilitate the development of managed care operations in rural areas. Regulatory reform will allow both models to compete. And though there are concerns that the advantage might fall to well-heeled managed care firms, the practical realities of rural health care suggest that cooperative ventures and hybrid approaches may result.

The need for compromise is strong in the health care sector. Ideas that may be embraced in the abstract, such as managed care, may create divisions in practice. Thus, while both the state hospital and medical associations have endorsed managed care, their ranks are far from consensus on the course of this reform. The West Virginia Hospital Association, for example, has a diverse membership base, some of whom are interested in private HMO arrangements, others who champion community-based networks, and others, no doubt, who straddle the fence of uncertainty. The state's physicians are also divided on the future of reform in West Virginia. The professional and trade associations that represent providers can act both as a venue for deliberation and a means of expressing policy preferences. Both institutional and individual providers are being forced to adapt to new conditions; we should expect that they will seek to play a role in influencing new arrangements.

From a practical perspective, a climate of cooperation will need to exist to effectively achieve managed care reform in West Virginia. The myth of the corporate juggernaut of managed care systems will likely be dispelled by implementation. The feasibility of establishing managed care arrangements will likely be tied directly to linkages that are forged with existing providers and their informal networks. The relationship between health care and public funding is so deeply embedded in West Virginia, be it in the form of support for public hospitals, rural health initiatives, funding for public health programs, or school clinics, that it is difficult to envision a health care system dictated solely by private corporations. From a political perspective, it is important to remember that these interests are well-entrenched in the state policy arena. Managed care transformation will no doubt be tempered by their champions in the statehouse.

The West Virginia Department of Health and Human Resources holds that community-based networks and private HMO operations are compatible. Indeed, the rural health care initiative, in particular, has been seen as necessary for creating conditions conducive to the establishing of private managed care arrangements.[45] This philosophy holds that the capacity-building effort of the initiative, such as encouraging the presence of providers in rural areas and enhancing coordination of public and private services, enables the evolution of private HMO arrangements. The state has also been sensitive to the potential for conflict between champions of private managed care and community-based health care systems in this time of transition. For example, in anticipation of Medicaid managed care, the state has sought to encourage public health officials to move out of the direct service delivery and concentrate more on epidemiology, sanitization, and water quality. But by the same measure, the state has encouraged private HMOs to contract out screening and diagnostic services with local health departments. To reinforce this transition, the state has changed funding mechanisms to discourage local public health departments from engaging in direct services. To preserve the options of providers in the face of change, the state's "any willing provider laws" enable leverage for providers to negotiate agreements with HMOs. The state has also sought to coordinate the move toward managed care on an interagency basis. For example, the state's Office of Aging has pursued feasibility studies on managed care arrangements for those needing long-term care.[46] An interagency council was created by the governor to foster coordination in implementing managed care programs now affecting state employees, workers compensation beneficiaries, and Medicaid clients.[47]

CONCLUSION

West Virginia has long faced serious challenges in funding and implementing its Medicaid program. Since the late 1980s the state has searched for long-term solutions aimed at holding in check expanding program costs and improving health care access for the state's poor and disadvantaged. In the early 1990s, social, political, and economic forces converged to provide a supportive context for efforts aimed at developing community-based networks for health care delivery. But with the defeat of the Clinton health care initiative, and in the face of a deepening Medicaid funding crisis in West Virginia, attention and priorities shifted to cost containment reforms. Encouraged by the federal government and emulating other states, West Virginia decided that one component of Medicaid reform would be the adoption of a managed care delivery system that relies heavily on private HMOs. The state has now moved into the demonstration phases of program conversion. If successful, the state intends to extend the program across West Virginia.

But the state's move to managed care poses risks for stake-holders in the health care sector. Such a move will upset existing program arrangements that convey distributive benefits to a wide array of health care providers in the state. The combined forces of funding cutbacks and a new model of service delivery create uncertainties for these established players. But the future is not secure for those solely interested in private managed care operations either. Regulatory and economic barriers pose challenges to expanding the Mountain Health Trust program to other parts of the state. This analysis suggests that short-term tensions may characterize relations between those advocating different models of Medicaid managed care reform. But the analysis also asserts that there are powerful political and practical reasons why divergent interests in West Virginia's health care community will likely cooperate in the future.

NOTES

1. I thank Nancy Adams for her valuable insights and comments in the development of this manuscript. The research assistance of Sara Walker is greatly appreciated.

2. Gregg Stone, "State's Poor to Be Enrolled in HMOs," *Charleston Gazette* (May 8, 1996): 1A and 9A; Gregg Stone, "Confusion Hinders Welfare HMO Program," *Charleston Gazette* (April 24, 1997): 1A and 9A.

3. Jennifer Bundy, "Medicaid Managers Embrace Managed Care to Cut Costs," *State Journal* 18 (September 1995): 19.

4. The figure for West Virginians without health insurance was reported by the West Virginia Hospital Association, "Senate Passes Health Insurance Reform," *Focus* 26 (April 1996): 1–2. In comparison to 20% of West Virginians being covered by Medicaid, in 1992 approximately 11.2% of the total U.S. population was covered by Medicaid; see U.S. Congress, House of Representatives, Committee on Ways and Means, *Overview of Entitlement Programs: 1994 Green Book* (Washington, D.C.: USGPO, July 1994), 787. According to Urban Institute figures, by 1994, the percentage of those in the United States covered by Medicaid had increased to approximately 12.5%, as stated by Leighton Ku of the Urban Institute in a presentation at a conference sponsored by the Council of State Governments on *Managing the New Federalism*, held in Lexington, Kentucky, May 10 and 11, 1996.

5. West Virginia Health Care Planning Commission, *Health Care Reform in West Virginia: A Shared Responsibility* (Charleston, W.Va.: West Virginia Health Care Planning Commission, 1992), 47.

6. West Virginia Hospital Association, *1996 Legislative Agenda* (Charleston, West Virginia, 1995): 1. It is far beyond the scope of this analysis to examine and discuss the Disproportionate Payment Share Hospital (DSH) system. Ostensibly, the program is aimed at compensating hospitals for care they provide to the under- or uninsured. However, a great deal of controversy has surrounded this element of the Medicaid program. In short, some observers suggest that both states and hospitals have benefited from federal payouts under the program through the use of creative financing techniques. In 1993, DSH payments accounted for approximately 14% of all Medicaid expenditures, according to Urban Institute calculations presented by Leighton Ku at a conference sponsored by the Council of State Governments on "Managing the New Federalism," held in Lexington, Kentucky, May 10 and 11, 1996. Reducing DSH payments has been suggested in recent federal-level Medicaid reform deliberations, but the likelihood of such cuts, given the clout of hospital associations and the interest of states in continuing such programs, is slight.

7. Bundy "Medicaid Managers," 19.

8. Council of State Governments, "Southern and Western States Potentially Face Larger Medicaid Reductions," *State Trends Bulletin* (November/December, 1995): 6–7.

9. "State Medicaid Shortfall Foreseen," *Martinsburg Journal* (October 17, 1995): B-7.

10. According to U.S. Congress figures, in an analysis of Medicaid payments by the states in a sixteen-year period spanning 1975 to 1991, Alaska, West Virginia, Florida, and Wyoming led the nation with the fastest rates of annual spending increases. U.S. Congress, Congressional Research Service and Committee on Energy and Commerce, Subcommittee on Health and the Environment, *Medicaid Source Book: Background Data and Analysis (A 1993 Update)* (Washington, D.C.: USGPO, 1993); 127.

11. Figures for 1994 and 1996 are from "State Medicaid Shortfall Foreseen," *Martinsburg Journal*, B-7. Figures for 1995 are from Fanny Seiler, "2 Agencies Project Shortages." *Charleston Gazette* (October 2, 1995): 7A.

12. Steven Heasley, "Medicaid Policy Considerations for Children," *West Virginia Governor's Cabinet on Children and Families Issue Brief* 1, Number 2 (1995).

13. West Virginia Hospital Association, "Medicaid Panel Cuts Target Hospitals," *Focus* 18 (December 1995): 1–2.

14. The figure for managed care enrollment in the state for 1995 is found in "Expert Says State Has Too Many Hospitals, Schools," *State Journal* (September 18, 1995): 16.

Figures for 1996 participation rate are found in West Virginia Hospital Association, "HMO Enrollment Hits 7% in West Virginia," *Focus* (April 25, 1997). The 7% figure stated in the title of the article is misleading, based as it is on 1990 population figures as opposed to 1996 population figures. Using 1996 population data, the actual participation rate in West Virginia stands at approximately 6%.

15. Quoted in Brad McElhinny, "PEIA Choice May Make Medicaid Managed-Care Move Easier," *Charleston Gazette* 27 (February 1995): 1A, 7A.

16. Stone, "State's Poor," 1A.

17. West Virginia Department of Health and Human Resources, *West Virginia Medicaid Managed Care Briefing Document* (September 1995); West Virginia Department of Health and Human Resources, *West Virginia's Section 1915(b) Waiver Request to Implement a Medicaid Managed Care Program* (August 1995).

18. In 1992, AFDC recipients accounted for 36% of the state's total Medicaid expenditures. See U.S. Congress, *Overview of Entitlement Programs*, 802.

19. West Virginia Department of Health and Human Resources, *West Virginia's Section 1915(b) Waiver Request to Implement a Medicaid Managed Care Program*, 32, 42–43. In the wake of short-term budget-cutting efforts by the Governor's Medicaid Crisis Panel, behavioral health services suffered significant funding decline. In 1996, funding for mental health services provided under Medicaid was decreased by 25% by the state. Support for institutions providing these services dropped from $30 million to $11 million for the year. See Phil Kabler, "Medicaid Cuts Created Crisis, Lawmakers Told," *Charleston Gazette* (June 11, 1996): 6A; Jack McCarthy, "Medicaid Service Maintained Despite Cuts," *Charleston Gazette* (June 7, 1996): 6B; Jack McCarthy, "Mental Health Centers Trying to Cope with Medicaid Cutbacks," *Charleston Gazette* (June 8, 1996): 5A.

20. West Virginia Department of Health and Human Resources, *West Virginia Medicaid Managed Care Briefing Document* (September 1995).

21. Ibid.

22. West Virginia Department of Health and Human Resources, *West Virginia's Section 1915(b) Waiver Request to Implement a Medicaid Managed Care Program*, 32–33.

23. Stone, "State's Poor," 9A. See also West Virginia Department of Health and Human Resources, *West Virginia Medicaid Managed Care Briefing Document*; and Automated Health Systems, Inc., "Frequently Asked Questions With Responses," mimeograph. Automated Health Systems will serve as the brokering firm for the Mountain Health Trust program.

24. Paul Owens, "Managed Care No Panacea, Lewis Says," *Charleston Daily Mail* (January 18, 1995): 1A, 6A; Paul Owens, "Managed Care Savings May Be Slow to Show," *Charleston Daily Mail* (July 11, 1995): 1A, 7A.

25. McElhinny, "PEIA Choice," 7A.

26. West Virginia Hospital Association, *1996 Legislative Agenda*: 4.

27. West Virginia Hospital Association. "HMO Enrollment Hits 7% in West Virginia," *Focus* (April 25, 1997): 2, 3. West Virginia Hospital Association, "HMOs Submit Mountain Care Applications," *Focus* (February 29, 1996): 2.

28. Stone, "State's Poor," 9A.

29. This information was provided in a telephone interview by the author with Ann Garcelon, Director of Communications, West Virginia Department of Health and Human Resources (June 11, 1996).

30. Ibid.

31. West Virginia Health Care Planning Commission: 48.

32. West Virginia Hospital Association, *Focus 2000: Strategic Plan* (Charleston: West Virginia Hospital Association, September 1994).

33. West Virginia Health Care Planning Commission: 1–15.

34. Ibid.: 1.

35. Ibid.: 40.

36. Paul Owens, "Caperton's Task Forces Show Little Success on Health Care," *Charleston Daily Mail* (July 6, 1995): 9A.

37. See, for example, Fanny Seiler, "State Medical Association Pushes 'Privatization of Medicaid' Plan," *Charleston Gazette* (January 4, 1994): 11B; Theresa Cox, "Medicaid Work Overwhelms Staff," *Charleston Daily Mail* (December 28, 1994): 1A, 11A; *Charleston Gazette*, "Abortion Muddle," editorial (June 5, 1993): 4A. Dawn Miller, "Judge Rejects Suit, Upholds Medicaid Tax," *Charleston Gazette* (December 28, 1994): 1A.

38. West Virginia Hospital Association, *1996 Legislative Agenda*: 2.

39. Seiler, "State Medical Association Pushes 'Privatization of Medicaid' Plan."

40. West Virginia Department of Health and Human Resources, *West Virginia's Section 1915(b) Waiver Request to Implement A Medicaid Managed Care Program*, 37–38.

41. Brent Cunningham and Paul Owens, "Medicaid Fight Drags On and On," *Charleston Daily Mail* (May 17, 1993): 1A, 11A; Paul Owens, "Hospitals Accept Truce on Medicaid," *Charleston Daily News* (May 18, 1993): 1A.

42. Lawrence Messina, "Court Asked to Terminate State Control of Medicaid," *Charleston Daily News* (February 9, 1994): 1D. The suit was eventually rejected by a state circuit court judge; see Miller, "Judge Rejects Suit," 1A.

43. "Medicaid Problems Overflow," *Charleston Daily Mail* (April 6, 1995): 9A.

44. West Virginia Hospital Association, *1996 Legislative Agenda*, 6.

45. This according to Ann Garcelon, Director of Communications, West Virginia Department of Health and Human Resources (telephone interview with author, July 2, 1996).

46. The West Virginia Office of Aging is exploring the possibilities of moving the elderly into a managed care system. Their initial analyses suggest there are many challenges to achieving such an objective. Among the major barriers identified is the absence of policy strategies aimed at addressing the unique needs of the aged and disabled in West Virginia. In addition, such factors as reluctance on the part of care providers to participate in a new system and the fragmented nature of long-term care policy arrangements and practices serve to complicate the development of managed care arrangements for the elderly. See West Virginia Department of Health and Human Resources, Office of Aging, *Introducing Managed Care to Long Term Care for the Elderly and Adult Disabled in West Virginia*, 1995.

47. West Virginia Hospital Association, "Interagency Council to Identify Areas for Collaboration," *Focus* (February 2, 1996): 5.

Selected Bibliography

BOOKS AND MONOGRAPHS

Aaron, Henry J. *Serious and Unstable Condition: Financing America's Health Care.* Washington, D.C.: The Brookings Institution, 1991.

Congressional Research Service. *Medicaid Source Book: Background Data and Analysis (A 1993 Update).* Washington, D.C.: U.S. Government Printing Office, 1993.

Coughlin, Teresa, Leighton Ku, and John Holahan. *Medicaid Since 1980: Costs, Coverage, and the Shifting Alliance Between the Federal Government and the States.* Washington, D.C.: Urban Institute Press, 1994.

Freund, Deborah A. *Medicaid Reform: Four Studies of Case Management.* Washington, D.C.: American Enterprise Institute, 1984.

Graig, Laurene A. *Health of Nations: An International Perspective on U.S. Health Care Reform,* 2nd ed., Washington, D.C.: Congressional Quarterly, Inc., 1993.

Holahan, John, Marilyn Moon, Pete W. Welch, and Stephen Zuckerman. *Balancing Access, Costs, and Politics: The American Context for Health Care Reform.* Washington, D.C.: The Urban Institute Press 1991.

Hurley, Robert E., Deborah A. Freund, and John E. Paul. *Managed Care in Medicaid: Lessons for Policy and Program Design.* Ann Arbor, Mich.: Health Administration Press, 1993.

Kaiser Commission. *Health Needs and Medicaid Financing: State Facts.* Washington, D.C.: Kaiser Commission, 1995.

Kaiser Commission on the Future of Medicaid. *Medicaid and Managed Care: Lessons from the Literature.* Menlo Park, Calif.: Henry J. Kaiser Family Foundation, March 1995.

Kaiser Commission on the Future of Medicaid. *Policy Brief: Medicaid and Managed Care.* Washington, D.C.: Kaiser Commission, 1995.

Kingdon, John W. *Agendas, Alternatives, and Public Policies.* New York: HarperCollins, 1984.

Liska, David, Karen Obermaier Marlo, Anuj Shah, and Alina Salganicoff. *Medicaid Expenditures and Beneficiareies: National and State Profiles and Trends, 1984–1994*, 2nd ed. Washington, D.C.: Kaiser Commission on the Future of Medicaid, 1994.

Raffel, Marshall W., and Norma K. Raffel. *The U.S. Health System: Origins and Functions*, 4th ed. Albany, N.Y.: Delmar Publishers, 1994.

Reagan, Michael D. *Curing the Crisis: Options for America's Health Care*. Boulder, Colo.: Westview Press, 1992.

Rowland, Diane et al. *Health Needs and Medicaid Financing: State Facts*. Washington, D.C.: Kaiser Commission on the Future of Medicaid, April 1995.

Sparer, Michael S. *Medicaid and the Limits of State Health Reform*. Philadelphia: Temple University Press, 1996.

Winterbottom, Colin, David Liska, and Karen Obermaier. *State-Level Databook on Health Care Access and Financing*, 2nd ed. Washington, D.C.: The Urban Institute, 1995.

ARTICLES

Alpha Center. "More for Less? Increasing Insurance Coverage Through Medicaid Waiver Programs." *State Initiatives in Health Care Reform* 10 (February 1995): 1–3.

Andersen, Elizabeth. "Administering Health Care: Lessons from the Health Care Financing Administration's Waiver Policy-Making." *Journal of Law and Politics* 10, no. 2 (Winter 1994): 215–262.

Bachman, Sara S., Stuart H. Altman, and Dennis F. Beatrice. "What Influences a State's Approach to Medicaid Reform?" *Inquiry* 25 (Summer 1988): 243–250.

Babbitt, Bruce, and Jonathon Rose. "Building a Better Mousetrap: Health Care Reform and the Arizona Program." *Yale Journal on Regulation* 3, no. 2 (Spring 1986): 243–282.

Baker, E. L. et al. "Health Care Reform and the Health of the Public." *Journal of the American Medical* Association 272, no. 16 (October 26, 1994).

Brecher, Charles. "Medicaid Comes to Arizona: A First Year Report on AHCCCS." *Journal of Health Politics, Policy and Law* 9, no. 3 (Fall 1984): 411–425.

Carey, T., K. Weiss, and C. Homer. "Prepaid versus Traditional Medicaid Plans: Lack of Effect on Pregnancy Outcomes and Prenatal Care." *HSR: Health Services Research* 26, no. 2 (June 1991).

Christianson, Jon B., Diane G. Hillman, and Kenneth R. Smith. "The Arizona Experiment: Competitive Bidding for Indigent Medical Care." *Health Affairs* (Fall 1983): 87–103.

Christianson, Jon B., Bradford L. Kirkman-Liff, Teddylen A. Guffey, and James R. Beeler. "Non-Profit Hospitals in a Competitive Environment: Behavior in the Arizona Indigent Care Experiment." *Hospital and Health Services Administration* (November 1987): 475–491.

Coughlin, Teresa, Leighton Ku, John Holahan, David Heslam, and Colin Winterbottom. "State Responses to Medicaid Spending Crisis: 1988–1992." *Journal of Health Politics, Policy and Law* 19, no. 4 (1994): 837–864.

Daniels, Mark R. "Implementing Policy Termination: Health Care Reform in Tennessee." *Policy Studies Review* 14, nos. 3/4 (1996): 353–374.

Daniels, Mark R. "Organizational Termination and Policy Continuation: Closing the Oklahoma Public Training Schools." *Policy Sciences* 28 (1995): 301–316.

Daniels, Mark R. "The Politics and Economics of Dependent Children's Mental Health Care Financing: The Oklahoma Paradox." *Journal of Health and Human Services Administration* 16, no. 2 (1993) 171–196.

Ellwood, Paul M., Jr., and George D. Lundberg. "Managed Care: A Work in Progress." *Journal of the American Medical Association* 276 (October 2, 1996): 1083–1086.

Ferrara, Chris, and Doug Bandow. "Finding an Alternative to Medicaid." *Journal of the Institute for Socioeconomic Studies* 9, no. 3 (Autumn 1984): 34–42.

Fisher, Rhona S. "Medicaid and Managed Care: The Next Generation?" *Academic Medicine* 69, no. 5 (May 1994): 317–322.

Fox, Daniel M. "Health Policy and the Politics of Research in the United States." *Journal of Health Politics, Policy and Law* 15 (Fall 1990): 481–499.

Freeman, Howard E., and Bradford Kirkman-Liff. "Health Care Under AHCCCS: An Examination of Arizona's Alternative to Medicaid." *Health Services Research* 20, no. 3 (August 1985): 245–266.

Freund, Deborah A. "Competitive Health Plans and Alternative Payment Arrangements for Physicians in the United States: Public Sector Examples." *Health Policy* 7 (1987): 163–173.

Gill, James M., and James J. Diamond. "Effect of Primary Care Referral on Emergency Department Use: Evaluation of a Statewide Medicaid Program." *Family Medicine* (March 1996): 1.

Gold, Rachel Benson, Susheela Singh, and Jennifer Frost. "The Medicaid Eligibility Expansions for Pregnant Women: Evaluating the Strength of State Implementation Efforts." *Family Planning Perspectives* 25 (1993): 196–207.

Golenski, John, and Stephen Thompson. "The Impossible Solution: Expanding Access to Health Care While Reducing Costs." *Stanford Law and Policy Review* 3 (Fall 1991): 73–80.

Grogan, Colleen M. "Hope in Federalism? What Can the States Do and What Are They Likely to Do?" *Journal of Health Politics, Policy and Law* 20, no. 2 (1995): 477–484.

Hackey, Robert S. "Regulatory Regimes and State Cost Containment Programs." *Journal of Health Politics, Policy and Law* 18 (Summer 1993): 491–502.

Hanson, Russell. "Health-Care Reform, Managed Competition, and Subnational Politics." *Publius: The Journal of Federalism* 24 (1994): 49–68.

Hillman, Diane G., and Jon B. Christianson. "Competitive Bidding as a Cost-Containment Strategy for Indigent Medical Care: The Implementation Experience in Arizona." *Journal of Health Politics, Policy and Law* 9, no. 3 (Fall 1984): 427–451.

Hoefler, James M., and Khi V. Thai. "Introduction to the Politics and Economics of Health Care Finance: A Symposium." *Journal of Health and Human Resources Administration* 16, no. 2 (1993): 115–197.

Holahan, John, Teresa Coughlin, Leighton Ku, Debra J. Lipson, and Shruti Rajan. "Insuring the Poor Through Section 1115 Medicaid Waivers." *Health Affairs* (Spring 1995): 199–216.

Holahan, John et al. "Explaining the Recent Growth in Medicaid Spending." *Health Affairs* 12, no. 3 (Fall 1993).

Hurley, Robert E., and Deborah A. Freund. "A Typology of Medicaid Managed Care."
    Medical Care 26, no. 8 (August 1988): 764–774.
Inglehart, John K. "Health Policy Report: Medicaid and Managed Care." *New England
    Journal of Medicine* 332, no. 25 (June 22, 1995): 1727–1731.
Kaplan, Robert M. "Value Judgement in the Oregon Medicaid Experiment." *Medical
    Care* 32 (November 1994): 975–988.
Kirkman-Liff, Bradford L., Jon B. Christianson, and Tracy Kirkman-Liff. "The Evolution
    of Arizona's Indigent Care System." *Health Affairs* 6, no. 4 (Winter 1987): 46–
    58.
Kirkman-Liff, Bradford L., Frank G. Williams, and L. A. Wilson II. "Medicaid and
    Captitated Competitive Contracting: The Arizona Experiment." *New England
    Journal of Human Services* (Summer 1985): 30–36.
McCall, Nelda, C. William Wrightson, Lynn Parringer, and Gordon Trapnell. "Managed
    Medicaid Cost Savings: The Arizona Experience." *Health Affairs* 13, no. 2
    (Spring 1994): 234–245.
McCombs, Jeffrey S., and Jon B. Christianson. "Applying Competitive Bidding to
    Health Care." *Journal of Health Politics, Policy and Law* 12, no. 4 (Winter
    1987): 703–722.
Oliver, Thomas R. "Analysis, Advice, and Congressional Leadership: The Physician
    Payment Review Commission and the Politics of Medicare." *Journal of Health
    Politics, Policy and Law* 18 (Spring 1993): 113–174.
Oliver, Thomas R. "Health Care Market Reform in Congress: The Uncertain Path from
    Proposal to Policy." *Political Science Quarterly* 106 (Fall 1991): 453–477.
Oliver, Thomas R., and Pamela Paul-Shaheen. "Translating Ideas into Actions: Entre-
    preneurial Leadership in State Health Care Reforms." *Journal of Health Politics,
    Policy and Law* 22 (June 1997).
Paringer, Lynn, and Nelda McCall. "How Competitive Is Competitive Bidding?" *Health
    Affairs* 10, no. 4 (Winter 1991): 220–230.
Peterson, Mark A. "Political Influence in the 1990s: From Iron Triangles to Policy
    Networks." *Journal of Health Politics, Policy and Law* 18, no. 2 (1993): 399–
    438.
Richards, Eric L. "Anti-Trust and the Future of Cost Containment Efforts in the Health
    Profession." *Nebraska Law Review* 62, no. 1 (1983): 49–85.
Schauffler, Helen Halpin, and Jessica Wolin. "Community Health Clinics under Managed
    Competition: Navigating Uncharted Waters." *Journal of Health Politics, Policy
    and Law* 21 (Fall 1996): 461–488.
Schlesigner, Mark, and David Mechanic. "Challenges for Managed Competition from
    Chronic Illness." *Health Affairs* 12 (1993 Supplement): 123–137.
Shi, Leiyu. "Public Health, Medical Care, and Mortality Rates." *Journal of Health Care
    for the Poor and Underserved* 6 (1995): 307–321.
Sisk, Jane E., Sheila A. Gorman, Anne Lenhard Reisinger, Sherry A. Glied, William H.
    DuMouchel, and Margaret M. Haynes. "Evaluation of Medicaid Managed Care:
    Satisfaction, Access, and Use." *Journal of the American Medical Association* 276
    (July 3, 1996): 50–55.
Sparer, Michael S. "Medicaid Managed Care and the Health Reform Debate: Lessons
    from New York and California." *Journal of Health Politics, Policy and Law* 21
    (Fall 1996): 433–460.

Williams, Frank G., David Phoenix, and Bradford L. Krikman-Liff. "The Prospects for Pre-Paid Long Term Care: The Arizona Medicaid Experiment." *Journal of Health Politics, Policy and Law* 14, no. 3 (Fall 1989): 549–563.

Wrightson, William. "Evaluation of the Arizona Health Care Cost Containment System." *Health Care Financing Review* 7, no. 2 (Winter 1985): 77–88.

CHAPTERS

Davis, Raymond G. "Public Health Policy: Perplexing Problems and Proximate Policies." In H. George Frederickson, ed., *Public Policy and the Two States of Kansas*. Lawrence: University of Kansas Press, 1994.

Hoadley, John F. "The Fruits of Reform: A New Payment Scheme." In Jonathan D. Moreno, ed., *Paying the Doctor: Health Policy and Physician Reimbursement*. New York: Auburn House, 1991.

Oliver, Thomas R. "Conceptualizing the Challenges of Public Entrepreneurship." In Chris E. Stout, ed., *The Integration of Psychological Principles in Policy Development*. Westport, Conn.: Praeger Publishers, 1996.

Index

About the Contributors

DAVID L. ARONSON is an assistant professor in the Department of Political Science, University of South Dakota. He has eight years' experience in hospital finance and twenty-five years in municipal government as Financial Officer. He has been with the University of South Dakota since 1992 and teaches classes in public administration. He received a Ph.D. in political science from Wayne State University, and Bachelor and Master of Public Administration degrees from the University of Michigan.

JAMES BOEX received a Master of Business Administration degree from the University of Akron and is Director, Office of Health Services, Organization and Research at Northeastern Ohio Universities College of Medicine.

DAVID BOND is a research associate at the Center for Governmental Research, Inc., in Rochester, New York. He was a major contributor to the CGR's 1995 collaborative research with the New York State Association of Counties, *Medicaid Cost Containment: Options for New York*. He works extensively with counties and municipalities in New York State on Medicaid funding and service delivery issues.

TERRY F. BUSS is chair, Department of Public Management, at the Sawyer School of Management, Suffolk University, in Boston. In summer 1997 he held a senior fellowship at the Congressional Research Service, Library of Congress, working on economic development policy for Congress. Prior to that he directed nation-wide technical assistance efforts for the U.S. Information Agency in Hungary and Russia from 1991 to 1997. He received two Fulbright Scholarships, both in Budapest, Hungary, at the School of Public Administration and University of Economics. He has published eleven books and more than 200 articles on a variety of public policy issues.

MARK R. DANIELS is an associate professor and coordinator of the Master of Public Administration program in the Department of Government and Public Affairs, Slippery Rock University of Pennsylvania. He worked for five years as Director of Human Resources, Training and Development for a national provider of child and adolescent mental health services. His research on Medicaid has appeared in *Policy Studies Review*, *Policy Sciences*, and *Journal of Health and Human Services Administration*. He is the author of *Terminating Public Programs: An American Political Paradox*.

RAYMOND G. DAVIS is chair of the Department of Health Services Administration and associate professor in the Department of Public Administration, University of Kansas. His research interests are in state policy reform initiatives including various forms of managed care to contain Medicaid costs. He presently chairs the board of trustees for Lawrence Memorial Hospital in Lawrence, Kansas.

AMY B. DROSKOSKI received her master's in public administration from the University of Delaware's Institute for Public Administration, where she worked on a survey of consumer attitudes about Delaware health care policy. She has spent time working at the Health Care Financing Administration on the review, implementation, and monitoring of Section 1115 Medicaid Managed Care Demonstrations. Ms. Droskoski is presently working on Medicaid and Medicare policy for the 105th Congress.

MARY ANN FELDHEIM is a Ph.D. candidate in the School of Public Administration, Florida Atlantic University–Fort Lauderdale and a visiting instructor at the University of Central Florida. She is a registered nurse with a Master of Science in Nursing, who is focusing her research on health care policy.

MICHAEL H. FOX is an assistant professor in the Department of Health Services Administration at the University of Kansas. Much of his research has involved physician and organizational behavior associated with state health policy initiatives. He worked with the Medicaid program as the Deputy Director of Policy and Health Statistics for the Maryland Department of Health and Mental Hygiene for seven years.

LEONARD H. FRIEDMAN is an assistant professor of Public Health and Coordinator of the Health Care Administration program in the Department of Public Health at Oregon State University. His research has examined the decision processes surrounding the acquisition of clinical technologies in hospitals. More recently, he has begun to explore the growth and development of integrated delivery networks in small markets and the influence of managed care on the growth of these systems.

KENT GARDNER leads the study of economic analysis at the Center for Governmental Research, Inc., in Rochester, New York. In his research, he explores in depth the relationship between public policy and economic vitality, and identifies ways to improve the efficiency and competitiveness of local and state economics. In this capacity he has done extensive research on New York State's health care system, particularly the effect of Medicaid on the health care industry and the state regional economies.

BRENDA GOLDSTEIN is the managed care coordinator for the Oregon Health Plan, where she is responsible for the oversight of managed care contracts between the state and prepaid health plans. She has been with the State of Oregon since the inception of the Oregon Health Plan. Ms. Goldstein received a master's degree in public health from Yale University.

MICHAEL HARRIS is an assistant professor in the Department of Political Science and MPA Program at Eastern Michigan University. He teaches courses in public policy and public administration. His current research interests include: comparative privatization policy; health care reform; political economy; and organizational adaptation to change.

ERIC D. JACOBSON is an assistant director of the University of Delaware's Institute for Public Administration and an assistant professor of Public Management. He has conducted numerous applied research projects in health policy and public economics. He is currently principal investigator of a survey research project intended to evaluate the quality of alternative health care delivery systems.

JOCELYN M. JOHNSTON is an assistant professor in the Department of Public Administration at the University of Kansas, where she teaches public finance, intergovernmental relations, and quantitative methods. Her research interests have focused on intergovernmental fiscal issues, including Medicaid policy and school finance. Currently, she is conducting research in the areas of privatization, property tax administration, and the implementation of social welfare policy reforms.

RHONDA S. KINNEY is an assistant professor in the Department of Political Science at Eastern Michigan University. She teaches courses on American political institutions and policy-making processes. Her research interests include women and the public policy process, health care reform, and institutional leadership and agenda-setting.

AARON KNIGHT has taught Texas politics for over ten years. His research interests include a broad array of policy and social justice issues. Currently he is studying the interplay between the unique political culture of the U.S.-Mexico border region and the pressing medical as well as social needs of its people.

RENE P. McELDOWNEY is an assistant professor in the health administration program at Auburn University. Her principal research interests include issues of health care economics, health care systems evaluation, and adaptive strategies of health care institutions. Her publications include works on the evaluation of mental health and substance abuse programs, Medicaid reform, physician supply, health care purchasing coalitions, the sociopolitical environment of international health care systems, physician autonomy, and British health care reform.

KAREN ANDERSON OLIVER received her A.B. from Princeton University. She earned an M.P.H. and Ph.D. in epidemiology and public health at Yale University, receiving a fellowship from the National Institute of Mental Health for her doctoral training. She has worked for William M. Mercer, Inc., on the design and evaluation of mental health benefits for private and public programs. From 1994 to 1997 she was Director of Evaluation in the Center for Health Program Development and Management at the University of Maryland Baltimore County. She is currently directing quality improvement and evaluation studies for Maryland Health Partners, which is providing administrative services for the state's new public mental health system.

THOMAS R. OLIVER received his bachelor's degree in human biology from Stanford University. He earned a master's degree in health administration from Duke University and a Ph.D. in political science from the University of North Carolina at Chapel Hill. He completed a postdoctoral fellowship in the Pew Health Policy Program at the University of California, San Francisco, and taught from 1991 to 1997 in the Policy Sciences Graduate Program at the University of Maryland Baltimore County. He is currently associate professor in the Department of Health Policy and Management at the Johns Hopkins University School of Hygiene and Public Health. His published research includes articles in the *New England Journal of Medicine*, *Political Science Quarterly*, *Stanford Law and Policy Review*, *Journal of Health Politics, Policy and Law*, and *Health Affairs*.

WILLIAM PARLE is currently an associate professor and head of the Department of Political Science at Oklahoma State University. A one-time hospital administrator, he has a long-standing interest in health care policy and health care reform.

L. CHRISTOPHER PLEIN is an assistant professor of Public Administration at West Virginia University. His research on such topics as agenda-setting, issue definition, and comparative policy and administration has been published in various edited books and in such journals as *Comparative Politics*, *Policy Studies Journal*, and *Science, Technology, and Human Values*. His research on health policy has concentrated on Medicaid reform, especially as it relates to policy design and implementation in West Virginia. Most recently, he has served on a task force, organized by the West Virginia chapter of the March of Dimes, to develop a profile of maternal and infant health needs in the state.

MICHELLE A. SAINT-GERMAIN is an associate professor at the Graduate Center for Public Policy and Administration at California State University, Long Beach. Her research interests include health policy and women's health, with an emphasis on older Hispanic women and breast cancer screening. She has studied these issues in Arizona, West Texas, and Southern California, as well as in Central America.

KHI V. THAI is a professor in the School of Public Administration, Florida Atlantic University–Fort Lauderdale. His research and teaching interests are in public budgeting, government accounting, and health care finance. In addition to numerous refereed articles and book chapters, he is co-editor of *Handbook on International Health Care Systems* (forthcoming), and editor of the *Journal of Public Budgeting and Accounting* (formerly *Public Budgeting and Financial Management*).

CAROL WATERS is an assistant professor of Political Science and Public Administration at Texas A&M International University. She obtained her MPA degree and Ph.D. at Texas Tech University. Prior publications include articles on health care policy and social service policy in Texas.

PATRICIA A. WILSON is an associate professor in the School of Public Administration and Urban Studies, San Diego State University. Her research interests include such topics as politics and power struggles in organizations, gerontology, health care issues, and violence in the workplace. She has published previously in many journals including *Public Administration Review*, *Journal of Public Management and Social Policy*, *The Public Manager*, *The International Journal of Public Administration*, and *The Journal of Management*. Dr. Wilson teaches public administration and public management theory to both undergraduate and graduate students.

RON WOOSLEY is currently a graduate student in the Department of Political Science at Oklahoma State University. His area of study is public administration with an interest in health care policy.

LAURA C. YANCER is a law student at the Ohio State University. She is currently working in the office of the Ohio Auditor, where she is helping to reform Ohio's auditing system. She has served as an intern for the National Council for Alternative Dispute Resolution in Washington, D.C., and as a researcher in the Department of Public Administration and Urban Studies at the University of Akron.

ISBN 0-86569-263-7

HARDCOVER BAR CODE